Mental health aspects of women's reproductive health

A global review of the literature

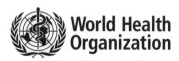 World Health Organization

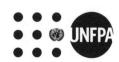 UNFPA

WHO Library Cataloguing-in-Publication Data

Mental health aspects of women's reproductive health : a global review of the literature

1.Mental health. 2.Mental disorders - complications. 3.Reproductive health services. 4.Reproductive behavior. 5.Women. I.World Health Organization. II.United Nations Population Fund.

ISBN 978 92 4 156356 7   (NLM classification: WA 309)

Contents

Photo credits

Cover   © River of Life Photo Competition (2004) WHO/ Liba Taylor
page 2   © WHO/ C. Gaggero
page 17   © River of Life Photo Competition (2004) WHO/ Joyce Ching
page 23   © WHO/ Yassir Abo Gadr
page 25   © River of Life Photo Competition (2004) WHO/ Dinesh Shukla
page 52   WHO/Maureen Dunphy
page 58   © River of Life Photo Competition (2004) WHO/ Abir Abdullah
page 69   © River of Life Photo Competition (2004) WHO/ Nathalie Behring-Chisholm
page 91   © River of Life Photo Competition (2004) WHO/ Masaru Goto
page 114   © 2000 Liz Gilbert/David and Lucile Packard Foundation, Courtesy of Photoshare
page 117   © River of Life Photo Competition (2004) WHO/ Douglas Engle
page 118   © River of Life Photo Competition (2004) WHO/ Veena Nair
page 129   © WHO photo
page 135   © River of Life Photo Competition (2004) WHO/ Cassandra Lyon
page 148   © River of Life Photo Competition (2004) WHO/ Katerini Storneg
page 152   © River of Life Photo Competition (2004) WHO/ Ahmed Afsar
page 165   © WHO photo

Acknowledgements

The World Health Organization, the Key Centre for Women's Health in Society, WHO Collaborating Centre, Australia, and the United Nations Population Fund wish to express their deep gratitude to the numerous experts who contributed to the development and finalization of this project starting with the main authors of this Review who are: Susie Allanson, Fertility Control Clinic, Wellington Parade, East Melbourne, Australia; Jill Astbury, School of Psychology, Victoria University, Australia; Mridula Bandyopadhyay, Mother & Child Health Research, Faculty of Health Sciences, La Trobe University, Australia; Meena Cabral de Mello, Department of Child and Adolescent Health and Development, World Health Organization; Jane Fisher, Key Centre for Women's Health in Society, WHO Collaborating Centre in Women's Health, University of Melbourne, Australia; Takashi Izutsu, Technical Support Division, United Nations Population Fund; Lenore Manderson, Key Centre for Women's Health in Society, WHO Collaborating Centre in Women's Health, University of Melbourne, Australia; Heather Rowe, Key Centre for Women's Health in Society, WHO Collaborating Centre in Women's Health, University of Melbourne, Australia; Shekhar Saxena, Department of Mental Health and Substance Dependence, World Health Organization; and Narelle Warren, Key Centre for Women's Health in Society, WHO Collaborating Centre in Women's Health, University of Melbourne, Australia.

The respondents of a mail survey who contributed directly or indirectly to the research evidence included in this Review are gratefully acknowledged. They are: Ahmed G Abou El-Azayem, Eastern Mediterranean Regional Council of the World Federation for Mental Health, Egypt; Mlay Akwillina, Reproductive Health Project, Tanzania; Mary Jane Alexander, Nathan Kline Institute for Psychiatric Research, USA; Faiza Anwar, Women's Health Educator, Australia; Victor Aparicio Basauri, WHO Collaborating Centre, Spain; Lara Asuncion Ramon de la Fuente, National Institute of Psychiatry, Mexico; Carlos Augusto de Mendonça Lima, Service Universitaire de Psychogériatrie, Switzerland; Christine Brautigam, Division for the Advancement of Women, United Nations; Jacquelyn C Campbell, Johns Hopkins University, USA; Amnon Carmi, International Center for Health Law and Ethics, Haifa University, Israel; Rebecca J Cook, University of Toronto, Canada; Dilbera, DAJA Organization, Macedonia; Mary Ellsberg, Violence and Human Rights Program at PATH, USA; Sofia Gruskin, Francois-Xavier Bagnoud Center for Health and Human Rights Harvard University School of Public Health, USA; Emma Margarita Iriarte, Tegucigalpa, Honduras; Els Kocken, WFP, Colombia; Pirkko Lahti, World Federation for Mental Health, Finland; Els Leye, International Centre for Reproductive Health, University Hospital, Belgium; Regine Meyer, Health & Population Section, GTZ, Germany; Alberto Minoletti, Ministerio de Salud, Chile; Jacek Moskalewicz, Institute of Psychiatry and Neurology, Poland; Vikram Patel, London School of Hygiene and Tropical Medicine, UK; Pennell Initiative, University of Manchester, UK; Ingrid Philpot, Ministry of Women's Affairs, New Zealand; Joan Raphael-Leff, Centre for Psychoanalytic Studies, University of Essex, UK; Tiphaine Ravenel Bonetti, Reproductive Health, Kathmandu, Nepal; Jacqueline Sherris, Reproductive Health, PATH, USA; Johanne Sundby, University of Oslo, Norway; Susan Weidman Schneider, LILITH Magazine, USA; and Susan Wilson, National Research Institute, Curtin University of Technology, Australia.

The following peer reviewers provided much constructive critical assessment during the long development phase: this work has benefited greatly from their comments, suggestions and generous advice. Natalie Broutet, Department of Reproductive Health and Research, World Health Organization; Meena Cabral de Mello, Department of Child and Adolescent Health, World Health Organization; Jane Cottingham, Department of Reproductive Health and Research, World Health Organization; Lindsay Edouard, Technical Support Division, United Nations Population Fund; Jane Fisher, Key Centre for Women's Health in Society, WHO Collaborating Centre in Women's Health, University of Melbourne, Australia; Sharon Fonn, University of the Witwatersrand, South Africa; Takashi Izutsu, Technical Support Division, United Nations Population Fund; Elise Johansen, Department of Reproductive Health and Research, World Health Organization; Paul Van Look, Department of Reproductive Health and Research, World Health Organization; Lenore Manderson, WHO Collaborating Centre for Women's Health, Department of

Public Health, The University of Melbourne, Australia; and Vikram Patel, London School of Hygiene and Tropical Medicine, UK, and Chairperson, Sangath, Goa, India; Arletty Pinel; Technical Support Division, United Nations Population Fund; Shekhar Saxena, Department of Mental Health and Substance Abuse, World Health Organization; Iqbal Shah, Department of Reproductive Health and Research, World Health Organization; Atsuro Tsutsumi, National Institute of Mental Health, Japan; Andreas Ullrich, Department of Chronic Diseases and Health Promotion, World Health Organization; and Effy Vayena, Department of Reproductive Health and Research, World Health Organization.

Hope Kelaher, WHO intern, provided much research assistance and Kathleen Nolan, Key Centre for Women's Health in Society, Australia, assisted with the editorial process. We are indebted to Pat Butler, WHO consultant for patiently editing this publication.

This production of this publication would not have been possible without the funding support extended by the United Nations Population Fund. For further information and feedback, please contact:

Key Centre for Women's Health in Society
WHO Collaborating Centre in Women's Health
School of Population Health
University of Melbourne
Australia
Tel: +61 3 8344 4333, fax: +61 3 9347 9824
email: enquiries-kcwhs@unimelb.edu.au
website: http://www.kcwh.unimelb.edu.au

Department of Mental Health and Substance Abuse
World Health Organization
Avenue Appia 20, 1211 Geneva 27, Switzerland
Tel: +41 22 791 21 11, fax: +41 22 791 41 60
email: mnh@who.int
website: http://www.who.int/mental-health

Department of Reproductive Health and Research
World Health Organization
Avenue Appia 20, 1211 Geneva 27, Switzerland
Tel: +41 22 791 4447, Fax: +41 22 791 4171
email: reproductivehealth@who.int
website: http://www.who.int/reproductive-health

Department of Child and Adolescent Health and Development
World Health Organization
Avenue Appia 20, 1211 Geneva 27, Switzerland
Tel: +41 22 791 3281, Fax: +41 22 791 4853
email: cah@who.int
website: http://www.who.int/child-adolescent-health

United Nations Population Fund
220 East 42nd Street, NY, NY 10017
Tel: 1-212-297-2706
email: izutsu@unfpa.org
website: http://www.unfpa.org

Foreword

The World Health Organization and the United Nations Population Fund in collaboration with the Key Centre for Women's Health in Society, in the School of Population Health at the University of Melbourne, Australia are pleased to present this joint publication of available evidence on the intricate relationship between women's mental and reproductive health. The review comprises the most recent information on the ways in which mental health concerns intersect with women's reproductive health. It includes a discussion of the bio-psycho-social factors that increase vulnerability to poor mental health, those that might be protective and the types of programmes that could mitigate adverse effects and promote mental health. This review is our unique contribution towards raising awareness on an emerging issue of major importance to public health. Its purpose is to provide information on the often neglected interlinks between these two areas so that public health professionals, planners, policy makers, and programme managers may engage in dialogue to consider policies and interventions that address the multiple dimensions of reproductive health in an integrated way.

A complete review would examine all mental health aspects of reproductive health and functioning throughout the lifespan for both men and women. However, the potential scope of the topic of reproductive mental health far outstrips the available evidence base. Most research into the mental health implications of reproductive health has focussed on a relatively small number of reproductive health conditions experienced worldwide and has investigated most usually, married women of reproductive age. A more comprehensive review is thus not possible yet. The focus on women in this review is not only because of the lack of evidence and data on men's reproductive mental health but also because reproductive health conditions impose a considerably greater burden on women's health and lives. The review comprises the most recent data from both high- and low-income countries on the ways in which women's mental health intersects with their reproductive health. The framework for analysis employed here is informed by two interconnected concepts: gender and human rights, especially reproductive rights.

Dramatic contrasts are apparent between industrialized and developing countries in terms of reproductive health services and status. These include access to contraception, antenatal care, safe facilities in which to give birth and trained staff to provide pregnancy, delivery and postpartum care; the diagnosis and treatment of sexually transmitted infections (STIs) including HIV, infertility treatment, and care for unsafe or unintended pregnancy. Around the world, reproductive health initiatives aim to address the complex of economic, sociodemographic, health status and health service factors associated with elevated risk of morbidity and mortality related to reproductive events during the life course. At present, the central contributing factors to disparities in reproductive health have been identified as: reproductive choice; nutritional and social status; co-incidental infectious diseases; information needs; access to health system and services and the training and skill of health workers. The most prominent risks to life are identified as those directly associated with pregnancy, childbirth and the puerperium, including haemorrhage, infection, unsafe abortion, pregnancy related illness and complications of childbirth. There is however, very limited consideration of mental health as a determinant of reproductive mortality and morbidity especially in the developing regions of the world.

Mental health problems may develop as a consequence of reproductive health problems or events. These include lack of choice in reproductive decisions, unintended pregnancy, unsafe abortion, sexually transmissible infections including HIV, infertility and pregnancy complications such as miscarriage, stillbirth, premature birth or fistula. Mental health is closely interwoven with physical health. It is generally worse when physical health including nutritional status is poor. Depression after childbirth is associated with maternal physical morbidity, including persistent unhealed abdominal or perineal wounds and incontinence.

Mental health is also governed by social circumstances. Women are at higher risk of mental health problems because they:

- carry a disproportionate unpaid workload of care for children or other dependent relations and household tasks;
- are more likely to be poor and not to be able to influence financial decision-making;
- are more likely to experience violence and coercion from an intimate partner than are men; and
- are less likely to have access to the protective factors of full participation in education, paid employment and political decision-making.

Health care behaviours including compliance with medical regimens such as anti-retroviral therapy (ARV) or appropriate use of contraceptives are diminished in the context of mental health problems. Poor mental health can be associated with risky sexual behaviour and substance abuse through impaired judgement and decision-making which can have dramatic consequences on reproductive health including heightened vulnerability to unintended pregnancy, STIs including HIV, and gender-based violence.

There is consistent evidence that women are at least twice as likely to experience depression and anxiety than men are. They are also more prone to self harm and suicide attempts, particularly if they have experienced childhood abuse or sexual or domestic violence. Adolescent girls with unplanned pregnancies are at elevated risk of suicide, as are women suffering from fistula, a childbirth injury caused by lack of emergency obstetric care. Suicide is a significant but often unrecognised contributor to maternal mortality, for example in Viet Nam, up to 14% of pregnancy-related deaths are by suicide. People living with HIV/AIDS have higher suicide rates, which stem from factors such as multiple bereavements, loss of physical and financial independence, stigma and discrimination, and lack of treatment, care and support.

More recently the adverse effects of poor maternal mental health have become the subject of renewed attention and concern because of increased awareness of the high rates of depression in mothers with small children in impoverished communities. About 10-15% of women in industrialized countries, and between 20-40 % of women in developing countries experience depression during pregnancy or after childbirth. Perinatal depression is one of the most prevalent and severe complications of pregnancy and childbirth. The effects of depression, anxiety and demoralization are amplified in the context of social adversity and poverty. These conditions have a pervasive adverse impact on women's health and wellbeing and caretaking capacity, with effects on the home environment, family life and parenting. They compromise women's capacity to provide sensitive, responsive and stimulating care, which is especially important for infants and children. Children of depressed mothers have poorer emotional, cognitive and social development than infants and children of non depressed mothers especially when the depression is severe and chronic and occurs in conjunction with other risks such as socioeconomic adversity. There is new evidence suggesting that maternal depression in developing countries may contribute to infant risk of growth impairment and illness through inadvertent reduced attention to and care of children's needs.

At present, the number of women having access to care that incorporates their mental health concerns is quite dismal. Even though the relationship between mental health problems and reproductive functions in women has fascinated the scientific community for some time, it is well recognized that mental health promotion, social change to prevent problems and develop acceptable treatments are under-investigated. This is particularly true for developing countries where the intersecting determinants of reproductive events or conditions and the mental health problems faced by women are simply not recognized. For example many women have questions and concerns about the psychological aspects of menstruation, contraceptive technologies, pregnancy, sexually transmitted infections, infertility and menopause. Feelings about hysterectomy or the loss or termination of a pregnancy may have a major impact on reproductive choices and well being. Sexual abuse is a frequent feature in the history of women with co-occurring mental health problems but is not addressed systematically. Survivors of gender-based violence commonly experience fear, anxiety, shame, guilt, anger and stigma; as a result, about a third of rape victims develop post traumatic stress disorder, the risk of depression and anxiety disorders increases three- to four-fold, and a proportion of women commit suicide. Other types of gender-based violence such as female genital mutilation (FGM), trafficking of girls/women, sexual abuse and forced marriage, commonly cause mental health problems. Besides encouraging the non tolerance of these practices, we must address the needs of those who are already victims and afflicted with these conditions.

Not only are feasible and cost effective interventions possible, but early detection and diagnosis of mental health problems can be undertaken by trained primary health care workers. Both simple psychological interventions such as supportive, interpersonal, cognitive-behavioural and brief solution focused therapies and when needed, psychotropic medications can be delivered through primary health care services for the treatment of many mental health problems. It has been shown, for example, that:

- the treatment of maternal depression can reduce the likelihood of maternal physical morbidity and mortality along with the likelihood of physical and mental or behavioural disorders in their children;
- the reduction of illicit drug-injection or the treatment of mood disorders can reduce the risk for HIV and AIDS and other STIs, unintended pregnancy and gender-based violence; and
- the treatment of depression, anxiety and trauma reactions results in better physical health, quality of life and social functioning of survivors of domestic violence.

Health care providers can involve the family, partner and peers in supporting women as agents of change in the family environment. The social environment, including health systems, and community organizations can be made more aware and receptive to the mental health problems of women and families. In many settings, culture-bound religious or other healing rituals which have shown to be effective can also play an important role.

Women's sexuality and reproductive health needs to be considered comprehensively with due consideration to the critical contribution of social and contextual factors. There is tremendous under-recognition of these experiences and conditions by the health professionals as well as by society at large. This lack of awareness compounded by women's low status has resulted in women considering their problems to be 'normal'. The social stigma attached to the expression of emotional distress and mental health problems leads women to accept them as part of being female and to fear being labeled as abnormal if they are unable to function.

The World Health Report 2005: Make Every Mother and Child Count (WHO, 2005) recognizes the importance of mental health in maternal, newborn and child health, especially as it relates to maternal depression and suicide, and of providing support and training to health workers for recognition, assessment and treatment of mothers with metal health problems. The International Conference on Population and Development (ICPD) Programme of Action and the Beijing Platform for Action urged member states to take action on the mental health consequences of gender-based violence and unsafe abortion in particular so that such major threats to the health and lives of women could be understood and addressed better. In addition, the mental health aspects of reproductive health are critical to achieving Millennium Development Goal (MDG) 1 on poverty reduction, MDG 3 on gender equality, MDG 4 on child mortality reduction, MDG 5 on improving maternal health and MDG 6 on the fight against HIV and AIDS and other communicable diseases. Moreover, humans are emotional beings and reproductive health can only be achieved when mental health is fully addressed as informed by the WHO's definition of health and the definition of right to health in the International Covenant of Economic, Social and Cultural Rights.

In response to these mandates, the present document has reviewed the research undertaken on a broad range of reproductive health issues and their mental health determinants/consequences over the last 15 years from both high- and low-income countries. Evidence from peer-reviewed journals has been used wherever possible but has been augmented with results of a specific survey initiated to gather state of the art information on reproductive and mental health issues from a variety of researchers and interested parties. Valuable data from consultant reports, national programme evaluations and postgraduate research work was also compiled, analyzed and synthesized.

Where evidence exists, suggestions have been made regarding the most feasible ways in which health authorities could advance policies, formulate programmes and reorient services to meet the mental health needs of women during their reproductive lives. Where gaps in the evidence are identified, recommendations are made about the areas and topics of research that need to be investigated. It is noteworthy that the evidence base everywhere, in both high- and low-income countries, has major gaps but there is a large divide between the amount of research undertaken and the health conditions chosen for research in low income compared with middle and high income countries. There is lack of information on chronic morbidities that are experienced disproportionately by women living in resource-poor and research-poor settings. It is important that lack of evidence and research on the mental health effects of such conditions predominantly affecting women in low income countries is not taken as implying that there are no mental health consequences of these conditions. All these facts justify the necessity of investigating and understanding the mental health determinants and consequences of reproductive health and the mechanisms through which the common mental health problems such as depression and anxiety disorders can be prevented and managed in low income countries as a matter of priority.

We hope that this review will draw attention to the substantial and important overlap between mental health and reproductive health, stimulate much needed additional research and assist in advocating for policy makers and reproductive health service providers to expand the scope of existing services to embrace a mental health perspective. Policy makers as well as service providers face a dual challenge: address the inseparable and inevitable mental health dimensions of many reproductive health conditions and improve the ways in which women are treated within reproductive health services, both of which have profound implications for mental as well as physical health. It is time that all reproductive health providers become sensitized to the fact that reproductive life events have mental health consequences and that without mental health there is no health.

Jill Astbury, Research Professor, School of Psychology, University of Victoria, Australia

Meena Cabral de Mello, Scientist, Department of Child and adolescent Health and Development, WHO

Jane Cottingham, Coordinator, Gender, Reproductive Rights, Sexual Health and Adolescence, WHO

Jane Fisher, Associate Professor, Key Center for Women's Health in Society, University of Melbourne, Australia

Takashi Izutsu, Technical Analyst, Technical Support Division, United Nations Population Fund

Arletty Pinel, Chief, Reproductive Health Branch, United Nations Population Fund

Shekhar Saxena, Department of Mental Health and Substance Abuse, WHO

Chapter 1

Overview of key issues

Jill Astbury

"Reproductive health is a state of complete physical, mental and social well-being and not merely the absence of disease or infirmity, in all matters relating to the reproductive system and to its functions and processes. Reproductive health therefore implies that people are able to have a satisfying and safe sex life and that they have the capability to reproduce and the freedom to decide if, when and how often to do so. Implicit in this last condition are the right of men and women to be informed and to have access to safe, effective, affordable and acceptable methods of family planning of their choice, as well as other methods of their choice for regulation of fertility which are not against the law, and the right of access to appropriate health-care services that will enable women to go safely through pregnancy and childbirth and provide couples with the best chance of having a healthy infant. In line with the above definition of reproductive health, reproductive health care is defined as the constellation of methods, techniques and services that contribute to reproductive health and well-being by preventing and solving reproductive health problems. It also includes sexual health, the purpose of which is the enhancement of life and personal relations, and not merely counselling and care related to reproduction and sexually transmitted diseases".

Programme of Action of the International Conference on Population and Development, para 7.2 (UNFPA, 1994)

Mental health as a component of reproductive health has generally been - and still is - inconspicuous, peripheral and marginal. The lack of attention it has received is unfortunate, given the significant contributions of both mental health and reproductive health to the global burden of disease and disability.

Of the ten leading causes of disability worldwide, five are neuropsychiatric disorders. Of these, depression is the most common, accounting for more than one in ten disability-adjusted life-years (DALYs) lost (Murray & Lopez, 1996). Depression occurs approximately twice as often in women as in men, and commonly presents with unexplained physical symptoms, such as tiredness, aches and pains, dizziness, palpitations and sleep problems (Katon & Walker, 1998; Hotopf et al., 1998). It is the most frequently encountered women's mental health problem and the leading women's health problem overall. Rates of depression in women of reproductive age are expected to increase in developing countries, and it is predicted that, by 2020, unipolar major depression will be the leading cause of DALYs lost by women (Murray & Lopez, 1996). More than 150 million people experience depression each year worldwide. Reproductive health programmes need to acknowledge the importance of mental health problems for women, and incorporate activities to address them in their services.

Reproductive health conditions also make a major contribution to the global burden of disability, particularly for women, accounting for

21.9% of DALYs lost for women annually compared with only 3.1% for men (Murray & Lopez, 1998). An estimated 40% of pregnant women (50 million per year) experience health problems directly related to the pregnancy, with 15% suffering serious or long-term complications. As a consequence, at any given time, 300 million women are suffering from pregnancy-related health problems and disabilities, including anaemia, uterine prolapse, fistulae (holes in the birth canal that allow leakage from the bladder or rectum into the vagina), pelvic inflammatory disease, and infertility (Family Care International, 1998). Further, more than 529 000 women die of pregnancy-related causes each year (WHO, 2006).

A global review of the interaction between reproductive health and mental health is potentially a vast undertaking, since each is in itself a large, specialized field of clinical, programmatic and research endeavours. Moreover, there are multiple points of intersection between mental health and reproductive health: for example, psychological issues related to pregnancy, childbirth and the postpartum period, and the mental health effects of violence, including sexual violence, adverse maternal outcomes, such as stillbirths and miscarriage, surgery on and removal of reproductive organs, sterilization, premarital pregnancies in adolescents, human immunodeficiency virus (HIV) infection and acquired immunodeficiency syndrome (AIDS), menopause and infertility (Patel & Oomman, 1999).

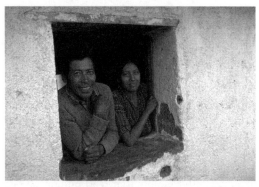

A complete review would examine all mental health aspects of reproductive health and functioning throughout the lifespan for both men and women. Such a review would consider in detail the relationships between mental and reproductive health at all levels, beginning with the individual and encompassing the effects of interpersonal relationships, and community and societal factors, including cultural values, mores

and laws. It would seek to explain the prevalence and severity of reproductive mental health problems and their intercountry variations. Such a review is impossible at present, because the necessary evidence is simply not available.

There are several possible reasons for the lack of a comprehensive database on reproductive mental health. First, the obvious lack of integration between mental health and reproductive health may reflect an enduring intellectual habit of mind-body dualism. The study of women's bodies and reproductive events has generally been rigidly separated from the study of their minds, including how women might think, feel and respond to these events and experiences. Second, efforts to examine the mental health implications of reproductive health have focused on a relatively small number of sexual and reproductive health conditions. For example, a Medline search for papers published between 1992 and March 2006 found more than 1500 papers on postnatal depression, but none on depression following vaginal fistula.

Third, there is a significant divide between the amount of research undertaken and the health conditions studied in low-income countries, compared with middle- and high-income ones. Chronic morbidities, including vesicovaginal fistula, perineal tears or poorly performed episiotomies, and uterovaginal prolapse, are much more common among women living in resource-poor and research-poor settings. It is important to bear in mind that the lack of evidence and research on the mental health effects of conditions that predominantly affect women in low-income countries does not imply that there are no mental health consequences of these conditions.

Fourth, the evidence base everywhere - in both high- and low-income countries - has significant gaps. Thus, the true impact on women's mental health of the multiple reproductive health conditions experienced over the course of their life cannot currently be ascertained.

The global burden of reproductive ill-health

Reproductive health conditions are estimated to account for between 5% and 15% of the overall disease burden, depending on the definition of reproductive health employed (Murray & Lopez, 1998). Even the higher figure is likely to be an underestimate, for several reasons. First, a number of conditions are not included in the calculations. These include fistulae, incontinence, uterine prolapse, menstrual disorders, non-sexually transmitted reproductive tract infections, female genital mutilation, and reproductive health morbidities associated with violence. Second, as Murray & Lopez (1996) note, there is a lack of data on the epidemiology of important non-fatal health conditions, such as those mentioned above, especially in low-income countries. Third, co-morbidities, such as the combination of poor mental and poor reproductive health, have not been assessed in terms of their contribution to DALYs. For example, suicidal ideation may be the outcome of a calamitous sequence of disabilities, initiated by obstructed labour resulting in organ prolapse or fistula; the calculation of burden of disease and disability in such a context is particularly difficult. Dependent co-disability, whereby one disability increases the likelihood of another developing, is extremely difficult to quantify (Murray & Lopez, 1996).

The available evidence on reproductive mental health conditions comes overwhelmingly from middle- and high-income countries, conveying the false impression that such conditions do not affect or concern women in low-income countries. Certain physical aspects of women's reproductive health, however, including fertility and its control, pregnancy, childbirth and lactation, receive significant attention in low-income countries, often in line with the narrow goals of population control policies. Unfortunately, the mental health effects of these reproductive health conditions are neither considered nor measured. The mental health and emotional needs of women are seen as being outside the scope of reproductive health services, which consequently provide no support or assistance in this regard. Even in Safe Motherhood Initiatives, "safety" is narrowly defined as physical safety, and the links between safe reproductive health care practices, treatments or services and the mental health of mothers are rarely considered. Mental health often appears to be considered an unaffordable "luxury" for women in resource-poor settings.

Another deficiency in the existing evidence base derives from the fact that research on reproductive health has predominantly been carried out on married women of childbearing age. Evidence on the reproductive health of single women, adolescent girls, and women past the age of childbearing is meagre. Moreover, men's reproductive health and the inter-relationships between women's and men's reproductive health are seriously underinvestigated.

Researchers' views

To augment the evidence obtained from peer-reviewed journals, to ascertain the extent of overlap between mental and reproductive health research, and to obtain further information on unmet research needs, a questionnaire was sent to 246 researchers around the world, working in either reproductive health or mental health. The questionnaire sought information about research being undertaken on the epidemiology, determinants and outcomes of reproductive health and mental health (Annex 1).

Respondents were asked to send copies of any relevant reports or publications to assist with the review, and to suggest which aspects of reproductive mental health required increased attention. Only 31 responses were received - a very low response rate of just over 12%. These responses supported the view that reproductive mental health is underinvestigated. Less than a quarter (8/31) of those who responded reported that they had investigated the impact of reproductive health on mental health, and only four had been involved in policy, programmes or services addressing both women's mental health and their reproductive health.

Just over half of the respondents (16/31) identified aspects of reproductive mental health that required increased attention. The two most important broad areas suggested for further inquiry were gender-based violence, specifically domestic violence (7/31), and maternal morbidity and gynaecological conditions generally (5/31). Within these areas, a number of concerns were raised, including access to safe abortion in the context of the threat of violence towards women seeking a termination of pregnancy, impairment of sexual health as a result of violence and abuse, and lack of control over contraceptive choice and the prevention of sexually transmissible infections, including HIV. Gynaecological topics requiring further investigation included unexplained vaginal discharge, fistula, cervical cancer prevention, and pregnancy-related issues, such as fear of childbirth, multiple pregnancies, and infertility. Premenstrual tension and menopause were mentioned as problems of the female reproductive cycle that warranted further investigation, and some respondents urged a stronger focus on adolescent health, sex education and high-risk behaviour in relation to both unwanted pregnancies and infections. One respondent urged that sexual enjoyment for women should be an objective of reproductive health programmes. Others commented on the importance of investigating all reproductive mental health topics with due regard to the psychosocial context in which they arose and an awareness of the additional problems faced by particular groups of women. Such groups included indigenous women, the elderly, the homeless, women living in rural or remote areas, persons with disabilities and those belonging to stigmatized or marginalized groups, including women with mental health problems who were also parents.

Women's views

Little research is available on women's own perceptions of their mental health or on their health priorities. For women themselves, mental health is critically important. One study reported that women's interest in mental health concerns actually outweighed their interest in reproductive health. Avotri & Walters (1999), in their study of women in the Volta region of Ghana, West Africa, found that psychosocial problems related to a heavy burden of work and a high level of worry predominated over reproductive health concerns. Women attributed their psychosocial distress to financial insecurity, financial and emotional responsibility for children, heavy workloads and a strict gender-based division of labour that put a disproportionate burden on them. In another study of HIV-positive women, mental health and well-being was the main focus of participants' concerns (Napravnik et al., 2000).

Focus and framework of the current review

The mental health aspects of women's reproductive health are the focus of this review, not only because of the lack of evidence on men's reproductive mental health but also because reproductive health conditions impose a considerably greater burden on women's health and lives.

To identify and reduce the emotional distress and poor mental health associated with the significant burden that reproductive health condi-

tions place on women, it is imperative to identify the relevant risk factors. The framework used for the analysis is informed by two interconnected concepts: gender and human rights, especially reproductive rights. Because of the inextricable relationship between health and human rights, the latter must be taken into account in any attempt to understand reproductive mental health. The public health goal of ensuring the conditions in which people can be healthy overlaps with the human rights goal of identifying, promoting and protecting the societal determinants of human well-being (Mann et al., 1999).

Gender analysis is necessary to elucidate how and why gender-based differences influence reproductive mental health. Areas for study include:

- risk and protective factors;
- access to resources that promote and protect mental and physical health, including information, education, technology and services;
- the manifestations, severity and frequency of disease, as well as health outcomes;
- the social and cultural determinants of ill-health/disease;
- the response of health systems and services;
- the roles of women and men as formal and informal health care providers.

Reproductive rights

Reproductive rights comprise a constellation of rights, established by international human rights documents, and related to people's ability to make decisions that affect their sexual and reproductive health (Sundari Ravindran, 2001). Two conferences in the 1990s were critical in promoting reproductive rights. The first was the International Conference on Population and Development (ICPD), held in Cairo in 1994, which produced a "Programme of Action" raising issues of reproductive rights and health concerning family planning, sexually transmitted diseases and adolescent reproductive health.. This was followed by the Fourth World Conference on Women (FWCW), in Beijing in 1995, which acknowledged women's right to have control over their sexuality, and articulated concepts of reproductive rights and health (Sundari Ravindran, 2001).

Reproductive rights include the basic rights of all couples and individuals to decide freely and responsibly the number, spacing and timing of their children, to have the information and means to do so, and to attain the highest possible standard of sexual and reproductive health. They also include their right to make decisions concerning reproduction free of discrimination, coercion and violence, as expressed in human rights documents (UNFPA, 1994 (para 7.3)).

All the major causes of death and disability associated with pregnancy, including haemorrhage, infection, eclampsia, obstructed labour and unsafe abortion, are potentially preventable or treatable (Berg et al., 2005). A denial of the right to timely and appropriate reproductive health care is a critical factor in increasing mortality and morbidity rates among women of reproductive age. Identifying and analysing violations of rights in relation to health contributes a new perspective to the socioeconomic and structural factors usually considered within a social model of health. Research that looks only at socio-economic indicators of risk fails to examine the "normative orders" that influence those indicators. The use of a rights-based approach offers a powerful lens to examine those normative orders and how they hamper women (in this instance) in realizing their right to good mental health in relation to reproduction (WHO, 2001).

Adding a gender and rights perspective helps to move away from a stereotyped conceptualization of reproductive health problems as "women's troubles". A gender and rights perspective moves beyond biological explanations of women's vulnerability to mental disorder to consider their vulnerability to a range of human rights violations. This vulnerability has little to do with biology and much to do with gender-based inequalities in power and resources. From a gender and rights perspective, improvements in women's reproductive mental health are contingent on the promotion and protection of women's human rights rather than the paternalistic protection of women as the "weaker sex". This perspective does not deny the role of biology; rather it considers how biological vulnerability interacts with, and is affected by, other sources of vulnerability including gender power imbalances, and how these can be remedied (WHO, 2001).

Although human rights violations are recognized as having a negative impact on mental health (Tarantola, 2001), there have been surprisingly few investigations of women's mental health, including reproductive mental health, in relation to their human rights (Astbury, 2001). Nevertheless, the higher risk of depression among women clearly underlines the importance of using a gender and rights perspective.

Gender, rights and reproductive mental health

The current review focuses on the common mental disorders, such as depression, anxiety and somatic complaints. This focus is based on the evidence that depression is the most important mental health condition for women worldwide and makes a significant contribution to the global burden of disease. Women suffer more often than men from the common disorders of depression and anxiety, both singly and as co-morbidities.

Reproductive rights include:

- the right to life;
- rights to bodily integrity and security of the person (against sexual violence, assault, compelled sterilization or abortion, denial of family planning services);
- the right to privacy (in relation to sexuality);
- the right to the benefits of scientific progress (e.g. control of reproduction);
- the right to seek, receive and impart information (informed choices);
- the right to education (to allow full development of sexuality and the self);
- the right to health (occupational, environmental);
- the right to equality in marriage and divorce;
- the right to non-discrimination (recognition of gender biases).

(Sundari Ravindran, 2001)

The gender-related nature of the most common mental disorders becomes even clearer when it is appreciated that high rates of depression, anxiety and co-morbidity are significantly linked to gender-based violence and socioeconomic disadvantage, situations that predominantly affect women (Astbury & Cabral de Mello, 2000). These same factors have pronounced negative impacts on a wide range of reproductive health conditions (Berer & Ravindran, 1999).

The current review does not attempt a comprehensive examination of reproductive mental health; rather it is a first step in bringing this important but neglected issue to the attention of a wide readership. Evidence indicates that depression is closely linked with a disproportionate exposure to risk factors, stressful life events, and adverse life experiences that are more common for women and that also affect their reproductive health (Patel & Oomman, 1999; Astbury & Cabral de Mello, 2000). If these risks serve as markers of multiple violations of women's human rights, it is imperative to name these violations. It is in their remedy that many risks for women's reproductive mental health will be eliminated or reduced.

This review addresses the following aspects of the reproductive health and mental health of women

- Mental health dimensions of pregnancy, childbirth and the postpartum period.
- Psychological aspects of contraception and elective abortion.
- Mental health consequences of miscarriage.
- Menopause and depression.
- Gynaecological morbidity and its impact on mental health.
- Mental health in the context of HIV/AIDS.
- Infertility and assisted reproduction.
- Mental health and female genital mutilation.

References

Astbury J (2001) Gender disparities in mental health. In: *Mental health: a call for action by world health ministers*. Geneva, World Health Organization.

Astbury J, Cabral de Mello M (2000) *Women's mental health: an evidence based review*. Geneva, World Health Organization.

Avotri JY, Walters V (1999) "You just look at our work and see if you have any freedom on earth": Ghanaian women's accounts of their work and health. *Social Science and Medicine*, 48:1123-1133.

Berer M, Ravindran TK, eds (1999) Safe motherhood initiatives: critical issues. *Reproductive Health Matters*. London: Blackwell Science.

Berg M et al (2005) Preventability of pregnancy-related deaths. Results of a statewide review. *Obstetrics and Gynecology*, 106:1228-1234.

Family Care International (1998) *Safe motherhood action agenda: priorities for the next decade*. A summary report of the Safe Motherhood Technical Consultation held in Sri Lanka, October 1997.

Hotopf M et al. (1998) Temporal relationships between physical symptoms and psychiatric disorder: results from a national birth cohort. *British Journal of Psychiatry*, 173:255-261.

Katon WJ, Walker EA (1998) Medically unexplained symptoms in primary care. *Journal of Clinical Psychiatry*, 59 (Suppl. 20): 15-21.

Mann JM et al. (1999) *Health and human rights*. In: Mann JM et al., eds, Health and human rights, New York and London, Routledge.

Murray CJL, Lopez AD (1996) *The global burden of disease*. Boston, Harvard School of Public Health (for the World Health Organization and the World Bank).

Murray CJL, Lopez AD (1998) *Health dimensions of sex and reproduction*. Boston, Harvard School of Public Health (for the World Health Organization and World Bank) (Global Burden of Disease and Injury Series, Vol. III).

Napravnik S et al. (2000) HIV-1 infected women and prenatal care utilization: Barriers and facilitators. *AIDS Patient Care & STDs*, 14: 411-420.

Patel V, Oomman NM (1999) Mental health matters too: gynaecological morbidity and depression in South Asia. *Reproductive Health Matters*, 7: 30-38.

Sundari Ravindran TK, ed. (2001) *Transforming health systems: gender and rights in reproductive health. A training curriculum for health programme managers*. Geneva, World Health Organization.

Tarantola D (2001) *Agenda item 10. Economic, Social and Cultural Rights*. Statement by Dr Daniel Tarantola, Senior Policy Advisor to the Director-General World Health Organization.

UNFPA (1994) *Programme of Action of the International Conference on Population and Development, Cairo*, 5-13 September 1994. New York, United Nations Population Fund.

WHO (2001) *Integration of the human rights of women and the gender perspective. Statement of the World Health Organization*. Geneva, 57th Session of the United Nations Commission on Human Rights, Agenda item 12.

WHO (2006) *Making a difference in countries: Strategic approach to improving maternal and newborn survival and health*. Geneva, World Health Organization (http://www.who.int/making_pregnancy_safer/publications/StrategicApproach2006.pdf).

Chapter

2

Pregnancy, childbirth and the postpartum period

Jane Fisher, Meena Cabral de Mello, Takashi Izutsu

In 1997, following a conference to address the gross disparities in maternal mortality rates between resource-poor and industrialized countries, a number of international organizations, including the World Health Organization, World Bank, and United Nations Population Fund, and government agencies established the Making Pregnancy Safer (Safe Motherhood) Initiative (Tinker & Koblinsky, 1993). Dramatic contrasts were apparent between industrialized and developing countries in terms of access to contraception, antenatal care, medical facilities for childbirth, and trained medical and nursing staff to provide pregnancy and obstetric health care. The multifaceted initiative aimed to address the complex economic, sociodemographic, health status and health service factors associated with an elevated risk of death related to pregnancy. Centrally important contributing factors were identified as: reproductive choice; nutritional status, co-existing infectious diseases; access to information; access to services; and training and skill of health workers (Lissner, 2001). The most prominent risks to life were identified as those directly associated with pregnancy, childbirth and the puerperium, including haemorrhage, infection, unsafe abortion, pregnancy illnesses, such as pre-eclampsia and gestational diabetes, and complications of delivery. The initiative, however, gave very limited consideration to mental health as a determinant of maternal mortality or morbidity

In the industrialized world, as pregnancy and childbirth have become safer and maternal mortality rates have declined, awareness has grown in the clinical and research communities of psychological factors associated with health in pregnancy, childbirth and the postpartum period. While there are historical references to disturbed behaviour associated with childbirth, it was not until the 1960s that systematic reports were published of elevated rates of admission to psychiatric hospital in the month after parturition (Robinson & Stewart, 1993). In 1964, Paffenberger reported the nature and course of psychoses following childbirth (Paffenberger, 1964) and in 1968 Pitt (1968) described an atypical depression observable in some women following childbirth. These reports stimulated the substantial research of the past four decades into the nosology of psychiatric illness associated with human reproduction. The determinants and adverse effects of poor mental health during pregnancy, childbirth and the postpartum year are now the subject of considerable attention and concern. The 2001 World Health Report was devoted to the burden of mental ill-health carried by individuals, families, communities and societies, and the need for accurate understanding of risk factors and prevalence in order to introduce effective prevention and treatment strategies (WHO, 2001). Most research has been conducted in Australia, Canada, Europe, and the United States of America; relatively little evidence is available from developing countries.

Mental health and maternal mortality

The predominant focus in endeavours to reduce maternal deaths has been on the direct causes of adverse pregnancy outcomes - obstructed labour, haemorrhage and infection - and on the health services needed to address them (Stokoe, 1991; Maine & Rosenfield, 1999; Goodburn & Campbell, 2001). Much less attention has been paid to mental health as a contributing factor to maternal deaths. In particular, violence - in the form of self-harm or of harm inflicted by others - during pregnancy or after childbirth has been under-recognized as a contributing factor to maternal mortality (Frautschi, Cerulli & Maine, 1994). The 2001 World Health Report identified a highly significant relationship between exposure to violence and suicide (WHO, 2001).

Despite close investigation, rates and determinants of suicide in pregnancy or after childbirth have proved difficult to determine, because of the extent to which the problem is underestimated or obscured in recording of causes of death or because systematic data are unavailable (Brockington, 2001). Socially stigmatized causes of death are less reliably recorded and probably under-reported (Radovanovic, 1994; Graham, Filippi & Ronsmans, 1996). Postmortem examinations after suicide do not always include the uterine examination necessary to confirm pregnancy and studies that have examined primary records in addition to death certificates have identified significant under-recognition (Weir, 1984; Brockington, 2001). Investigations of suicide in women often fail to report pregnancy status or consider it as an explanatory factor (Hjelmeland et al., 2002; Pearson et al., 2002; Hicks & Bhugra, 2003). There are substantial apparent intercountry variations in rates of suicide. Maternal mortality data combine records of deaths occurring during pregnancy and up to 42 days after the end of a pregnancy and, in many settings, specific data regarding suicide or parasuicide in pregnancy are unavailable. In industrialized countries, there is generally an excess of male to female deaths by suicide (Brockington, 2001). However, in the countries of South and East Asia for which data are available, the ratio is reversed, especially among younger women, who have suicide rates up to 25% higher than men (Lee, 2000; Ji, Kleinman & Becker, 2001; Phillips, Li & Zhang, 2002). Overall, suicide accounted for 50-75% of all deaths in women aged 10-19 years in a 10-year period in Vellore,

Southern India (Aaron et al., 2004). In these settings, women often have more limited educational opportunities than men, less access to financial resources and control of expenditure, restricted autonomy and greater likelihood of being threatened with violence. It is suggested that these gender disparities are linked to poorer mental health and higher risk of despair and consequent self-harm (Brockington, 2001; Ji, Kleinman & Becker 2001; Batra, 2003; Fikree & Pasha, 2004; Kumar, 2003). Completion of suicide in South and East Asia is related in part to the lethality of the method of self-harm, in particular self-poisoning by pesticides and herbicides, which are readily accessible in rural farming communities (Pearson et al., 2002; Fleischman et al., 2005).

It has been argued that pregnancy is a period of stable mood and relative emotional well-being and that pregnant women are, therefore, at lower risk of suicide than non-pregnant women (Marzuk et al., 1997; Sharma, 1997). In industrialized countries, rates of suicide in pregnancy have declined over the past 50 years, a change attributed to the increased availability of contraception, affordable and accessible services for the termination of pregnancy, and reduction in the stigma associated with births to unmarried women (Kendell, 1991; Frautschi et al., 1994).

> Summary reviews have found that suicide in pregnancy is not common; however, when it happens, it is primarily associated with unwanted pregnancy or entrapment in situations of sexual or physical abuse or poverty (Brockington, 2001; Frautschi, Cerulli & Maine, 1994).

Suicide is disproportionately associated with adolescent pregnancy, and appears to be the last resort for women with an unwanted pregnancy in settings where reproductive choice is limited; for example, where single women are not legally able to obtain contraceptives, and legal pregnancy termination services are unavailable (Appleby, 1991; Frautschi, Cerulli & Maine, 1994). Young women who fear parental or social sanction, or who lack the financial means to pay for an abortion, or who cannot obtain a legal abortion may attempt to induce abortion themselves. Women who do this by self-poisoning, use of instruments, self-inflicted trauma, or herbal and folk remedies are at increased risk of death by misadventure (Smith, 1998). Investigations in three districts in Turkey found that suicide was one of the five leading causes of death among women of reproductive age, and was associated with age under 25 years and being unmarried; pregnancy status was not reported (Tezcan & Guciz Dogan, 1990). Ganatra & Hirve (2002), in a population survey of mortality associated with abortion in Maharashtra, India, found that death rates from abortion-related complications was disproportionately higher among adolescents, because they were more likely than older women to use untrained service providers. In addition, a number of adolescents had committed suicide to preserve the family honour without seeking abortion. Young women from minority ethnic groups are at increased risk of suicide in pregnancy (Church & Scanlan, 2002).

There has been relatively limited investigation of suicide after childbirth, but in industrialized countries reported rates are lower than expected, and usually associated with severe depression or postpartum psychosis (Appleby, Mortensen & Faragher, 1998). Attachment to the infant appears to reduce the risk of suicide in mothers of newborns (Appleby, 1991), but population-based comparisons indicate that the rate of suicide among women who have just given birth is not significantly different from the general female suicide rate (Oates, 2003a). Maternal suicide is associated with a heightened risk of infanticide (Brockington, 2001). Confining assessment of maternal mortality to the first 6 weeks postpartum probably leads to underestimation of maternal mortality from suicide, which may occur much later in the postpartum period (Yip, Chung & Lee, 1997).

The British Confidential Enquiries into Maternal Deaths found that maternal deaths from psychological causes, most usually suicide, were at least as prevalent as deaths from hypertensive disorders of pregnancy when data collection was extended to twelve months postpartum, and that, overall, suicide was the leading cause of maternal death (Department of Health, 1999).

Suicide in combination with other deaths attributable to psychiatric problems, particularly substance abuse, accounted for 28% of maternal deaths in the United Kingdom in 1997-99 - more than any other single cause (Oates, 2003b). In Sweden, teenage mothers aged under 17 years were found to be at elevated risk of premature death, including suicide, and alcohol abuse compared with mothers aged over 20 years (Otterblad Olausson et al., 2004). The deaths were not only associated with severe mental illness, but were also related to domestic violence and the complications of substance abuse. Two large data linkage studies found that, compared with childbirth, miscarriage and, more strongly, pregnancy termination were associated with increased suicide risk in the following year, especially among unmarried, young women of low socioeconomic status. These findings were attributed to either a risk factor common to both depression and induced abortion, most probably domestic violence, or depression associated with loss of pregnancy (Gissler & Hemminki, 1999; Gissler, Hemminki & Lonnqvist, 1996; Reardon et al., 2002).

There have been very few systematic studies of suicide after childbirth in developing countries. In a detailed classification of cause of 2882 deaths during pregnancy or up to 42 days postpartum, in three provinces in Viet Nam in 1994-1995, the leading cause (29%) was external events, including accidents, murder and suicide. Overall 14% of the deaths were by suicide (Hieu et al., 1999). Lal et al. (1995) reviewed 219 deaths among 9894 women who had given birth in three rural areas of Haryana, India, in 1992, and found that 20% were due to suicide or accidental burns. Granja, Zacarias & Bergstrom (2002), in a review of pregnancy-related deaths at Maputo Central Hospital, Mozambique, in 1991-1995, found that 9 of 27 (33%) deaths not attributable to pregnancy or coincidental illness were by suicide. Seven of the nine suicide deaths were in women aged less than 25 years. In the United Kingdom, the report of the Confidential Enquiries into Maternal Deaths recommended that all maternal deaths should be classified as occurring by violent or non-violent means (Department of Health, 1999). The Centers for Disease Control and Prevention and the American College of Obstetricians and Gynecologists now recommend that the definition of maternal death should include any death of a woman while she is pregnant or within one calendar year of termination of the pregnancy, and that these should be classified as to whether or not they occurred by violent means (American College of Obstericians and Gynecologists, 2003).

Although completed suicide may be rare, parasuicide - thoughts of suicide and attempts to self-harm - is up to 20 times more common (Brockington, 2001). Parasuicide is more prevalent in women than men in most countries. It is associated with low education and socioeconomic status, but predominantly with childhood sexual and physical abuse, and sexual and domestic violence (Brockington, 2001; Stark & Flitcraft, 1995). In pregnancy, suicidal ideation and attempts at self-harm are significantly more common in women with a history of childhood sexual abuse than those without such a history (Bayatpour, Wells & Holford, 1992; Farber, Herbert & Reviere, 1996). Women with a history of sexual and physical abuse in childhood are also more likely that those without such a history to have attempted suicide prior to pregnancy (Farber, Herbert & Reviere, 1996). Past physical abuse is itself a risk factor for pregnancy in adolescence (Adams & East, 1999). Both unwanted pregnancy and parasuicide are more common in adolescents without a psychiatric history who have experienced physical or sexual "dating violence" (Silverman et al., 2001). In addition, women who attempt suicide in pregnancy are significantly more likely to have been subject to domestic violence (Stark & Flitcraft, 1995), and suicide attempts by self-poisoning are most likely to occur in the early weeks of an unwelcome pregnancy (Czeizel, Timar & Susanszky, 1999).

Appleby & Turnbull (1995) found that rates of self-harm treated in hospital in the first postnatal year were low in the United Kingdom, and argue that maternal concerns for infant wellbeing are protective. The Edinburgh Postnatal Depression Scale (EPDS), a widely used screening and research instrument, has a specific item assessing the presence and intensity of suicidal ideation (Cox, Holden & Sagovsky, 1987). Most studies using this instrument have not presented data specifically related to this item, but one of the scale's developers (Holden, 1991; Holden, 1994) has reported that women who are severely depressed commonly have a positive score on it. There is a small emerging body of literature on postpartum parasuicide in developing countries, which suggests that it is not uncommon. Rahman & Hafeez (2003) report that more than one-third (36%) of mothers caring for young children and living in refugee camps in the North West Frontier Province of Pakistan had a mental disorder and that 91% of these women had suicidal thoughts. Fisher et al. (2004) found that, among a consecutive cohort of 506 women attending infant health clinics six weeks postpartum in Ho Chi Minh City, Viet Nam, 20% acknowledged thoughts of wanting to die.

Intense grief reactions can accompany pregnancy loss and may increase parasuicide rates. Parasuicide rates are 93 times higher in the year after treatment for ectopic pregnancy than among non-pregnant age-matched controls; this is interpreted as a response to the loss of the pregnancy and the potential loss of fertility as well as damage to self-regard, and recovery from unanticipated surgery (Farhi, Ben-Rafael & Dicker, 1994). Although no systematic evidence is currently available, Adamson (1996) has suggested that parasuicide and suicide may also be consequences of the profound distress that accompanies vesicovaginal fistula in women in some developing countries.

Maternal deaths by inflicted violence

Deaths of women during pregnancy or within 42 days of termination of pregnancy, from causes not related to or aggravated by the pregnancy or its management, are termed pregnancy-related deaths. Deaths from inflicted violence have been underascertained in standard recording of maternal mortality, which is limited to pregnancy and the first 42 days postpartum. Violence-related maternal deaths are under-reported in routine data collection and are often inaccurately regarded as incidental or chance events (Granja, Zacarias & Bergstrom, 2002)

A number of meticulous studies, using detailed scrutiny of primary health, coroner's court and hospital records in addition to death certificates, have had remarkably consistent findings (Dannenberg et al., 1995; Fildes et al., 1992; Gissler & Hemminki, 1999; Horon & Cheng, 2001; Parsons & Harper, 1999). Fildes et al. (1992) found that the leading cause of death during pregnancy or after childbirth in one American county (accounting for 46.3% of pregnancy-related deaths) was trauma, including homicide (57% of them) and suicide (9%). Dannenberg et al. (1995) reported that 39% of deaths of pregnant or newly delivered women in New York City were not directly related to the pregnancy, 63% of which were by homicide and 13% by suicide; women from minority ethnic groups were at heightened risk. In the county of Maryland, USA, Horon & Cheng (2001) found that 20% of all pregnancy-related deaths were by homicide, which was the leading cause of such deaths in 1993-1998. Pregnancy was not recorded on 50% of the death certificates, so linkage of multiple vital records was essential for accurate identification. Parsons & Harper (1999) found that 51% of non-maternal deaths in North Carolina followed domestic violence, and that obstetric care providers were not aware of the severe risks faced by these individuals. Gissler & Hemminki (1999) reported that one-third of deaths in Finland in the year after childbirth or termination of pregnancy were attributable to homicide, more commonly following induced abortion than a live birth. Otterblad Olausson et al. (2004) showed that violence inflicted on adolescent mothers contributed to increased premature mortality later in life, compared with older mothers.

In developing countries, intimate partner violence or violence from other family members is associated with increased maternal mortality, although systematic representative international studies are unavailable. Granja, Zacarias & Bergstrom (2002) found that 37% of pregnancy-related deaths in their investigation in Mozambique were by homicide and 22% were accidents. Batra (2003), in describing deaths from burning among young married women in India, noted that 47.8% of the deaths were suicide, with torture by in-laws the most common explanatory factor.

In general, these studies concluded that maternal mortality could be accurately ascertained only if causes of death were expanded to include deaths due to violence inflicted by self or others.

Mental health and antenatal morbidity

In contrast to the substantial investigations of women's psychological functioning after childbirth, relatively little research has been devoted specifically to mental health during pregnancy (Llewellyn, Stowe & Nemeroff, 1997). Research has generally focused on the risks for the fetus of poor maternal mental health, in terms of adverse alterations to the intrauterine environment, risky

behaviours, in particular substance abuse, failure to attend antenatal clinics, and increased risk of adverse obstetric outcome. Conventionally, pregnancy has been regarded as a period of general psychological well-being for women, with a lower rate of hospital admissions for psychiatric illness (Oppenheim, 1985; Kendell, Chalmers & Platz, 1987), reduced risk of suicide (Marzuk et al., 1997) and lower rates of panic disorder (Sharma, 1997). However, Viguera et al. (2002) reported that risk of recurrence of bipolar affective disorder was not diminished in pregnancy.

Depression in pregnancy

Llewellyn et al. (1997) suggest that certain symptoms of depression, including appetite change, lowered energy, sleep disturbance and reduced libido, are considered "normal" in pregnancy and their psychological significance is therefore underestimated. A range of psychosocial factors has been associated with depression in pregnancy, including unwanted conception, unmarried status, unemployment and low income (Pajulo et al., 2001; Zuckerman et al., 1989). Certain early experiences within the family of origin, in particular recalled conflict and divorce, appear to increase depressive symptoms and contribute to reduced personal resources (Bernazzani et al., 1997). Three sources of support appear to influence mood in pregnancy: the woman's own parents, in particular her mother; her partner; and her wider social group, including same-age peers (Berthiaume et al., 1996; Brugha et al., 1998; Pajulo et al., 2001).

Despite the impression of well-being in pregnancy, comparable rates of depressive symptoms have been found among pregnant and non-pregnant women. Large systematic studies have shown that rates of depression in late pregnancy are as high or higher than rates of postpartum depression (Zuckerman et al., 1989; Da Costa et al., 2000; Evans et al., 2001; Josefsson et al., 2001).

Only a few studies of the prevalence of antenatal depression in South and East Asian, African or South American countries are available. Chen et al. (2004) surveyed pregnant women attending antenatal clinics at a Singapore obstetric hospital, and reported that 20% had clinically significant depressive symptoms. Young women and women with complicated pregnancies were at elevated risk. Lee et al. (2004a) found that 6.4% of 157 Hong Kong Chinese women in advanced pregnancy were depressed. Fatoye, Adeyemi & Oladimeji (2004) found higher rates of depressive and anxious symptoms in pregnant women than in matched non-pregnant women in Nigeria. Depression was associated with having a polygamous partner, a previous termination of pregnancy, and a previous caesarean birth. In a small study of 33 low-income Brazilian women, Da Silva et al. (1998) found that 12% were depressed in late pregnancy, and that depression was associated with insufficient support from the partner and lower parity. Chandran et al. (2002) interviewed a consecutive cohort of 359 women registered for antenatal care in a rural community in Tamil Nadu, India, and found that 16.2% were depressed in the last trimester. Rahman, Iqbal & Harrington (2003) established that 25% of pregnant women attending services in Kahuta, a rural community in Pakistan, were depressed in the third trimester of pregnancy. Risk was increased among the poorest women and those experiencing coincidental adverse life events.

Anxiety in pregnancy

There has been a widely held belief that anxiety in pregnancy is harmful to the fetus and contributes to adverse obstetric outcomes. The incidence of anxiety disorders is the same in pregnant women and those who are not pregnant (Diket & Nolan, 1997). Subclinical levels of anxiety vary normally through pregnancy, with peaks in the first and third trimester, and are specifically focused on infant health and well-being and childbirth (Lubin, Gardener & Roth, 1975; Elliott et al., 1983). Anxiety in pregnancy is higher among younger, less well-educated women of low socioeconomic status (Glazer, 1980). Elevated anxiety may have adaptive value as a maturational force in impelling women to prepare for a major life transition (Astbury, 1980). In a detailed and comprehensive review, Istvan (1986) concluded that there was little evidence to support the contention that, in humans, maternal stress or anxiety influenced either neonatal health or obstetric outcome. He commented further that previous research had failed to account for the complex interactive effects of poverty, age and reproductive choice in attributing poor pregnancy outcomes to women's mental health. However, recent investigations have revisited the issue, with suggestions that mater-

nal anxiety in pregnancy has adverse effects on birth weight (Texiera, Fisk & Glover, 1999) and on later behavioural and emotional problems in the children (Glover et al., 2002; Glover & O'Connor, 2002; O'Connor, Heron, & Glover, 2002; O'Connor et al., 2002). These recent studies have been criticised because, in assessing anxiety in the last trimester of pregnancy, they failed to take into account the mother's knowledge of the health and development of her baby acquired through antenatal care. Anxiety is likely to be higher in women who know that their infant's intrauterine development is compromised (Perkin, 1999). Sjostrom et al. (2002) found that maternal anxiety did not affect fetal movements or fetal heart rate in late pregnancy. Brooke et al. (1989) demonstrated that smoking in pregnancy was the main determinant of low birth weight and that psychological and social factors had no direct effect independent of smoking.

Pregnant women are generally encouraged to modify their self-care and personal habits to ensure optimal maternal and fetal health. This includes advice to alter their diet, avoid alcohol, stop smoking cigarettes, gain a specified amount of weight, exercise (but not to excess), rest, relax and have regular health checks. The evidence for some of this advice is poor, and the recommendations have been criticised for failing to take into account personal circumstances and social realities (Lumley & Astbury, 1989). It is difficult for women to ensure adequate nutrition for themselves if they are poor or have restricted access to shared resources (Nga & Morrow, 1999). Smoking and substance abuse in pregnancy are associated with depression arising from conflict in marital and family relationships, domestic violence and financial concerns (Kitamura et al., 1996; Bullock et al., 2001; Pajulo et al., 2001). Women who smoke in pregnancy have poorer nutritional intake (Haste et al., 1990). Both physical and sexual abuse are predictive of substance abuse in pregnant adolescents (Bayatpour, Wells & Holford, 1992). Pregnant women who are dependent on opiates and have a co-morbid diagnosis of post-traumatic stress disorder (PTSD) are more likely than those without PTSD to have a history of sexual abuse and to have experienced severe conflict in their family of origin (Moylan et al., 2001). Poorer health in pregnancy and delay in accessing antenatal care are linked to insufficient social support (Webster et al., 2000).

In addition to social factors, participation in prenatal genetic screening and diagnosis can also generate anxiety (Green, 1990a). This occurs independently of the results of the test, and is worse if there is a long interval between the test and the result becoming available (Green, 1990a). The anxiety can be modified by skilled genetic counselling and psychosocial support, but may persist (Keenan et al., 1991). Although screening may be beneficial, anxieties are unnecessarily aroused by false-positive results for women whose fetus is actually healthy. Normal results in follow-up tests do not always provide effective reassurance (Marteau et al., 1992). False-negative results of prenatal screening, encouraging parents to believe they are giving birth to a healthy child, have a modest adverse effect on parental adjustment, which may still be evident 2-6 years after the birth (Hall, Bobrow & Marteau, 2000). In the past decade, research has focused on the determinants of informed, autonomous decision making and uptake of services, but not on the emotional consequences of participation in prenatal genetic screening and diagnosis. There is currently no evidence of the psychological impact of increased surveillance during pregnancy on the overall experience of pregnancy and the postnatal period. Systematic investigations are difficult because services are changing rapidly.

Termination of pregnancy for fetal abnormality is relatively rare, but can have significant and lasting psychological consequences (Green, 1990a). There is little social understanding or support for either parents or the health professionals involved (Kolker & Burke, 1993). Hunfeld et al. (1997) compared 27 women with a history of late pregnancy loss (after 20 weeks) due to fetal abnormality, who subsequently had a live birth, with 27 mothers of newborns without such a history. Those with prior pregnancy loss had significantly greater anxiety and depression than women without such a history; this was interpreted as re-evoked grief about the previous loss. They also perceived their infants as having more problems and were more anxious about infant care (Hunfeld, Wladimiroff & Passchier, 1994; Hunfeld et al., 1997). Prenatal screening and diagnosis can now be carried out early in pregnancy, and little is known about the psychological consequences of first trimester termination of pregnancy for fetal abnormality. Most research on first-trimester abortion has focused on those carried out for social reasons, after which psychological morbidity is low (Adler, 2000). Termination of a planned and wanted pregnancy is likely to have a different meaning, and research findings for one group cannot be generalized to the other. Decision-making about first-trimester abortion for fetal abnormality is complicated by the fact that many affected pregnancies, if left, will terminate spontaneously (McFadyen et al., 1998). There is no evidence on the psychological aspects of forced termination of pregnancy, or pregnancy termination associated with sex selection, in settings with restrictions on family size and a preference for male children.

Cultural preferences and mental health in pregnancy

In many cultures, there is a preference for sons rather than daughters; the psychological consequences of this for pregnant women have not been systematically investigated. Country-level sex ratios are skewed in favour of males in China, India and the Republic of Korea (Fathalla, 1998; Bandyopadhyay, 2003). Clinicians can use techniques such as ultrasound, amniocentesis, and chorionic villus sampling to determine fetal sex, and female fetuses may subsequently be aborted selectively (Kristof, 1993). Although legislation prohibits this practice, it is known to persist. Women can be blamed for sex determination and may not be able to make a free choice about continuing or terminating a pregnancy (Fathalla, 1998; Bandyopadhyay, 2003). The birth of a daughter was found to contribute independently to postpartum depression in women in India and Pakistan (Patel, Rodrigues & DeSouza, 2002; Chandran et al., 2002; Rahman, Iqbal & Harrington., 2003); it is therefore reasonable to speculate that mental health during pregnancy may also be adversely affected by the family and social reaction to the conception of a daughter.

Inflicted violence and mental health in pregnancy

Violence is estimated to occur in between 4% and 8% of pregnancies (Petersen et al., 1997), although higher rates have been reported: 11% in South Carolina between 1993 and 1995 (Cokkinides et al., 1999); 13.5% in an American prenatal care programme (Covington et al., 2001); 15.7% among women attending an antenatal clinic in a hospital in Hong Kong, China (Leung et al., 1999); and 22% among women attending a routine antenatal clinic in Nagpur, India (Purwar et al., 1999).

Women who are the victims of domestic violence during pregnancy, including verbal aggression and minor and severe physical abuse, are significantly more likely to rate their relationship with their male partner as poor (Cloutier et al., 2002). Investigations have focused on the links between violence and adverse maternal and neonatal outcomes, with relatively little emphasis to date on mental health (Petersen et al., 1997; Shumway et al., 1999). However Muhajarine & D'Arcy (1999) found that women who had experienced physical abuse in pregnancy reported higher stress and more coincidental adverse life events, while Webster, Chandler, & Battistutta (1996) reported that they were more likely to be taking antidepressant medication than women who had not experienced violence. Stewart & Cecutti (1993) found that abused women in a range of prenatal care settings were significantly more emotionally distressed than non-abused women.

Eating disorders and pregnancy

There has been much less exploration of other psychological conditions in pregnancy. However, there is evidence that women with an eating disorder - anorexia nervosa or bulimia nervosa - may be unwilling to disclose these conditions during routine care. They are at increased risk of miscarriage and intrauterine growth retardation, and may have co-morbid depression and anxiety (Franko & Spurrell, 2000).

Mental health and postpartum morbidity

In becoming a mother, a woman often has to relinquish her autonomy, personal liberty, occupational identity, capacity to generate an income, and social and leisure activities in favour of caring for the infant. The adaptation to her new required roles, major responsibilities, moving from being in the childless generation to the parent generation, increased unpaid workload and, for some, harm to bodily integrity through unexpected adverse reproductive events places great demands both on individual psychological resources and on existing relationships. Psychological disequilibrium is normal during life transitions and in adapting to change, and

there is continuing theoretical consideration of the extent to which perinatal psychological disorder should be regarded as a normal process. However, there is now substantial evidence that women's mental health can be compromised by childbirth and that some women experience psychiatric illness. Debate continues about whether psychiatric illnesses occurring in pregnancy or after childbirth are clinically distinct from those observed at other phases of the life cycle, and of the relative etiological contributions of biological and psychosocial factors. There is now a consistent view that psychological disturbance following childbirth can be conceptualized as fitting one of three distinct conditions, of differing severity: transient mood disturbance, depression and psychotic illness.

Postpartum blues or mild transient mood disturbance

Maternity, third day or postpartum blues are a phenomenon occurring in up to 80% of women in the days immediately following childbirth (Pitt, 1973; Kennerley & Gath, 1986). The syndrome is characterized by a range of symptoms, most commonly a lability of mood between euphoria and misery, heightened sensitivity, tearfulness often without associated sadness, restlessness, poor concentration, anxiety and irritability (Yalom et al., 1968; Stein, 1982). Disturbed sleep (Wilkie & Shapiro, 1992), feelings of unreality and detachment from the baby have also been reported (Robinson & Stewart, 1993). There have been a small number of specific transcultural studies of the nature and incidence of postpartum blues, which have reported rates in non-Anglophone countries ranging from 13% to 50% (Howard, 1993; Kumar, 1994). Sutter et al. (1997) reported a rate of 42.5% in a sample of French mothers. Very limited evidence is available about postpartum blues in developing countries. Davidson (1972) reported that 60% of newly delivered women in Jamaica were tearful or sad, while Ghubash & Abou-Saleh (1997) found that 24.5% of Arab women met the criteria for a clinical case of psychiatric morbidity using the WHO Self Reporting Questionnaire on the second day after birth.

> The birth of an infant demands a dramatic adaptation by women.

The coincidence of the maternity blues with the major hormonal changes associated with parturition has led investigators to look for a biological basis to the condition, but findings are generally inconsistent (Robinson & Stewart, 1993; Steiner, 1998). Similarly, there is no consistent evidence for the contribution of parity (Kendell et al., 1981), obstetric factors (Condon & Watson, 1987; Oakley, 1980), hospital or home as place of delivery (Kendell et al., 1981; Pop et al., 1995), or personal or family history of mood disorder (O'Hara et al., 1991) to the incidence or severity of the condition. The distress peaks between three and five days postpartum, and usually resolves spontaneously without specialist intervention. However, in some women a more persistent and severe depression develops. There is some evidence that the more severe symptoms of blues, including early self-reports of feeling depressed, having thoughts about death or being unable to stop crying, predict later development of depression (O'Hara et al., 1991; Sutter et al., 1997). Steiner's (1998) summary review concluded that the evidence base was insufficient to predict, diagnose, prevent, treat or give prognostic indicators for the maternity blues.

Postpartum psychotic illness

A very small group of women (approximately 1 or 2 per 1000) develop an acute psychosis within the first month postpartum; this is the most severe psychiatric illness associated with childbirth. Relative lifetime risk and incidence are usually calculated in terms of psychiatric admissions for treatment of psychotic illness after childbirth. The risk for women of experiencing a psychotic illness is highly elevated for the first thirty days postpartum and remains elevated, but at a lower rate, for two years following childbirth (Kendell, Chalmers & Platz, 1987; McNeil & Blenow, 1988). Clinical characteristics include acute onset and extreme affective variation, with mania and elation as well as sadness, thought disorder, delusions, hallucinations, disturbed behaviour and confusion (Marks et al., 1992; Pfuhlmann, Stoeber & Beckmann, 2002; Scottish Intercollegiate Guidelines Network, 2002). Postpartum psychoses are most accurately construed as episodes of cycloid affective illness; rates of schizophrenic psychotic episodes are not elevated postnatally (Brockington, Winokur & Dean, 1982; Kendell, Chalmers & Platz, 1987; Brockington, 1992; Kumar, 1994; Pfuhlmann, Stoeber & Beckmann, 2002). Although treat-

ment is similar, there is a divergence of views as to whether puerperal psychotic episodes in an individual with an existing diagnosis of bipolar affective disorder should be understood to be the same as first episodes following childbirth (Pfuhlmann, Stoeber & Beckmann, 2002). Risk of recurrence after subsequent pregnancies is between 51% and 69% (Pfuhlmann, Stoeber & Beckmann, 2002).

There is continuing conjecture about the relative contributions of biological and psychosocial etiological factors to the development of postpartum psychoses and the possibilities of meta-analysis to elucidate this are restricted by methodological limitations in existing studies (Pfuhlmann, Stoeber & Beckmann, 2002). However, the timing of onset of the illness, family history and molecular genetic studies support an underlying biological etiology, with childbirth as the precipitating factor (Pfuhlmann, Stoeber & Beckmann, 2002). Postpartum psychosis has been associated with primiparity, personal or family history of affective psychosis, unmarried status and perinatal death of an infant (Kendell, 1985; Kendell, Chalmers & Platz, 1987). The contribution of obstetric factors is not clear, but there is some evidence that caesarean delivery increases the risk of postpartum psychosis and of relapse after subsequent births (Kendell et al., 1981; Nott, 1982; McNeil & Blenow, 1988). Puerperal and non-puerperal episodes of psychosis are predicted most strongly by a history of psychotic episodes and by marital difficulties (Marks et al., 1992).

Systematic international comparisons of the prevalence, clinical characteristics and course of postnatal psychotic illnesses, including in developing countries, are not available. However, in all countries in which studies have been conducted, psychotic illnesses following childbirth have been identified (Howard, 1993; Kumar, 1994). Investigations of women admitted to hospital with postpartum mental illness in countries outside Western Europe and North America report higher rates of puerperal psychosis. Schizophrenia is reported more commonly than affective illness in those settings, but these patterns may reflect intercountry differences in diagnostic criteria (Howard, 1993; Kumar, 1994). Both Howard (1993) and Kumar (1994) highlighted the higher incidence in developing countries of puerperal psychoses associated with organic illness, including confusional states related to fever from infections or to poor nutrition. Ndosi & Mtawali (2002) described a case series of 86 women who developed psychosis within six weeks of giving birth in the United Republic of Tanzania; the incidence rate of 3.2 per 1000 was approximately double that reported in industrialized countries. Most of the women were young and primiparous; co-existing anaemia and infectious illnesses were common and 80% of the illnesses were categorized as organic psychoses.

There is much less evidence about the complex reproductive mental and physical health needs of women with pre-existing chronic severe mental illness (Kumar, Hipwell & Lawson, 1994). Although people with schizophrenic illnesses appear to have reduced fertility and smaller families, this effect is less marked for women than for men, and many are parents (McGrath et al., 1999; Nimgaonkar, 1998; Nimgoankar et al., 1997). Among those with severe chronic mental illness, frequency of sexual activity may be normal, but contraceptive use may be lower and autonomous reproductive decision-making compromised (Thomas et al., 1996; Cole, 2000). The multiple psychosocial difficulties experienced by those with severe chronic mental illnesses can have adverse effects on the formation of mother-infant attachment. The children of parents with psychiatric illnesses are at increased risk of neglect or inadequate care and the later development of psychopathology (Kumar, Hipwell & Lawson, 1994; Nimgoankar et al., 1997; Oates, 1989; Cole, 2000).

Postpartum depression

Over the lifespan, on average, women experience major depression between 1.6 and 2.6 times more often than men. This difference is most apparent in the life phase of caring for infants and young children (Epperson, 1999; Astbury, 2001). Depression arising after childbirth has attracted substantial research interest in the past 40 years, and there is now an extensive literature on its nature, prevalence, prediction, course and associations with risk and protective factors.

Postpartum depression is a clinical and research construct used to describe an episode of major or minor depression arising after childbirth (Cox, 1994; Epperson, 1999; Paykel, 2002). The International Classification of Diseases (ICD 10) (WHO, 1992) does not have a specific diagnostic

category of postpartum depression, and classifies depression after childbirth as a depressive episode of either mild (four symptoms), moderate (five symptoms), or severe (at least five symptoms, with agitation, feelings of worthlessness or guilt or suicidal thoughts or acts). Although onset within one month of giving birth is specified for an episode to be labelled as postpartum depression in the fourth edition of the Diagnostic and Statistical Manual of Mental Disorders (DSM IV) (American Psychiatric Association 1994), it is not distinguished nosologically from depressive episodes in general (Cramer, 1993; Paykel, 2002).

While there is debate about whether depression following childbirth is a clinically distinct condition, there is consistent evidence that 10-15% of women in industrialized countries will experience non-psychotic clinical depression in the year after giving birth, with most developing it in the first five weeks postpartum (Cox, Murray & Chapman, 1993; O'Hara & Swain, 1996; Epperson, 1999). Severe depression, needing inpatient treatment, occurs in 3-7% of women after childbirth (O'Hara & Zekoski, 1988).

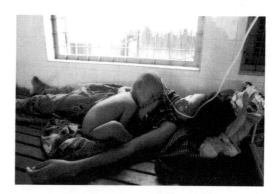

It is still not clear whether postnatal depression is a continuation of an existing state, or first occurs after delivery. There is also a lack of clarity over how long the postpartum period should be considered to last, and therefore for how long after delivery a depression can be regarded as specifically postnatal in onset (Cooper & Murray, 1997; Paykel, 2002). There is a clustering of new cases around childbirth, which is argued to be distinctive (Cramer, 1993). DSM IV specifies within a month of parturition, but Nott (1987) found that the highest incidence of new cases occurred 3-9 months postpartum. Chaudron et al. (2001) demonstrated that 5.8% of cases of depression identified at four months postpartum were not apparent at one month. Most conceptualizations take a categorical approach, in which individuals are classified as satisfying the criteria for a clinical case, or are regarded as well. Some authors, however (Green, 1998; Romito, 1989; Fisher, Feekery & Rowe-Murray, 2002), argue that adjustment processes, including transient dysphoria and symptoms of depression, can be observed in most women postpartum, and that a continuum of emotional well-being or a broad spectrum of adjustment experiences may be a more accurate conceptualization. Mood in the first year after childbirth is dynamic and determined by multiple factors (Gjerdingen & Chaloner, 1994; Evans et al., 2001). In practice, it is common for any episode of depression during this period to be regarded as linked to the birth (Scottish Intercollegiate Guidelines Network, 2002). Postpartum depression is of serious public health concern because of its demonstrated adverse consequences on the development of maternal confidence and the cognitive, emotional and social development of their infant (Murray, 1997; Murray et al., 1999).

Postpartum depression is characterized by the persistent presence for at least two weeks of cognitive and affective symptoms including: low mood, guilt, despondency, self-deprecation, anhedonia, impaired concentration, irritability, elevated anxiety, rumination and social withdrawal. The somatic symptoms of sleep and appetite disturbance are also present, but are not uncommon in normal postpartum adjustment (Campbell & Cohn, 1991).

Biological risk factors for postpartum depression

The causes of depression in the postpartum period are still the subject of controversy, debate and research. Broadly, the arguments concern the relative contributions of biological and psychosocial factors. The evidence for a biological contribution is derived from a number of sources. Biochemical hypotheses hold that the dramatic hormonal changes that follow childbirth and are involved in lactation may precipitate or maintain depression (Hendrick, Altshuler & Suri, 1998; Epperson, 1999). Links between postpartum depression and a history of premenstrual mood change or increased familial vulnerability to affective illness and alcohol dependence are cited in support of a biological etiology (Stowe & Nemeroff, 1995). However, summary and systematic reviews have concluded that, although some women may be particularly psychologically vulnerable to hormonal change, a direct link between hormones or other neurochemicals and postpartum depression has not yet been demonstrated (Robinson & Stewart, 1993; Hendrick, Altshuler & Suri, 1998; Scottish Intercollegiate Guidelines Network, 2002).

Two medical conditions may contribute to altered mood after childbirth. The incidence of abnormal thyroid function is higher in the first six months postpartum (7% versus 3% in the wider population) (Hendrick, Altshuler & Suri, 1998; Epperson, 1999). Although most women with postpartum depression have normal thyroid function, fatigue, lowered mood and impaired volition have been associated with hypothyroidism, while agitation and excessive weight loss are linked to hyperthyroidism. Postpartum haemorrhage and lactation are associated with iron deficiency anaemia, which contributes to fatigue and lowered mood (Epperson, 1999). These conditions are often under-recognized.

Psychosocial risk factors for postpartum depression

The prevalence of schizophrenia and bipolar affective disorder, for which there is evidence of genetic vulnerability, is similar in men and women. Patel (2005) argues cogently that sex differences in the prevalence of depression and anxiety cannot be attributed to "over-simplistic biological or hormonal explanations for the female excess because few biological parameters show this degree of variability". He concludes that women's vulnerability to depression is attributable to social, economic and cultural factors beyond individual control. Evidence that a range of psychological, social and economic factors contribute to postpartum depression is more substantial than that for biological explanatory models. Nevertheless, associations between risk factors and conditions cannot be interpreted as causal links, and there is a general view that postpartum depression is unlikely to be attributable to a single cause, but is probably the outcome of the interaction of a number of risk and protective factors (Cramer, 1993; O'Hara & Swain, 1996; Wilson et al., 1996; Beck, 2001; Scottish Intercollegiate Guidelines Network, 2002).

A personal history of mood disorder, previous psychiatric hospitalization, and anxious or depressed mood in pregnancy are consistently found to be predictive of postpartum depression (O'Hara et al., 1991; Webster et al., 1994; O'Hara & Swain, 1996; Wilson et al., 1996; Beck, 2001; Scottish Intercollegiate Guidelines Network, 2002). Although this phenomenon is widely observed, the factors that contribute to disturbed affect in women are not well understood. Studies consistently assess prevalence of psychiatric illness, in particular mood disorder and alcohol dependence in the family of origin (Stowe & Nemeroff, 1995), and report elevated rates in those with postpartum depression. However, histories of abuse or exposure to violence have rarely been considered or assessed. Poor parental care, especially poor maternal care and neglect in childhood (Boyce, Hickie & Parker, 1991; Boyce et al., 1998; Douglas, 2000), and childhood sexual and physical abuse (Buist & Barnett, 1995; Buist & Janson, 2001) contribute to adult depression and appear to be associated with postpartum mood disorders. Women who have been sexually abused in childhood have increased anxiety about their own children's safety and feel inhibited in providing intimate parenting to their infants (Douglas, 2000).

A poor relationship between the woman and her partner is now regarded as a major predictor of depression after childbirth (Romito, 1989; O'Hara & Swain, 1996; Cooper & Murray, 1997; Beck, 2001; Scottish Intercollegiate Guidelines Network, 2002). The problems in this relationship have been variously conceptualized as: increased marital conflict (Kumar & Robson, 1984); men being less available after delivery, and providing insufficient practical support (O'Hara, 1986) or poor emotional support (Paykel et al., 1980; Dimitrovsky, Perez-Hirshberg & Istkowitz, 1987); poor adjustment or unhappiness (Webster et al., 1994); low satisfaction (Beck, 2001); insufficient involvement in infant care (Romito, 1989); and holding rigid traditional sex role expectations (Wilson et al., 1996). The relationship with the partner also appears to significantly affect the time taken to recover (Gjerdingen & Chaloner, 1994). Very similar findings have emerged from transcultural studies. A poor quality of marital relationship - variously described as inability to confide in an intimate partner or lack of support, or arguments and tension in the relationship - is centrally related to women's mental health postpartum, and

has been found to distinguish depressed from non-depressed women in Hong Kong, China (Chan et al., 2002), India (Chandran et al., 2002; Rodrigues et al., 2003), Pakistan (Rahman, Iqbal & Harrington, 2003), Brazil (Da Silva et al., 2003) and Viet Nam (Fisher et al., 2004).

Some authors have suggested that depressed women are more likely to be irritable and socially withdrawn, and that for this reason they may be difficult for their partners to relate to, or may be providing less care for their partners, or may perceive their relationship as poor (Cramer, 1993). Boyce, Hickie & Parker (1991) stated that a woman who is depressed postnatally "may be particularly incapable of evoking additional care and support from her partner" or "may tend to choose a partner incapable of providing care or to behave in a way which elicits uncaring responses from her intimate". The alternative proposition - that the behaviour of male partners contributes to maternal depression - has not usually been considered.

Although there have been some investigations into whether men's mental health might also be adversely affected by childbirth, overall there has been much less systematic examination of perinatal psychological functioning in men than in women. Marks & Lovestone (1995) postulated that men may feel excluded from the intimate relationship between mother and infant, and themselves become depressed or anxious. Men are not at elevated risk of psychotic illness after the birth of a baby (Marks & Lovestone, 1995). Rates of depression among men in the postpartum period appear to be low: less than 5% among Portuguese fathers 12 weeks postpartum (Areias et al., 1996); 1.2% among Irish fathers six weeks postpartum (Lane et al., 1997); 3% among fathers in the Avon Longitudinal Study of Pregnancy and Childhood (Deater-Deckard et al., 1998); and 2.8% among Australian fathers four months postpartum (Matthey et al., 2000). In one study, severe postpartum intrusive stress symptoms were found in 9% of mothers and 2% of fathers (Skari et al., 2002). Condon, Boyce & Corkindale (2004) conducted one of the first-ever systematic prospective studies of men's psychological well-being, involving 312 first-time fathers. They found that the greatest level of psychological symptoms was during mid-pregnancy, and that there was actually some improvement in mood by three months postpartum. Overall, only 1.9% of the sample had a clinically significant score on the EPDS at three months after the birth. The authors suggest that distress may be expressed in other ways, perhaps as increased alcohol use or irritability, but that men actually experience little mood change during the period of their partner's pregnancy and after the birth. Matthey et al. (2001) suggest that distress may be under-reported by men, and that screening instruments may require different cut-off scores to detect clinically significant symptoms in men and in women.

Violence against women by their intimate partners has been described as "the most prevalent ... gender-based cause of depression in women" (Astbury, 2001). Criticism, coercion, control, humiliation, and verbal or physical violence by an intimate partner on whom the woman is dependent, is causally linked to depression and anxiety (Astbury, 2001). Unfortunately, most research on the etiology of postpartum depression has not assessed the effect of coercion, intimidation and violence by the intimate partner. Boyce, Hickie & Parker (1991), Schweitzer, Logan & Strassberg (1992), and Matthey et al. (2000), using the Intimate Bonds Measure (Wilhelm & Parker, 1988), found that women whose partnerships were characterized by high levels of control and low levels of care were at increased risk of postpartum depression. However, fear of intimidation and actual experience of abuse were not ascertained. A prospective cohort study of 838 parturient Chinese women in Hong Kong, China (Leung et al., 2002), using the Abuse Assessment Screen, found that 16.6% had been abused in the previous year. Among women who had experienced domestic violence, higher scores on the EPDS were reported 2-3 days after delivery, 1-2 days after discharge from hospital, and six weeks postpartum than among those with no experience of violence. There was no difference between the two groups of women in terms of sociodemographic factors, although the abused women were more likely to report that their pregnancy had been unplanned. Women admitted to an early parenting service were significantly more likely to be depressed if they had experienced an act of physical violence in the previous year, or if they percieved their partners as critical and coercive (Fisher, Feekery & Rowe-Murray, 2002). Stewart & Robinson (1996), in a review of the literature on violence, identified a tendency to promote the idea of "female masochism ... [suggesting] that women are in some

way responsible for their own victimisation". The literature has generally failed to acknowledge or examine the social factors, including financial dependence and desire to maintain the integrity of their relationship, that prevent women from leaving violent relationships.

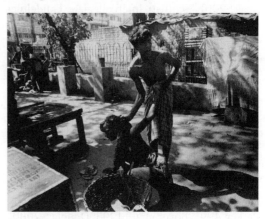

Broader social factors are also associated with depression after childbirth. Poor social support, including having few friends or confiding relationships and lack of assistance in crises, is related to postpartum depression. General dissatisfaction with available support, rather than specific characteristics or number or quality of relationships, appears to be relevant (Boyce et al., 1998; Beck, 2001; Scottish Intercollegiate Guidelines Network, 2002). Postpartum depression has been found to be more common among young mothers and single women (Paykel et al., 1980; Feggetter, Cooper, & Gath, 1981; Webster et al., 1994). Having a first child at over 30 years of age has also been implicated (Dennerstein, Lehert & Riphagen, 1989; Astbury et al., 1994; Chaudron et al., 2001), and it is possible that women who have babies at a different time than most of their peers have social needs that are not met. Social disruption associated with recent immigration or relocation, especially if compounded by being unable to speak the local language and understand and obtain local services, also heightens the risk of difficulties in adjusting to parenthood (Howard, 1993; Webster et al., 1994; Fisher et al., 2002; Parvin, Jones & Hull, 2004).

International studies have also found that a lack of practical assistance from family, including dedicated care during the early postpartum period, is more commonly reported by women who are depressed than those who are not depressed (Mills, Finchilescu & Lea, 1995; Chandran et al., 2002; Inandi et al., 2002; Rahman, Iqbal &

Harrington, 2003; Rodrigues et al, 2003; Fisher et al., 2004; Lee et al., 2004). If this practical dedicated support is available from a supportive and uncritical person, it is psychologically protective (Rahman, Iqbal & Harrington, 2003; Fisher et al., 2004; Lee et al., 2004b). Problematic relationships with the partner's family, especially critical coercion from the mother-in-law, have been found to be more common among women who are depressed in both qualitative (Rodrigues et al., 2003;) and survey investigations (Chandran et al., 2002; Inandi et al.,, 2002; Rahman, Iqbal & Harrington, 2003; Fisher et al., 2004; Lee et al., 2004b).

Although some have argued that socioeconomic status is not associated with postpartum depression (Paykel et al., 1980), this claim has not been tested accurately since young, poorly educated women in low-status occupations are less likely to be recruited to, and retained in, studies. Women receiving obstetric care in the private health care sector - who are likely to be of higher socioeconomic status - consistently have a better mood in pregnancy and the postpartum year than those receiving care in the public sector (Kermode, Fisher & Jolley, 2000). Groups found to be more likely to be depressed include: parturient women who are unemployed or in low-status unskilled occupations (Zelkowitz & Milet, 1995; Righetti-Veltema et al., 1998; Chaudron et al., 2001; Rubertsson et al., 2005); those who do not have a job to return to after a period of maternity leave (Warner et al., 1996); and those who have to resume employment sooner than desired or work for more hours than desired (Gjerdingen & Chaloner, 1994). Social disadvantage exerts pervasive adverse effects that may not be distinguishable in settings where poverty is endemic. However, there is consistent evidence that maternal mental health is directly affected by poverty in resource-poor countries (Cooper et al., 2002). Limited education reduces women's access to paid occupations and secure employment. Women living in poverty and experiencing economic difficulties, who have low education and no access to employment that allow them time to care for their infant, are more likely to be depressed (Chandran et al., 2002; Inandi et al., 2002; Rodrigues et al., 2003; Fatoye, Adeyemi & Oladimeji, 2004; Fisher et al., 2004).

Adverse life events coincidental with childbirth, such as bereavement, serious illness in the family, conflict with friends, or serious financial problems, can make the psychological adjustment to parenthood more difficult and distressing (Kumar & Robson, 1984; O'Hara and Swain, 1996; Boyce et al., 1998; Beck, 2001; Scottish Intercollegiate Guidelines Network, 2002). In developing countries, bereavement or serious illness in the family, the partner not having an income, housing difficulties, crowded living conditions and lack of privacy are associated with higher rates of maternal depression (Chandran et al., 2002; Patel et al., 2002; Rahman, Iqbal & Harrington, 2003; Fisher et al., 2004). The distress associated with an unwanted or unwelcome pregnancy does not necessarily diminish during pregnancy, can persist postpartum, and be associated with depression (Kumar & Robson, 1984; Warner et al., 1996; Scottish Intercollegiate Guidelines Network, 2002). The contribution of sexual violence or forced intercourse to unwanted pregnancy and depression has not been examined.

Certain aspects of personality are also implicated in the propensity to become depressed, particularly at times of major life transition, including childbirth. These include: heightened sensitivity to the opinions of others; over-eagerness to please; lack of assertiveness and timidity, obsessiveness; and excessive worrying (Boyce, Hickie & Parker, 1991; Boyce & Mason, 1996; Grazioli & Terry, 2000; Scottish Intercollegiate Guidelines Network, 2002). A meta-analysis by Beck (2001) identified low self-esteem as an independent risk factor for postpartum depression. However, the familial, social and cultural factors that contribute to personality development in women, including a propensity to be uncomplaining, compliant, and unassertive and to have a low sense of entitlement, have not been considered in relation to these findings.

Physical health and postpartum depression

The contribution of intrapartum experiences to postpartum mood has been considered, using two approaches. Some investigators have constructed composite scores to assess cumulative exposure to obstetric interventions, and then correlated the scores with later mood (Oakley, 1980; Elliott et al., 1984; Astbury et al., 1994). Others have examined the impact of particular procedures. In general there is no correlation between cumulative exposure to obstetric procedures and mood (Elliott et al., 1984; Astbury et al., 1994), but there is consistent evidence that certain modes of delivery - particularly instrumental intervention in vaginal birth (e.g. forceps) and caesarean surgery - can have adverse psychological consequences (Green, 1990b; Campbell & Cohn, 1991; Boyce & Todd, 1992; Hannah et al., 1992; Brown & Lumley, 1994; Fisher, Astbury & Smith, 1997; O'Neill, Murphy & Greene, 1990). These have been variously conceptualized as depression, disappointment, grief and dissatisfaction; however, mode of delivery does not appear to contribute independently to postpartum depression when other risk factors are taken into account (Johnstone et al., 2001). Emergency surgery during childbirth, in particular caesarean section, can induce acute stress reactions and disrupt the first encounter between mother and infant (Fisher, Astbury & Smith, 1997; Righetti-Veltema et al., 1998; Rowe-Murray & Fisher, 2001, 2002). There is emerging evidence that childbirth events can lead to post-traumatic stress disorders, but the effect is not direct and appears to be moderated by quality of care and of personal support (Ayers and Pickering, 2001). In addition to being associated with prolonged physical recovery and fatigue, surgery can also compromise the development of maternal confidence (Garel et al., 1990; Brown & Lumley, 1994; Rowe-Murray & Fisher, 2001).

Poor physical health after childbirth contributes to poor mental health (Gjerdingen & Chaloner, 1994; Brown, 1998). Physical problems related to the birth can persist for months and are often undiagnosed and untreated (Gunn et al., 1998). Not breastfeeding has been associated with increased likelihood of postpartum depression (Warner et al., 1996; Eberhard-Gran et al., 2002) and may be an early indicator of vulnerability (Eberhard-Gran et al., 2002). The effects of length of stay in hospital after childbirth on physical and psychological recovery are equivocal. Profound fatigue is widespread among mothers of newborns (Brown, 1998), but is often considered normal or trivial, despite its adverse impact on daily functioning (Milligan et al., 1996). Excessive tiredness has been regarded as symptomatic of depression (Stowe & Nemeroff, 1995), but an alternative view is that it is associated with the unrecognized and unpaid workload of caring for a newborn baby. Exhaustion may lead to depression in women whose workload is neither acknowledged nor shared (Fisher, Feekery & Rowe-Murray, 2002).

Large community surveys have not found an effect of early discharge from maternity hospital (Brown, 1998; Thompson et al., 2000), but 20% of women admitted to a residential service for treatment of early parenting difficulties considered that their maternity stay had been too short (Fisher et al., 2002).

Premature birth and the birth of an infant with disabilities are highly distressing events that can lead to depression (Calhoun & Calhoun, 1980; Kumar & Robson, 1984). Women with a multiple gestation have increased risk of ill-health, pregnancy loss and premature or operative birth, all of which are associated with anxiety in pregnancy. Because of the competing and major demands of caring for more than one infant, multiple births are also associated with increased risk of postpartum depression and complicated grief reactions (Fisher & Stocky, 2003).

Infant factors and maternal mental health

Investigations of both infant development and mother-infant interaction have presumed that infants are essentially normative and that variations in developmental outcomes primarily reflect parenting factors (Murray & Cooper, 1997). Cross-sectional cohort comparisons have found that mothers who are depressed are significantly more likely to report excessive infant crying and disturbed infant sleep and feeding than mothers who are not depressed (Milgrom, Westley, & McCloud, 1995; Armstrong et al., 1998a; Righetti-Veltema et al., 2002). Some authors have interpreted this as indicating that the behaviour of depressed mothers increases the likelihood of disturbed infant behaviour (Milgrom, Westley & McCloud, 1995; Righetti-Veltema et al., 2002). However, others acknowledge that the care of an unsettled, crying infant, who resists soothing and has deregulated sleep, undermines maternal confidence and well-being and may be relevant to the onset of maternal depression and to disturbances in mother-infant interaction. These inter-relationships have not yet been well conceptualized and are generally under-investigated, but evidence is emerging that they may be more significant than has previously been acknowledged (Cramer, 1993; Murray & Cooper, 1997; Armstrong et al., 1998b).

Babies are born with distinguishable variations in intrinsic characteristics or temperament, and these exert a significant effect on the infant's interactions with the environment, especially with caregivers (Oberklaid et al., 1984). Nine dimensions of infant temperament have been identified in comprehensive interview- and observation-based rating studies of large samples of infants: motor activity; regularity of sleeping and feeding patterns; response to unfamiliar people or stimuli; ease of adaptation to change; intensity of emotional reactions; threshold to reaction; overall mood; distractibility; and persistence (Oberklaid et al., 1984; Sanson et al., 1987). Infants are more temperamentally difficult when they: have little rhythm in sleeping and feeding patterns; are easily aroused; have difficulty in adapting to changes in the environment; and react with great intensity. Hopkins, Campbell & Marcus (1987) compared 25 depressed mothers of six-week-old babies with 24 non-depressed mothers of the same age, socioeconomic status and religious affiliation. They found that the infants of the depressed mothers had more neonatal complications and were less adaptable and fussier than those of the mothers who were not depressed.

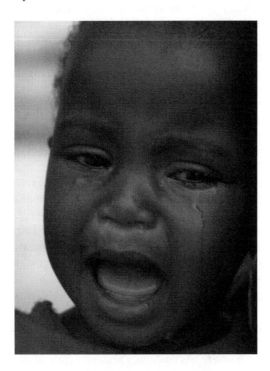

Infant crying is highly arousing to carers, but there is wide individual variation in the amount and intensity of infant crying and fussing in the first year of life (Lehtonen & Barr, 2000). Contemporary advice on infant care encourages mothers to trust their intuition and do what feels appropriate. They are told to distinguish their infant's cries, and discern whether these are indicating pain, hunger, a startle reaction or fatigue. However, there is little empirical support for the notion that cries are in fact specific or distinguishable, and in reality parents have to use other contextual and behavioural cues to decode them (Craig, Gilbert-Macleod & Lilley, 2000). Mothers most often attribute infant cries to hunger, and the widespread contemporary advice to "feed on demand" may promote the notion that babies only cry when hungry (Craig, Gilbert-Macleod & Lilley, 2000). Excessive prolonged crying is often presumed to be because of gastrointestinal pain, but gastrointestinal pathology is rarely found on clinical investigation. Inconsolable crying, deregulated behaviour and resistance to soothing are usually difficult to explain, and are now thought to be early indicators of a difficult temperament (Barr & Gunnar, 2000). Up to 25% of mothers of 4-6-month-old infants report that their babies cry for more than three hours a day (Beebe, Casey & Pinto-Martin, 1993). Mothers can feel ineffective and helpless caring for an inconsolable infant. Confidence can diminish rapidly and they are less likely to experience their infants as a source of positive reinforcement (Beebe, Casey & Pinto-Martin, 1993). Excessive infant crying is associated with earlier cessation of breastfeeding, frequent changes of infant formula, maternal irritability, poor mother-infant relationship, deterioration in the familial emotional environment, and heightened risk of infant abuse (Wolke, Gray & Meyer, 1994; Lehtonen & Barr, 2000). Infant feeding difficulties, including refusal of breast or bottle, frequent small feeds, and multiple overnight waking for feeds, frequently occur in conjunction with deregulated sleep and persistent crying (Barber et al., 1997). Parents of inconsolable infants receive less positive reinforcement from the infant, such as laughing or responding to soothing, and have greater exposure to the negative stimulus of infant crying. This can reduce their confidence in their ability to parent, and may increase the likelihood of postpartum depression (Mayberry & Affonso, 1993). It is not surprising that longitudinal studies have shown that infant sleep problems precede maternal depression (Lam, Hiscock & Wake, 2003)

Cultural specificity of postpartum mood disturbance

There is debate about whether the ways depression and other mood disturbances are expressed are universal or culturally determined (Jenkins, Kleinman, & Good, 1991). In cultures in which discussion of emotions is proscribed, or in which distress is associated with shame or stigma, depression may be manifested as non-specific somatic symptoms (Ng, 1997). It has been argued that culturally prescribed ritual forms of peripartum care for women are psychologically protective (Cox, 1996; Howard, 1993; Manderson, 1981; Stern & Kruckman, 1983). Socially structured peripartum customs are characterized as providing dedicated care, an honoured status, relief from normal tasks and responsibilities, and social seclusion for the mother and her newborn (Howard, 1993; Kumar, 1994; Stern & Kruckman, 1983). Stern & Kruckman (1983) concluded that ethnographic studies in cultures where such customs were observed showed little evidence of postpartum depression.

More recent studies have used validated screening and diagnostic tools to investigate whether postpartum depression is a culture-bound condition. While there is still debate about appropriate methods of measurement, it appears that - if the complexities of translation, literacy levels and familiarity with test-taking are taken into account - structured interviews and screening instruments, such as the Edinburgh Postnatal Depression Scale, can be used cross-culturally (Clifford et al., 1999; Laungani, 2000; Small, 2000).

A number of studies have compared peripartum experiences, rates of depression, and risk factors in groups of different ethnicity living in industrialized countries. Fuggle et al. (2002) examined small groups of Bangladeshi women living in London and Dhaka with English women, and found an overall rate of depression of 11.5%, with no difference between groups. Matthey, Barnett, & Elliot (1997) reported that there were no differences in scores in the clinical range on the EPDS between Vietnamese, Arabic and Anglo-Celtic women living in south-west Sydney. Despite some variation in the ranking of the contribution of different risk factors by ethnic group (Stuchbery, Matthey, & Barnett, 1998), the risk factors identified as relevant to all groups were highly consistent. They were: inability to confide in the partner and insufficient practical support from the partner (Matthey, Barnett & Elliot, 1997; Stuchbery, Matthey & Barnett, 1998) or from parents or the wider social circle (Fuggle et al., 2002).

Studies using structured clinical interviews or screening questionnaires have been conducted in a range of non-English-speaking countries, to establish the incidence and correlates of clinically significant depressive symptoms in the early postpartum period. In Europe, the following incidence rates were found: 8.7% in Malta (Felice et al., 2004); 14% in Iceland (Thome, 2000); 9% in Italy and 11% in France (Romito, Saurel-Cubizolles & Lelong, 1999); 11.4% in Sweden and 14.5% in Finland (Affonso et al., 2000); and 29.7% in Spain (based on clinical case criteria in the General Health Questionnaire (GHQ)) (Escriba et al., 1999). In Singapore, 3.5% of postpartum women satisfied the criteria for a clinical case, but 86% had some depressive symptoms three months postpartum (Kok, Chan & Ratnam, 1994); in Hong Kong, China, 13.5% of postpartum women had a diagnosable psychiatric illness (Lee et al., 2001); and in Japan the incidence was 17% (Yamashita et al., 2000). In Israel, Glasser et al. (1998) found that 22.6% of women had EPDS scores in the clinical range at six weeks postpartum.

Some comparable investigations have been undertaken in resource-poor countries; these are summarized in Table 2.1. Contrary to previous beliefs, very high rates of depression - 2-3 times those in industrialized countries - were observed. There is little evidence to support the notion that women in developing countries do not experience depression (Moon Park & Dimigen, 1995; Patel & Andrew, 2001; Fisher et al., 2004)). The finding of high rates of postpartum depression in developing country contexts challenges the anthropological view that ritual postpartum care protects women. It appears that this assertion may be an oversimplification and warrants more comprehensive and detailed investigation . Even where it is culturally prescribed, ritual may not be available to all women (Inandi et al, 2002; Fisher et al., 2004). Observation of postpartum rituals, including lying over heat, wearing warm clothes and using cotton swabs in the ears to protect the body against "cold", and taking herbal preparations, was no less common among Vietnamese women who were depressed than among those who were not (Fisher et al, 2004).

Still, increased care that provides dedicated, practical support for a defined period, especially from the woman's family of origin, may be protective (Moon Park & Dimigen, 1995; Rodrigues et al., 2003; Lee et al., 2004). In contrast, ritual care that imposes control and restricts the woman's autonomy might actually be harmful (Chan et al., 2002; Fisher et al., 2004; Lee et al., 2004b).

While differences in instruments, sampling and method of data collection may have contributed to the range of rates of depression found, questions assessing psychological state were meaningful and recognizable to women in these studies (Fisher et al., 2004). In countries where most women give birth without being attended by a skilled health worker, hospital-based samples are highly biased and likely to under-represent the experiences of the poorest women. For example, in East Africa, only 32.5% of women give birth attended by health professionals, while in West Africa the figure is 39.7%; many of these take place in community clinics, and are accessible only to relatively wealthy women (WHO, 2005). Most women in these settings give birth at home, assisted either by family members or by traditional birth attendants. It is probable, therefore, that the city hospital-based samples used by Cox (1983) in Kampala (Uganda), Aderibigbe, Gureje & Omigbodun (1993) in Ibadan (Nigeria), and Regmi et al. (2002) in Kathmandu (Nepal) represent relatively advantaged women whose rates of poor mental health are likely to be similar to those of women in rich countries. There are striking similarities between the risk factors for depression identified in these investigations and those that are well established in the industrialized world.

The first is that a poor quality of relationship with the intimate partner is consistently found to distinguish depressed from non-depressed women postpartum (Mills, Finchilescu & Lea, 1995; Chan et al., 2002; Chandran et al., 2002; Rahman, Iqbal & Harrington, 2003; Rodrigues et al., 2003; Da Silva et al., 2003; Fisher et al., 2004). This relationship is variously described as inability to confide in, or lack of support from, the partner, or arguments and tension in the relationship. Intimate partner violence has not been specifically assessed in most investigations of risk factors for postnatal depression. However, Patel et al. (2002) demonstrated unequivocally that women who are exposed to intimidation or

physical violence from a partner are at greatly increased risk of becoming depressed after childbirth. Wider family relationships are also implicated, but as yet the evidence available is limited. However, problematic relationships with the partner's family, especially critical coercion from a mother-in-law, have been reported to be more common among women who are depressed in both qualitative investigations (Rodrigues et al., 2003) and survey investigations (Chandran et al., 2002; Inandi et al., 2002; Rahman, Iqbal & Harrington, 2003; Fisher et al., 2004). In addition, a lack of practical assistance from the family, including dedicated care during the early postpartum period, is more commonly reported by women who are depressed than those who are not depressed (Mills, Finchilescu & Lea, 1995; Chandran et al., 2002; Inandi et al., 2002; Rahman, Iqbal & Harrington, 2003; Rodrigues et al., 2003; Fisher et al., 2004). If practical dedicated support is available, it is psychologically protective (Rahman, Iqbal & Harrington, 2003; Fisher et al., 2004).

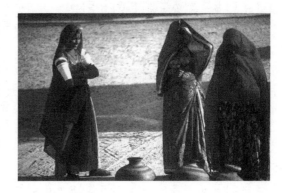

There is consistent evidence that maternal mental health is also influenced by socioeconomic factors (Cooper et al., 2002). Limited education reduces women's access to paid occupations and secure employment. Women living in poverty and experiencing economic difficulties, who have low education and no access to employment that allows them time to care for their infant are more likely to be depressed (Chandran et al., 2002; Inandi et al., 2002; Rodrigues et al., 2003; Fatoye, Adeyemi & Oladimeji, 2004; Fisher et al., 2004).

Coincidental adverse life events, including bereavement or serious illness in the family, the partner not having an income, housing difficulties, crowded living conditions and lack of privacy are also associated with higher rates of

Table 2.1 Postpartum mental health in developing countries

Authors	Sample	Setting	Measures	Results
Cox, 1983	183 parturient women	Kasangati Hospital, Kampala, Uganda	Goldberg's Standardised Psychiatric Interview, 3 months postpartum	10% depressive illness, 3 anxiety disorders
Aderibigbe, Gureje & Omigbodun, 1993	162 pregnant women	University College Hospital, Ibadan, Nigeria	General Health Questionnaire 28, Psychiatric Assessment Schedule at 6–8 weeks postpartum	14% postpartum psychiatric caseness
Ghubash & Abou-Saleh, 1997	Consecutive cohort of 95 parturient women	New Dubai Hospital, United Arab Emirates	EPDS score ≥12 on day 7, and Present State Examination score ≥ 5 at 8 and 30 weeks postpartum	24.5% (of which 17.8% was depression) on day 7; 15.8% at week 8
Nhiwatiwa, Patel & Acuda, 1998	Consecutive cohort of 500 pregnant women	Periurban settlement, Zimbabwe	Shona Symptom Questionnaire, Revised Clinical Interview Schedule	16% met criteria for psychiatric case (85% of which was depression)
Cooper et al., 1999	147 parturient women	Obstetric clinics in Khayelitsha, a periurban township, South Africa	Structured clinical interview for DSM IV, 2 months postpartum	34.7% major depression
Inandi et al., 2002	2514 women who had given birth in the previous year	Women selected systematically from villages in five relatively undeveloped provinces of eastern and central Turkey	EPDS score >12	27.2%
Regmi et al., 2002	Consecutive sample of 100 postapartum women and 40 non-postpartum women	Hospital postnatal clinic, Kathmandu, Nepal. Comparison group of nurses and their friends	EPDS score >12 and DSM-IV structured clinical interview, 2–3 months postpartum	Prevalence of depression: 12% in postpartum women and 12.5% in comparison group
Patel, Rodrigues & De Souza, 2002	Consecutive cohort of 270 pregnant women	District hospital, Goa, India	General Health Questionnaire 12, EPDS and Revised Clinical Interview Schedule, 6–8 weeks and 6 months postpartum	23% depressive disorder at 6–8 weeks postpartum
Chandran et al., 2002	Cohort of 359 pregnant women	Tamil Nadu, India	EPDS score >12, 6–12 weeks postpartum	11%
Rahman, Iqbal & Harrington, 2003	Consecutive cohort of 632 pregnant women	Southern Kahuta, Pakistan	WHO Schedule for Clinical Assessment in Neuropsychiatry and structured questionnaires, in late pregnancy and 12 weeks postpartum	28% depressive disorder 12 weeks postpartum
Rahman et al., 2003	Consecutive cohort of 172 mothers and infants	Immunization clinic, Rawalpindi, Pakistan	WHO Self-reporting Questionnaire - 20, Assets Questionnaire, and structured questionnaires, 9 months postpartum	40% met SRQ-20 criteria for clinically significant mental distress
Fisher et al., 2004	Consecutive cohort of 506 women	Immunization clinics at Hung Vuong Obstetrics and Gynaecology Hospital and Maternal and Child Health and Family Planning Centre, Ho Chi Minh City, Viet Nam	Structured interview including EPDS, 6 weeks postpartum	32.7% (EPDS score >12)

maternal depression (Chandran et al., 2002; Patel et al., 2002; Rahman, Iqbal & Harrington, 2003; Fisher et al., 2004). Social support from peers, including companionship and opportunities to confide, has not been systematically assessed in many of these studies; however, Mills, Finchilescu & Lea (1995) and Rahman, Iqbal & Harrington (2003) demonstrated that women who lacked it were more likely to be depressed.

A comprehensive assessment of the links between reproductive experiences and mental health in developing countries is not yet available, However, evidence is emerging that women who have adverse obstetric experiences, including operative birth, poor postpartum health and difficulties in breastfeeding, are more likely to report depressive symptoms in the immediate postpartum period (Mills, Finchilescu & Lea, 1995; Fatoye, Adeyemi & Oladimeji, 2004; Fisher et al., 2004).

There are also some risk factors that appear to be more common in cultural contexts where women face restrictions related to strong gender-role expectations. Lack of reproductive choice, including about use of contraceptive, contributes to unwanted pregnancy, which in a number of these investigations was associated with a greater likelihood of depression (Inandi et al., 2002; Fisher et al., 2004). In cultures with a strong preference for sons, giving birth to a daughter was consistently associated with depression (Patel et al., 2002; Inandi et al., 2003; Fatoye, Adeyemi & Oladimeji, 2004), particularly for women who had already given birth to a daughter (Rahman, Iqbal & Harrington, 2003). The social and psychological complexities faced by women caring for an infant while living in their parents-in-law's multigenerational household have not been systematically examined. It is known that autonomy, especially in regard to household finances, is linked to mental health. Power disparities between a woman and her mother-in-law may restrict her autonomy, especially during the period of increased dependence that follows childbirth; this may contribute to poor mental health (Chan et al., 2002; Chandran et al., 2002; Lee et al., 2004b).

The focus on postpartum depression has excluded consideration of other relevant expressions of psychological distress in women after childbirth. In particular, relatively little attention has been devoted to the nature and prevalence of postnatal anxiety disorders, despite evidence of substantial co-morbidity with depression (Barnett & Parker, 1986; Stuart et al., 1998). The relevance of post-traumatic stress disorders to mental health in pregnancy, and the potential of childbirth and other reproductive events to evoke post-traumatic stress reactions, remain underexplored (Fisher, Astbury & Smith, 1997; Wijma, Soderquist & Wijma, 1997; Boyce & Condon, 2001). Research into the determinants of postpartum onset of panic disorder, and the links between maternal experience and a history of an eating disorder, are only now being considered.

Maternal mental health, infant development and the mother-infant relationship

Depression after childbirth, through its negative impact on the mother's interpersonal functioning, disrupts the quality and sensitivity of the mother-infant interaction. This can have adverse effects on the emotional, cognitive and social development of the infant. Postnatal depression reduces the sensitivity, warmth, acceptance and responsiveness of the mother to her infant (Murray et al., 1996a).

At the same time, the infant's own sensitivity to its interpersonal environment, including the lowered mood and social behaviour of the mother, exacerbates the effect of reduced maternal sensitivity. An infant is less likely to form a secure emotional attachment if the mother is depressed or insensitive (Murray, 1992; Murray & Cooper, 1997). Examinations of the behaviour of infants in face-to-face interactions with their depressed mothers have reported fewer positive facial expressions, more negative expressions and protest behaviour, higher levels of withdrawal and avoidance, more fussing, and an absence of positive affect (Field et al., 1990). Two-month-old infants whose mothers were depressed had higher rates of disrupted behaviour and were more likely to avoid contact with their mothers than comparison infants (Murray et al., 1996a). Effects are more marked in socioeconomically disadvantaged populations, in particular among adolescents and those who are single. In lower-risk populations, there are fewer differences in the mother-infant interactions of depressed and non-depressed mothers (Campbell, Cohn, & Meyers, 1995; Murray et al., 1996a). The link between postnatal depression and impairment of the mother-infant relationship has been reported in middle- and high-income countries, such as the United Kingdom (Murray, 1992; Murray & Cooper, 2003) and the United States of America (Field et al., 1990), and in a low-income cohort in South Africa (Cooper et al., 1999).

Independently of the adverse effects of poverty, crowded living conditions and infectious diseases, maternal depression contributes to infant failure to thrive in resource-poor settings (Patel et al., 2004). Patel, Desouza & Rodrigues (2003) examined the impact of maternal depression 6-8 weeks postpartum on the subsequent growth and development of infants in Goa, India. Compared with controls, infants of depressed mothers were more than twice as likely to be underweight at six months of age (30% versus 12%) and three times more likely to be short for age (25% versus 8%). They also had significantly lower mental development scores, even after adjustment for birth weight and maternal education (Patel, Desouza & Rodrigues, 2003). Anoop et al. (2004), in a case-control study in a rural community in Tamil Nadu, India, found that infants whose weight was 50-80% of the expected weight for age were significantly more likely to have a mother who was depressed than infants of normal weight.

These effects do not necessarily remit when maternal mood improves. There is consistent evidence of poorer cognitive development in preschool-age children of mothers who were depressed postnatally (Lyons-Ruth et al., 1986; Murray, 1992; Murray et al., 1996). Young boys whose mothers were depressed postnatally were found to have poorer cognitive development and to display more antisocial behaviour, overactivity and distractibility compared with boys whose mothers were not postnatally depressed (Cogill et al., 1986; Murray et al., 1996b; Sinclair & Murray, 1998).

Hay et al. (2001) examined the long-term consequences of maternal depression in a community sample of 132 11-year-old children from south London, whose mothers had completed psychiatric interviews three months postpartum. Children, especially boys, whose mothers had been depressed had significantly lower intelligence scores, and a higher rate of special educational needs, including difficulties in mathematical reasoning and visuomotor performance,

and more attentional problems than those whose mothers had been well (Hay et al., 2001). Possible confounders, such as parental intelligence, social disadvantage and later mental health problems in the mothers, did not alter the effect of maternal postnatal depression on the children's intellectual status. Luoma et al. (2001) assessed a group of school-age children whose mothers had been depressed, according to the EPDS, antenatally, postnatally or currently. They found that depression present both during pregnancy and after childbirth was strongly predictive of behavioural problems in the children at 8-9 years of age. The worst child outcomes were predicted by a combination of prenatal and recurrent maternal depression (Luoma et al., 2001).

A meta-analysis of nine studies (Tatano Beck, 1998) found small but significant adverse effects of maternal postpartum depression on the cognitive and emotional development of children older than one year. However, other investigators have found no association between postnatal depression and adverse child development in women who are socially advantaged (Murray et al., 1996b). When social adversity is taken into account, statistical differences between depressed and non-depressed groups often disappear (Murray et al., 2003). Hay et al. (2001) found that breastfed children of women who had been depressed postpartum did not have verbal or mathematical cognitive deficits. Similarly, Sharp et al. (1995) found that breastfeeding was a reliable predictor of intellectual functioning in three-year-old children, as measured by the McCarthy Scales of Children's Abilities. These findings on the importance of breastfeeding for cognitive development are important, because mothers who are depressed are more likely to stop breastfeeding early (Cooper, Murray & Stein, 1993).

The sensitivity of fathers is also a crucial mediating factor. Sensitive fathers reduce the impact of maternal depression and reduced responsiveness, especially for temperamentally reactive infants. Conversely, maternal sensitivity is reduced and risk of depression is increased if the partner behaves aggressively either during pregnancy or postpartum (Leung et al., 1999; Crockenberg & Leerkes, 2003). In general, the long-term adverse effects of maternal depression on child cognitive outcomes are mostly confined to socioeconomically disadvantaged groups, and are worse for boys.

Most of the research into the impact of maternal postnatal depression on child development has been done in developed countries. The recent findings in developing countries of the close relationship between the mental health of mothers and the physical and mental development of their children are of vital importance to both child health and maternal and reproductive health programmes, especially in areas with high rates of poor infant growth.

Prevention and treatment of maternal mental health problems

In spite of the high prevalence of perinatal mood disorders, there is relatively little systematic data about the efficacy of prevention and treatment strategies (Boath & Henshaw, 2001; Lumley & Austin, 2001). Most mild depression in the postpartum year resolves as mothers gain more experience and their confidence grows. However, more severe depression can persist, becoming chronic or recurring from time to time (Cooper & Murray, 1995).

A range of interventions to prevent the development of depression have been tested in randomized controlled trials; most have had only a modest or negligible effect. Screening questionnaires administered during pregnancy to identify women at risk of becoming depressed after childbirth have low positive predictive values, and reviewers have concluded that there is insufficient evidence to introduce screening as part of routine antenatal care (Lumley & Austin, 2001). "Preparation-for-parenthood" groups for women during pregnancy did not prevent postpartum depression, except when partners were included in at least one session (Gordon & Gordon, 1960; Elliot et al., 2000). Although the quality of a woman's relationships, in particular with her partner, is central to her emotional well-being during pregnancy and after childbirth, most interventions have not involved family members. A single session during the postpartum hospital stay, in which women could talk with a midwife about their experience of caesarean or forceps-assisted delivery, did not reduce the rate of depression (Small et al., 2000). Two recent systematic reviews have concluded that the research base on preventive interventions is extremely limited, and there is currently no compelling evidence to support the introduction of any of the interventions that have been tested in primary prevention trials (Lumley & Austin, 2001; Scottish Intercollegiate Guidelines Network, 2002).

There have been a number of randomized controlled trials of treatments for postnatal depression, but many are limited because of high rates of loss to follow-up, a short follow-up period, or potential bias because most eligible respondents refused to participate (Hoffbrand, Howard, & Crawley, 2001; Ray & Hodnett, 2001). Both pharmacological and psychological treatments have been found to reduce the severity of symptoms and the duration of depression (Appleby, Koren, & Sharp, 1999). Decisions about prescribing pharmacological treatments - usually antidepressant medication - have to be weighed against the potential harm to the fetus or infant, as the drug may be transmitted through the placenta and in breast milk. Most women prefer a non-pharmacological approach (O'Hara & Swain, 1996). Psychological approaches, combining problem-solving strategies, supportive empathic listening, and opportunities to focus on past and present relationships, either in groups or individually, are more effective than routine care in reducing depression. A randomized trial comparing non-directive counselling, cognitive behavioural therapy, psychodynamic therapy and routine primary care found short-term improvements in maternal mood with all treatments; however, only psychodynamic therapy significantly reduced depression (Cooper et al., 2003). None of the benefits of treatment were evident by nine months postpartum; treatment did not prevent subsequent episodes of depression; and in the long term the benefits were not superior to spontaneous remission (Cooper et al., 2003). MacArthur et al. (2002) demonstrated that specifically trained community health visitors could provide care for mothers of newborns that led to reduced rates of depression at four months postpartum compared with women cared for by

While identification and effective treatment of perinatal psychological disturbance are important, there is an equally vital need to reduce the risk factors that render women vulnerable to depression and anxiety. Reduction of poverty, attention to the human rights of reproductive choice, personal safety and equality of access to education, and occupational conditions that acknowledge women's multiple roles and provide secure and family-friendly employment can help ensure good mental health during pregnancy, in childbirth, and while caring for a newborn baby.

health visitors who had not been trained. Short-term benefits were also apparent in the pilot test of a randomized trial of increased peer support for women at high risk of developing depression (Dennis, 2003). Teaching mothers how to soothe their infants and settle them to sleep, either in clinics or during home visits, improved maternal mood (Armstrong et al., 1999, 2000; Hiscock & Wake, 2002). In Taiwan, China, women who attended weekly support group meetings had lower scores on the Beck Depression Inventory, less perceived stress and improved perception of interpersonal support than controls who did not attend group meetings (Chen et al., 2000). It is generally agreed that a team approach, involving primary care providers, allied health workers and specialist mental health practitioners, as well as a range of health facilities, is needed (Brockington, 1992; Barnett & Morgan, 1996).

While there have been a number of trials of treatments for postnatal depression, relatively few have been designed to improve developmental outcomes for the child. Murray et al. (2003), in a comparison of home visits by professional health visitors trained to provide one of three psychotherapies to depressed mothers of newborns, found that non-directive counselling fostered more sensitive mother-infant interactions among those who were experiencing social adversity than psychodynamic or cognitive behavioural therapies. At four months, mothers who received counselling reported fewer difficulties in various aspects of their relationship with their infant, such as play, separation and management of infant needs for attention, compared with those who received routine primary care. This benefit was sustained in more positive maternal reports of infant emotional and behavioural functioning at 18 months. However, there was no significant impact of any of the treatments on cognitive development or emotional and behavioural adjustment at home or in school when the children reached 5 years of age (Murray et al., 2003).

In conclusion, mental health is inextricably linked to maternal mortality and morbidity, but has been generally neglected in initiatives to improve maternal health. In the field of perinatal mental health, a disproportionate emphasis has been placed on identifying the correlates and consequences of poor maternal mental health, and much less on exploring the contribution of paternal, familial or social factors, with an increased risk of misattribution of causality and victim-blaming (Wilson et al., 1996)

Summary

Future research

1. Research attention has focused disproportionately on mental health after childbirth, compared with mental health during pregnancy, which warrants more comprehensive investigation.

2. There is increasing evidence about the predictors, prevalence and correlates of poor postpartum mental health in developing countries, but investigations have yet to be conducted in some of the poorest countries.

3. The contribution of maternal mental health to maternal mortality should be ascertained, covering events up to one year postpartum.

4. Interventions to prevent the development of psychopathology after childbirth have focused almost exclusively on women. Emerging evidence suggests that strategies involving partners may be more effective, but these need to be designed and appropriately evaluated.

5. Randomized controlled trials are needed of treatments for depression, during pregnancy and after childbirth that are suitable for use in primary care settings.

6. Investigations of infant development following maternal depression should ascertain and control for the contribution of social adversity.

7. The contribution of intimate partner violence and coercion to women's perinatal mental health has been neglected and warrants inclusion in future investigations.

Policy

1. Risk factors for poor mental health should be ascertained as part of routine primary perinatal health care.

2. Mental health is integral to safe motherhood, and should be included in all future initiatives, programmes and recommendations for standard care.

Services

1. All health professionals in perinatal and maternal and infant services should have the skills needed to assess psychological well-being and provide comprehensive, psychologically informed care.

2. Assessment of risk factors for poor reproductive mental health should be routine in perinatal health care. These include: past personal or family history of psychiatric illness or substance abuse; past personal history of sexual, physical or emotional abuse; current exposure to intimate partner violence or coercion; current social adversity; coincidental adverse life events; and unsettled infant behaviour or developmental difficulties.

3. Specialist perinatal mental health services require an understanding of the contribution of denial of human rights to poor mental health.

References

Aaron R et al. (2004) Suicides in young people in rural southern India. *Lancet*, 363, 1117-1118.

Adams JA, East PL (1999) Past physical abuse is significantly correlated with pregnancy as an adolescent. *Journal of Pediatrics and Adolescent Gynaecology*, 12: 133-138.

Adamson P (1996) Commentary: a failure of imagination. In: *The Progress of Nations 1996*, New York, UNICEF.

Aderibigbe YA, Gureje O, Omigbodun O (1993) Postnatal emotional disorders in Nigerian Women: a study of antecedents and associations. *British Journal of Psychiatry*, 163, 645-650.

Adler NE (2000) Abortion and the null hypothesis. *Archives of General Psychiatry*, 57: 785-786.

Affonso D et al. (2000) An international study exploring levels of postpartum depressive symptomatology. *Journal of Psychosomatic Research*, 49(3): 207-216.

American College of Obstetricians and Gynecologists (2003) *Violence against women, drawing the line*. Washington, American College of Obstetricians and Gynecologists.

American Psychiatric Association (1994) *Diagnostic and statistical manual of mental disorders, fourth edition (DSM IV)*. Washington, DC.

Anoop S et al. (2004) Maternal depression and low maternal intelligence as risk factors for malnutrition in children: a community based case-control study from South India. *Archives of the Diseases of Childhood*, 89: 325-29.

Appleby L (1991) Suicide during pregnancy and in the first postnatal year. *British Medical Journal*, 302(6769): 126-27.

Appleby L, Koren G, Sharp D (1999) Depression in pregnant and postnatal women: an evidence-based approach to treatment. *British Journal of General Practice*, 49(447): 780-782.

Appleby L, Mortensen PB, Faragher B (1998) Suicide and other causes of mortality after postpartum psychiatric admission. *British Journal of Psychiatry*, 173(9): 209-211.

Appleby L, Turnbull G (1995) Parasuicide in the first postnatal year. *Psychological Medicine*, 25(5): 1087-1090.

Areias MEG et al. (1996) Comparative incidence of depression in women and men, during pregnancy and after childbirth: validation of the Edinburgh Postnatal Depression Scale in Portuguese Mothers. *British Journal of Psychiatry*, 169(1): 30-35.

Armstrong K et al. (1998a) Childhood sleep problems: association with prenatal factors and maternal distress/depression. *Journal of Paediatrics and Child Health*, 34, 263.

Armstrong K et al. (1998b) Sleep deprivation or postnatal depression in later infancy: separating the chicken from the egg. *Journal of Paediatrics and Child Health*, 34, 260.

Armstrong KL et al. (1999) A randomized controlled trial of nurse home visiting to vulnerable families with newborns. *Journal of Paediatrics and Child Health*, 35(3): 237-44.

Armstrong KL et al. (2000) Promoting secure attachment, maternal mood and child health in a vulnerable population: a randomised controlled trial. *Journal of Paediatrics and Child Health*, 36: 555-562.

Astbury J (1980) The crisis of childbirth: can information and childbirth education help? *Journal of Psychosomatic Research*, 24: 9-13.

Astbury J (2001) Gender disparities in mental health. In: *Mental Health: A call for action by World Health Ministers*. Geneva, World Health Organization: 73-92.

Astbury J et al. (1994) Birth events, birth experiences and social differences in postnatal depression. *Australian Journal of Public Health*, 18(2): 176-184.

Ayers S, Pickering AD (2001) Do women get posttraumatic stress disorder as a result of childbirth? A prospective study of incidence. *Birth* 28: 111-118

Bandyopadhyay M (2003) Missing girls and son preference in rural India: looking beyond popular myth. *Health Care for Women International*, 24, 910-926.

Barber C et al. (1997) Using a breastfeeding prevalence survey to identify a population for targeted programs. *Canadian Journal of Public Health*, 88(4): 242.

Barnett B, Morgan M (1996) Postpartum psychiatric disorder: who should be admitted to which hospital? *Australian and New Zealand Journal of Psychiatry*, 30: 709-714.

Barnett B, Parker G (1986) Possible determinants, correlates and consequences of high levels of anxiety in primiparous mothers. *Psychological Medicine*, 16: 177-185.

Barr R, Gunnar M (2000) Colic: the transient reactivity hypothesis. In: Barr R, Hopkins B, Green J (eds). *Crying as a sign, a symptom and a signal*. London, MacKeith Press

Batra A (2003) Burn mortality: recent trends and sociocultural determinants. *Burns*, 29: 270-275.

Bayatpour M, Wells RD, Holford S (1992) Physical and sexual abuse as predictors of substance use and suicide among pregnant teenagers. *Journal of Adolescent Health*, 13: 128-132.

Beck CT (1999) Maternal depression and child behaviour problems: a meta-analysis. *Journal of Advanced Nursing*, 29(3): 615-622.

Beck CT (2001) Predictors of postpartum depression: an update. *Nursing Research*, 50(5): 275-285.

Beebe S, Casey R, Pinto-Martin J (1993) Association of reported infant crying and maternal parenting stress. *Clinical Pediatrics*, 32: 15-19.

Bernazzani O et al. (1997) Psychosocial factors related to emotional disturbances during pregnancy. *Journal of Psychosomatic Research*, 42(4): 391-402.

Berthiaume M et al. (1996) Correlates of gender role orientation during pregnancy and the postpartum. *Sex Roles*, 35(11/12): 781-800.

Bertolote J et al. (2005) Suicide attempts, plans and ideation in culturally diverse sites: the WHO SUPRE-MISS community survey. *Psychological Medicine*, 35: 1457-1465.

Boath E, Henshaw C (2001) The treatment of postnatal depression: a comprehensive literature review. *Journal of Reproductive and Infant Psychology*, 13(3): 215-248.

Boyce P, Condon JT (2001) Psychological debriefing: providing good clinical care means listening to women's concerns. *British Medical Journal*, 322(7291): 928.

Boyce P, Hickie I, Parker G (1991) Parents, partners or personality? Risk factors for post-natal depression. *Journal of Affective Disorders*, 21: 245-255.

Boyce P, Mason C (1996) An overview of depression-prone personality traits and the role of interpersonal sensitivity. *Australian and New Zealand Journal of Psychiatry*, 30: 90-103.

Boyce PM, Todd AL (1992) Increased risk of postnatal depression after emergency caesarean section. *Medical Journal of Australia*, 157 (3 August): 172-174.

Boyce P et al. (1998) Psychosocial factors associated with depression: a study of socially disadvantaged women with young children. *Journal of Nervous and Mental Diseases*, 186(1): 3-11.

Brockington I (2001) Suicide in women. *International Clinical Psychopharmacology*, 16: S7-S19.

Brockington I, Winokur G, Dean C (1982) Puerperal psychosis. In: Brockington I, Kumar R, eds., *Motherhood and mental illness*, London, Academic Press: 37-69.

Brockington IF (1992) Disorders specific to the puerperium. *International Journal of Mental Health*, 21(2): 41-52.

Brooke O et al. (1989) Effects on birthweight of smoking, alcohol, caffeine, socioceconomic factors and psychosocial stress. *British Medical Journal*, 298: 795-801.

Brown S (1998) Maternal health after childbirth: results of an Australian population based survey. *British Journal of Obstetrics and Gynaecology*, 105: 156-161.

Brown S, Lumley J (1994) Satisfaction with care in labor and birth: a survey of 790 Australian women. *Birth*, 21(1): 4-13.

Brugha TS et al. (1998) The Leicester 500 Project. Social support and the development of postnatal depressive symptoms, a prospective cohort survey. *Psychological Medicine*, 28(1): 63-79.

Buist A, Barnett B (1995) Childhood sexual abuse: A risk factor for postpartum depression? *Australian and New Zealand Journal of Psychiatry*, 29: 604-608.

Buist A, Janson H (2001) Childhood sexual abuse, parenting and postpartum depression–a 3-year follow-up study. *Child Abuse and Neglect*, 25: 909-921.

Bullock LFC et al. (2001) Retrospective study of the association of stress and smoking during pregnancy in rural women. *Addictive Behaviors*, 26: 405-413.

Calhoun M, Calhoun L (1980) The psychological impact of having a handicapped baby. In: Selby J et al., eds., *Psychology and human reproduction*, New York, The Free Press: 127-144.

Campbell S, Cohn J (1991) Prevalence and correlates of postpartum depression in first-time mothers. *Journal of Abnormal Psychology*, 100(4): 594-599.

Campbell SB, Cohn JF, Meyers T (1995) Depression in first time mothers: mother-infant interaction and depression chronicity. *Developmental Psychology*, 31: 349-357.

Chan SW et al. (2002) A qualitative study of the experiences of a group of Hong Kong Chinese women diagnosed with postnatal depression. *Journal of Advanced Nursing*, 39: 571-579.

Chandran M et al. (2002) Post-partum depression in a cohort of women from a rural area of Tamil Nadu, India. Incidence and risk factors. *British Journal of Psychiatry*, 181: 499-504.

Chaudron LH et al. (2001) Predictors, prodromes and incidence of postpartum depression. *Journal of Psychosomatic Obstetrics and Gynaecology*, 22(2): 103-112.

Chen CH et al. (2000) Effects of support group intervention in postnatally distressed women. A controlled study in Taiwan. *Journal of Psychosomatic Research*, 49: 395-399.

Chen H et al. (2004) Depressive symptomatology in pregnancy. A Singaporean perspective. *Social Psychiatry and Psychiatric Epidemiology*, 39: 975-979.

Church S, Scanlan M (2002) Suicide: The unspoken consequence of mental illness during pregnancy and childbirth. *The Practising Midwife*, 5(8): 22-25.

Clifford C et al. (1999) A cross-cultural analysis of the use of the Edinburgh Postnatal Depression Scale (EPDS) in health visiting practice. *Journal of Advanced Nursing*, 30(3): 655-664.

Cloutier S et al. (2002) Physically abused pregnant women's perceptions about the quality of their relationships with their male partners. *Women and Health*, 35(2-3): 149-163.

Cogill S et al. (1986) Impact of postnatal depression on cognitive development in young children. *British Medical Journal*, 292: 1165-1167.

Cokkinides V et al. (1999) Physical violence during pregnancy: maternal complications and birth outcomes. *Obstetrics and Gynecology*, 93(5): 661-666.

Cole M (2000) Out of sight, out of mind: Female sexuality and the care plan approach in psychiatric inpatients. *International Journal of Psychiatry in Clinical Practice*, 4(4): 307-310.

Condon J, Watson T (1987) The maternity blues: exploration of a psychological hypothesis. *Acta Psychiatrica Scandinavica*, 76: 164-171.

Condon JT, Boyce P, Corkindale CJ (2004) The First-Time Fathers Study: a prospective study of the mental health and wellbeing of men during the transition to parenthood. *Australian and New Zealand Journal of Psychiatry,* 38: 56-64.

Cooper P, Murray L, Stein A (1993) Psychosocial factors associated with the early termination of breastfeeding. *Journal of Psychosomatic Research*, 37: 171-176.

Cooper PJ, Murray L (1995) Course and recurrence of postnatal depression: evidence for the specificity of diagnostic concept. *British Journal of Psychiatry*, 166(2): 191-195.

Cooper PJ, Murray L (1997) Prediction, detection, and treatment of postnatal depression. *Archives of Diseases in Childhood*, 77: 97-98.

Cooper PJ et al. (1999) Post-partum depression and the mother-infant relationship in a South African peri-urban settlement. *British Journal of Psychiatry*, 175: 554-558.

Cooper PJ et al. (2002) Impact of a mother-infant intervention in an indigent peri-urban South African context. *British Journal of Psychiatry*, 180: 76-81.

Cooper PJ et al. (2003) Controlled trial of the short and long term effect of psychological treatment of post-partum depression. Impact on maternal mood. *British Journal of Psychiatry*, 182: 412-419.

Covington D et al. (2001) Preterm delivery and the severity of violence during pregnancy. *Journal of Reproductive Medicine*, 46(12): 1031-1039.

Cox J (1983) Postnatal depression: a comparison of African and Scottish women. *Social Psychiatry* 18: 25-28.

Cox J (1996) Perinatal mental disorder - a cultural approach. *International Review of Psychiatry*, 8: 9-16.

Cox J, Murray D, Chapman G (1993) A controlled study of the onset, duration and prevalence of postnatal depression. *British Journal of Psychiatry*, 163: 27-31.

Cox JL (1994) Introduction and classification dilemmas. In: Cox JL, Holden J, eds., *Perinatal psychiatry: use and misuse of the Edinburgh Postnatal Depression Scale*. London, Gaskell.

Cox JL, Holden JM, Sagovsky R (1987) Detection of postnatal depression. Development of the 10-item Edinburgh Postnatal Depression Scale. *British Journal of Psychiatry*, 150: 782-786.

Craig K, Gilbert-Macleod C, Lilley C (2000). Crying as an indicator of pain in infants. In: Barr R, Hopkins B, Green J, eds., *Crying as a sign, a symptom and a signal*. London, MacKeith Press.

Cramer B (1993) Are postpartum depressions a mother-infant relationship disorder? *Infant Mental Health Journal*, 14(4): 283-297.

Crockenberg SC, Leerkes EM (2003) Parental acceptance, postpartum depression and maternal sensitivity: mediating and moderating processes. *Journal of Family Psychology*, 17:80-93.

Czeizel AE, Timar L, Susanszky E (1999) Timing of suicide attempts by self-poisoning during pregnancy and pregnancy outcomes. *International Journal of Gynaecology and Obstetrics*, 65: 39-45.

Da Costa D et al. (2000) Psychosocial correlates of prepartum and postpartum depressed mood. *Journal of Affective Disorders*, 59: 31-40.

Dannenberg AL et al. (1995) Homicide and other injuries as causes of maternal death in New York City, 1987 through 1991. *American Journal of Obstetrics and Gynaecology*, 172(5): 1557-1564.

Davidson J (1972) Post-partum mood change in Jamaican women: a description and discussion on its significance. *British Journal of Psychiatry*, 121: 659-663.

Da Silva V et al. (1998) Prenatal and postnatal depression among low income Brazilian women *.Brazilian Journal of Medical and Biological Research*, 31: 799-804.

Deater-Deckard K et al. (1998) Family structure and depressive symptoms in men preceding and following the birth of a child. *American Journal of Psychiatry*, 155(6): 818-823.

Dennerstein L, Lehert P, Riphagen F (1989) Postpartum depression - risk factors. *Journal of Psychosomatic Obstetrics and Gynaecology*, 10(suppl): 53-65.

Dennis CL (2003) The effect of peer support on postpartum depression: A pilot randomized controlled trial. *Canadian Journal of Psychiatry*, 48: 115-124.

Department of Health (1999) *Report of the Confidential Enquiries into Maternal Deaths*. London, Department of Health.

Diket AL, Nolan TE (1997) Anxiety and depression: diagnosis and treatment during pregnancy. *Obstetrics and Gynecology Clinics of North America*, 24(3): 535-558.

Dimitrovsky L, Perez-Hirshberg M, Istkowitz R (1987) Depression during and following pregnancy: quality of family relationships. *Journal of Psychology*, 12(3): 213-218.

Douglas AR (2000) Spotlight on practice. Reported anxieties concerning intimate parenting in women sexually abused as children. *Child Abuse and Neglect*, 24(3): 425-434.

Eberhard-Gran M et al. (2002) Depression in postpartum and non-postpartum women: prevalence and risk factors. *Acta Psychiatrica Scandiniavica*, 106: 426-433.

Elliott SA et al. (1983) Mood change during pregnancy and after the birth of a child. *British Journal of Clinical Psychology*, 22: 295-308.

Elliott S et al. (1984) Relationship between obstetric outcome and psychological measures in pregnancy and the postnatal year. *Journal of Reproductive and Infant Psychology*, 2: 18-32.

Elliot SA et al. (2000) Promoting mental health after childbirth: a controlled trial of primary prevention of postnatal depression. *British Journal of Clinical Psychology*, 39(3): 223-241.

Epperson N (1999) Postpartum major depression: detection and treatment. *American Family Physician*, 59(8): 2247-2254.

Escriba V, Mas R, Romito P, Saurel-Cubizoles MJ. (1999) Psychological distress of new Spanish mothers. *European Journal of Public Health*, 9: 294-299

Evans J et al. (2001) Cohort study of depressed mood during pregnancy and after childbirth. *British Medical Journal*, 323(7307): 257-260.

Farhi J, Ben-Rafael Z, Dicker D (1994) Suicide after ectopic pregnancy. *New England Journal of Medicine*, 330(10): 714.

Farber EW, Herbert SE, Reviere SL (1996) Childhood abuse and suicidality in obstetrics patients in a hospital-based urban prenatal clinic. *General Hospital Psychiatry*, 18: 56-60.

Fathalla M (1998) The missing millions. *People Planet*, 7: 10-11.

Fatoye F, Adeyemi A, Oladimeji B (2004) Emotional distress and its correlates among Nigerian women in late pregnancy. *Journal of Obstetrics and Gynaecology*, 24: 504-509.

Feggetter G, Cooper P, Gath D (1981) Non-psychotic psychiatric disorders in women one year after childbirth. *Journal of Psychosomatic Research*, 25(5): 369-372.

Felice E et al. (2004). Prevalence rates and psychosocial characteristics associated with depression in pregnancy and postpartum women in Malta. *Journal of Affective Disorders*, 82: 297-301.

Field T et al. (1990) Behavior state matching and synchrony in mother-infant interactions in non-depressed versus depressed dyads. *Developmental Psychology*, 26: 7-14.

Fikree FF, Pasha O (2004) Role of gender in health disparity: the South Asian context. *British Medical Journal*, 328(7443): 823-826.

Fildes J et al. (1992) Trauma: the leading cause of maternal death. *Journal of Trauma*, 32(5): 643-645.

Fisher J, Astbury J, Smith A (1997) Adverse psychological impact of operative obstetric interventions: a prospective study. *Australian and New Zealand Journal of Psychiatry*, 31: 728-738.

Fisher JRW et al. (2002) Nature, severity and correlates of psychological distress in women admitted to a private mother-baby unit. *Journal of Paediatrics and Child Health*, 38: 140-145.

Fisher JRW, Feekery CJ, Amir LH, Sneddon M. (2002) Health and social circumstances of women admitted to a private mother baby unit. *Australian Family Physician* 31: 39-58.

Fisher JRW, Stocky, AJ (2003) Maternal perinatal mental health and multiple births: implications for practice. *Twin Research*, 6(6): 506-513.

Fisher J et al. (2004) Prevalence, nature, severity and correlates of postpartum depressive symptoms in Vietnam. *BJOG: An International Journal of Obstetrics and Gynaecology*, 111: 1353-1360.

Franko DL, Spurrell EB (2000) Detection and management of eating disorders during pregnancy. *Obstetrics and Gynaecology*, 96(6): 942-946.

Frautschi S, Cerulli A, Maine D (1994) Suicide during pregnancy and its neglect as a component of maternal mortality. *International Journal of Gynaecology and Obstetrics*, 47: 275-284.

Fuggle P et al. (2002) Screening for postnatal depression in Bengali women: preliminary observations from using a translated version of the Edinburgh Postnatal Depression Scale (EPDS). *Journal of Reproductive and Infant Psychology*, 20(2): 71-82.

Ganatra B, Hirve S (2002) Induced abortion among adolescent women in rural Maharashtra, India. *Reproductive Health Matters*, 10: 76-85.

Garel M et al. (1990) Psychosocial consequences of caesarean childbirth: a four-year follow-up study. *Early Human Development*, 21: 105-114.

Gazmararian JA et al. (2000) Violence and reproductive health: current knowledge and future research directions. *Maternal and Child Health Journal*, 4(2): 79-84.

Ghubash R, Abou-Saleh MT (1997) Postpartum psychiatric illness in Arab culture: prevalence and psychosocial correlates. *British Journal of Psychiatry*, 171: 65-68.

Gissler M, Hemminki E (1999) Pregnancy-related violent deaths. *Scandinavian Journal of Public Health*, 27(1): 54-55.

Gissler M, Hemminki E, Lonnqvist J (1996) Suicides after pregnancy in Finland, 1987-94: register linkage study. *British Medical Journal*, 313: 1431-1434.

Gjerdingen DK, Chaloner KM (1994) The relationship of women's postpartum mental health to employment, childbirth, and social support. *Journal of Family Practice*, 38(5): 465-473.

Glasser S et al. (2000). Postpartum depression in an Israeli cohort: demographic, psychosocial and medical risk factors. *Journal of Psychosomatic Obstetrics and Gynecology*, 21:99-108.

Glazer G (1980) Anxiety levels and concerns among pregnant women. *Research in Nursing and Health*, 3(3): 107-113.

Glover V, O'Connor T (2002) Effects of antenatal stress and anxiety: implications for development and psychiatry. *British Journal of Psychiatry*, 180: 389-391.

Glover V et al. (2002) Mechanisms by which maternal mood in pregnancy may affect the development of the fetus. *Journal of Affective Disorders*, 68(1): 96.

Goodburn E, Campbell O (2001) Reducing maternal mortality in the developing world; sector-wide approaches may be the key. *British Medical Journal*, 322(7291): 917-920.

Gordon RE, Gordon KK (1960) Social factors in prevention of postpartum emotional problems. *Obstetrics and Gynecology*, 15: 433-437.

Graham WJ, Flilippi VGA, Ronsmans C (1996) Demonstrating programme impact on maternal mortality. *Health Policy and Planning*, 11(1): 16-20.

Granja A, Zacarias E, Bergstrom S (2002) Violent deaths: the hidden face of maternal mortality *BJOG: an International Journal of Obstetrics and Gynaecology*, 109: 5-8.

Grazioli R, Terry DJ (2000) The role of cognitive vulnerability and stress in the prediction of postpartum depressive symptomology. *British Journal of Clinical Psychology*, 39(4): 329-347.

Green J (1990a) Prenatal screening and diagnosis: some psychological and social issues. *British Journal of Obstetrics and Gynaecology*, 97: 1074-1076.

Green J (1990b) "Who is unhappy after childbirth?" Antenatal and intrapartum correlates from a prospective study. *Journal of Reproductive and Infant Psychology*, 8: 175-183.

Green JM (1998) Postnatal depression or perinatal dysphoria? Findings from a longitudinal community-based study using the Edinburgh Postnatal Depression Scale. *Journal of Reproductive and Infant Psychology*, 16: 143-155.

Gunn J et al. (1998) Does an early postnatal check-up improve maternal health: results from a randomised trial in Australian general practice? *British Journal of Obstetrics and Gynaecology*, 105: 991-997.

Hall S, Bobrow M, Marteau T (2000) Psychological consequences for parents of false negative results on prenatal screening for Down's syndrome: retrospective interview study. *British Medical Journal*, 320: 407-412.

Hannah P et al. (1992) Links between early post-partum mood and post-natal depression. *British Journal of Psychiatry*, 160: 777-780.

Haste F et al. (1990) Nutrient intakes during pregnancy: observations on the influence of smoking and social class. *American Journal of Clinical Nutrition*, 51(1): 29-36.

Hay DF et al. (2001) Intellectual problems shown by 11-year-old children whose mothers had postnatal depression. *Journal of Child Psychology and Psychiatry*, 42(7): 871-889.

Hendrick V, Altshuler L, Suri R (1998) Hormonal changes in the postpartum and implications for postpartum depression. *Psychosomatics*, 39(2): 93-101.

Hicks M, Bhugra D (2003) Perceived causes of suicide attempts by UK South Asian women. *American Journal of Orthopsychiatry*, 73: 455-462.

Hieu D et al. (1999) Maternal mortality in Vietnam in 1994 -1995. *Studies in Family Planning*, 30(4): 329-338.

Hiscock H, Wake M (2002) Randomised controlled trial of behavioural infant sleep intervention to improve infant sleep and maternal mood. *British Medical Journal*, 324(7345): 1062-1065.

Hjelmeland H et al. (2002) Why people engage in parasuicide: a cross-cultural study of intentions. *Suicide and Life-Threatening Behaviour*, 32: 380-393.

Hoffbrand S, Howard L, Crawley H (2001) Antidepressant drug treatment for postnatal depression. *Cochrane Database of Systematic Reviews*, 2(CD002018).

Holden J (1991) Postnatal depression: its nature, effects, and identification using the Edinburgh Postnatal Depression Scale. *Birth*, 18(4): 211-220.

Holden J (1994) Can non-psychotic depression be prevented? In: Cox J, Holden J, eds., *Perinatal psychiatry. The use and misuse of the Edinburgh Postnatal Depression Scale*. London, Gaskell: 55-81.

Hopkins J, Campbell S, Marcus M (1987) Role of infant-related stressors in postpartum depression. *Journal of Abnormal Psychology*, 96(3): 237-241.

Horon IL, Cheng D (2001) Enhanced surveillance for pregnancy-associated mortality - Maryland, 1993-1998. *Journal of the American Medical Association*, 285(11): 1455-1459.

Howard R (1993) Transcultural issues in puerperal mental illness. *International Review of Psychiatry*, 5: 253-260.

Hunfeld J, Wladimiroff J, Passchier J (1994) Pregnancy termination, perceived control, and perinatal grief. *Psychological Reports*, 74: 217-218.

Hunfeld JAM et al. (1997) Trait anxiety, negative emotions, and the mothers' adaption to an infant born subsequent to late pregnancy loss: A case-control study. *Prenatal Diagnosis*, 17(9): 843-851.

Inandi T et al. (2002) Risk factors for depression in the postnatal first year, in eastern Turkey. *International Journal of Epidemiology* 31: 1201-1207.

Istvan J (1986) Stress, anxiety and birth outcomes: a critical review of the evidence. *Psychological Bulletin*, 100(3): 331-348.

Jenkins J, Kleinman A, Good B (1991) Cross-cultural studies of depression. In: Becker J, Kleinman A, eds., *Psychosocial aspects of depression*. New Jersey, Lawrence Erlbaum and Associates.

Ji J, Kleinman A, Becker A (2001) Suicide in contemporary China: a review of China's distinctive suicide demographics in their sociocultural context. *Harvard Review of Psychiatry*, 9: 1-12.

Johnstone S et al. (2001) Obstetric risk factors for postnatal depression in urban and rural community samples. *Australian and New Zealand Journal of Psychiatry*, 35(1): 69-74.

Josefsson A et al. (2001) Prevalence of depressive symptoms in late pregnancy and postpartum. *Acta Obstetrica et Gynecologica Scandiniavica*, 80: 251-255.

Keenan K et al. (1991) Low level of maternal serum alpha-fetoprotein: its associated anxiety and the effects of genetic counseling. *American Journal of Obstetrics and Gynecology*, 164: 54-56.

Kendell R (1985) Emotional and physical factors in the genesis of puerperal mental disorders. *Journal of Psychosomatic Research*, 29(1): 3-11.

Kendell RE (1991) Suicide in pregnancy and the puerperium. *British Medical Journal*, 302: 126-127.

Kendell RE, Chalmers JC, Platz C (1987) Epidemiology of puerperal psychosis. *British Journal of Psychiatry*, 150: 662-673.

Kendell R et al. (1981) Mood changes in the first three weeks following childbirth. *Journal of Affective Disorders*, 3(4): 317-326.

Kennerley H, Gath D (1986) Maternity blues reassessed. *Psychiatric Developments*, 1: 1-17.

Kermode M (1999) *Health insurance status and mood during pregnancy and following birth: A longitudinal study of multiparous women.* Melbourne, University of Melbourne.

Kitamura T et al. (1996) Psychosocial study of depression in early pregnancy. *British Journal of Psychiatry*, 168(6): 732-738.

Kok LP, Chan PSL, Ratnam SS (1994) Postnatal depression in Singapore women. *Singapore Medical Journal*, 35: 33-35.

Kolker A, Burke BM (1993) Grieving the wanted child: ramifications of abortion after prenatal diagnosis of abnormality. *Health Care of Women International*, 14(6): 513-526.

Kristof N (1993) China: ultrasound abuse in sex selection. *Women's Health Journal*, Oct-Dec, 16-17.

Kumar R (1994) Postnatal mental illness: a transcultural perspective. *Social Psychiatry and Psychiatric Epidemiology*, 29: 250-264.

Kumar V (2003) Burnt wives - a study of suicides. *Burns*, 29: 31-35.

Kumar RC, Hipwell AE, Lawson C (1994) Prevention of adverse effects of perinatal maternal mental illness on the developing child. In: Cox JL, Holden J, eds., *Perinatal psychiatry: use and misuse of the Edinburgh Postnatal Depression Scale*. London, Gaskell.

Kumar R, Robson K (1984) A prospective study of emotional disorders in childbearing women. *British Journal of Psychiatry*, 144: 35-47.

Lam P, Hiscock H, Wake M (2003). Outcomes of infant sleep problems: a longitudinal study of sleep, behavior, and maternal well-being. *Pediatrics*, 111(3): E203.

Lane A et al. (1997) Postnatal depression and elation among mothers and their partners: prevalence and predictors. *British Journal of Psychiatry*, 171(12): 550-555.

Laungani P (2000) Postnatal depression across cultures: conceptual and methodological considerations. *International Journal of Health Promotion and Education*, 38(3): 86-94.

Lee DTS et al. (2001) A psychiatric epidemiological study of postpartum Chinese women. *American Journal of Psychiatry*, 158(2), 220-226.

Lee D et al. (2004a) A prevalence study of antenatal depression among Chinese women. *Journal of Affective Disorders*, 82: 93-99.

Lee DT et al. (2004b) Ethnoepidemiolgy of postnatal depression. Prospective multivariate study of sociocultural risk factors in a Chinese population in Hong Kong. *British Journal of Psychiatry*, 184: 34-40.

Lee S (2000) In China, suicide in young women is a problem too. *British Medical Journal*, 321: 636-637.

Lehtonen L, Barr R (2000). 'Clinical pies' for etiology and outcome in infants presenting with early increased crying. In: Barr R, Green J, eds., *Crying as a sign, a symptom and a signal*, London, MacKeith Press.

Leung W et al. (1999) The prevalence of domestic violence against pregnant women in a Chinese community. *International Journal of Gynaecology and Obstetrics*, 66(1): 32-30.

Leung WC et al. (2002) Domestic violence and postnatal depression in a Chinese community. *International Journal of Gynecology and Obstetrics*, 79(2): 159-166.

Lissner C (2001) *Safe Motherhood Needs Assessment version 1.1*. Geneva, World Health Organization.

Llewellyn AM, Stowe ZM, Nemeroff CB (1997) Depression during pregnancy and the puerperium. *Journal of Clinical Psychiatry*, 58(15): 26-32.

Lubin B, Gardener S, Roth A (1975) Mood and somatic symptoms during pregnancy. *Psychosomatic Medicine*, 37(2): 136-146.

Lumley J, Astbury J (1989) Advice for pregnancy. In: Chalmers I, Enkin M, Keirse M, eds., *Effective care in pregnancy and childbirth*, Oxford, Oxford University Press.

Lumley J, Austin M-PV (2001) What interventions may reduce postpartum depression. *Current Opinion in Obstetrics and Gynaecology*, 13: 605-611.

Luoma I et al. (2001) Longitudinal study of maternal depressive symptoms and child well-being. *Journal of the American Academy of Adolescent Psychiatry*, 40: 1367-1374.

Lyons-Ruth K et al. (1986) The depressed mother and her one year old infant: environment, interaction, attachment and infant development. In: Tronick EZ, Field T, eds., *Maternal depression and infant disturbance. New directions for child development*. San Francisco, Jossey-Bass.

MacArthur C et al. (2002) Effects of redesigned community postnatal care on women's health 4 months after birth: a cluster randomised controlled trial. *Lancet*, 359: 378-385.

Maine D, Rosenfield A (1999) The Safe Motherhood Initiative: why has it stalled? *American Journal of Public Health*, 89(4): 480-482.

Manderson L (1981) Roasting, smoking and dieting in response to birth: Malay confinement in cross-cultural perspective. *Social Science and Medicine*, 15B: 509-520.

Marks M, Lovestone S (1995) The role of the father in parental postnatal mental health. *British Journal of Medical Psychology*, 68: 157-168.

Marks MN et al. (1992) Contribution of psychological and social factors to psychotic and non-psychotic relapse after childbirth in women with previous histories of affective disorder. *Journal of Affective Disorders*, 29: 253-264.

Marteau T et al. (1992) The psychological effects of false-positive results in prenatal screening for fetal abnormality: a prospective study. *Prenatal Diagnosis*, 12: 205-214.

Marzuk PM et al. (1997) Lower risk of suicide during pregnancy. *American Journal of Psychiatry*, 154(1): 122-123.

Matthey S, Barnett BE, Elliot A (1997) Vietnamese and Arabic women's responses to the Diagnostic Interview Schedule (depression) and self-report questionnaires: cause for concern. *Australian and New Zealand Journal of Psychiatry*, 31: 360-369.

Matthey S et al. (2000) Paternal and maternal depressed mood during the transition to parenthood. *Journal of Affective Disorders*, 60: 75-85.

Matthey S et al. (2001) Validation of the Edinburgh Postnatal Depression Scale for men, and comparison of item endorsement with their partners. *Journal of Affective Disorders*, 64: 175-184.

Mayberry L, Affonso D (1993) Infant temperament and postpartum depression: a review. *Health Care for Women International*, 14: 201.

McFadyen A et al. (1998) First trimester ultrasound screening: carries ethical and psychological implications. *British Medical Journal*, 317(7160): 694-695.

McGrath JJ et al. (1999) The fertility and fecundity of patients with psychoses. *Acta Psychiatrica Scandinavica*, 99(6): 441-446.

McNeil T, Blenow G (1988) A prospective study of postpartum psychoses in a high-risk group. Relationship to birth complications and neonatal abnormalities. *Acta Psychiatrica Scandinavica*, 78(4): 478-484.

Milgrom J, Westley D, McCloud P (1995) Do infants of depressed mothers cry more than other infants? *Journal of Paediatric and Child Health*, 31: 218.

Milligan R et al. (1996) Postpartum fatigue: clarifying a concept. *Scholarly Inquiry for Nursing Practice: An International Journal*, 10(3): 279-291.

Mills EP, Finchilescu G, Lea SJ (1995) Postnatal depression - an examination of psychosocial factors *South Africa Medical Journal*, 85: 99-105.

Moon Park E-H, Dimigen G (1995) A cross-cultural comparison: postnatal depression in Korean and Scottish mothers. *Psychologia*, 38: 199-207.

Moylan PL et al. (2001) Clinical and psychosocial characteristics of substance-dependent pregnant women with and without PTSD. *Addictive Behaviors*, 26: 469-474.

Muhajarine N, D'Arcy C (1999) Physical abuse during pregnancy: prevalence and risk factors. *Canadian Medical Association Journal*, 160(7): 1007-1111.

Murray L (1992) The impact of postnatal depression on infant development. *Journal of Child Psychology and Psychiatry*, 33: 543-561.

Murray L, Cooper P, eds. (1997) *Postpartum depression and child development*. London, The Guilford Press.

Murray L, Cooper PJ (2003) The impact of postpartum depression on child development. In: Goodyer L, ed. *Aetiological mechanisms in developmental psychopathology*, Oxford, Oxford University Press.

Murray L et al. (1996a) The impact of postnatal depression and associated adversity on early mother infant interactions and later infant outcome. *Child Development*, 67: 2512-2516.

Murray L et al. (1996b) The cognitive development of 5-year old children of postnatally depressed mothers. *Journal of Child Psychology and Psychiatry*, 37: 927-935.

Murray L et al. (1996c) The role of infant factors in postnatal depression and mother-infant interactions. *Developmental Medicine and Child Neurology*, 38: 109-119.

Murray L et al. (1999) The socioemotional development of 5-year-old children of postnatally depressed mothers. *Journal of Child Psychology and Psychiatry*, 40(8): 1259-1271.

Murray L et al. (2003) Controlled trial of the short and long term effect of psychological treatment of post partum depression. *British Journal of Psychiatry*, 182: 420-427.

Ndosi N, Mtawali M (2002) The nature of puerperal psychosis at Muhimbili National Hospital: its physical co-morbidity, associated main obstetric and social factors. *African Journal of Reproductive Health*, 6(1): 41-49.

Ng HC (1997) The stigma of mental illness in Asian cultures. *Australian and New Zealand Journal of Psychiatry*, 31: 382-390.

Nga D, Morrow M, ed. (1999) *Nutrition in pregnancy in rural Vietnam: Poverty, self-sacrifice and fear of obstructed labour*. Oxford, Blackwell Science (*Reproductive Health Matters*, special edition).

Nhiwatiwa S, Patel V, Acuda W (1998) Predicting postnatal mental disorder with a screening questionnaire: a prospective cohort study from Zimbabwe. *J Epidemiol Community Health* 52: 262-266.

Nimgaonkar V (1998) Reduced fertility in schizophrenia: here to stay? *Acta Psychiatrica Scandinavica*, 98(5): 348-353.

Nimgoankar V et al. (1997) Fertility in schizophrenia: results from a contemporary US cohort. *Acta Psychiatrica Scandinavica*, 95(5): 364-369.

Nott P (1987) Extent, timing and persistence of emotional disorders following childbirth. *British Journal of Psychiatry*, 151: 523-527.

Nott PN (1982) Psychiatric illness following childbirth in Southampton: a case register study. *Psychological Medicine*, 12: 557-561.

Oakley A (1980) *Women confined: towards a sociology of childbirth*. Oxford, Martin Robertson.

Oates M (1989) Management of major mental illness in pregnancy and the puerperium. *Clinical Obstetrics and Gynaecology*, 3(4): 791 -804.

Oates M (2003a) Suicide: the leading cause of maternal death *British Journal of Psychiatry*, 183: 279-281.

Oates M (2003b) Perinatal psychiatric disorders: a leading cause of maternal morbidity and mortality. *British Medical Bulletin*, 67: 219-229.

Oberklaid F et al. (1984). Temperament in Australian infants. *Australian Paediatric Journal*, 20: 181.

O'Connor T, Heron J, Glover V (2002) Antenatal anxiety predicts child behavioral / emotional problems independently of postnatal depression. *Journal of the American Academy of Child and Adolescent Psychiatry*.

O'Connor TG et al. (2002) Maternal antenatal anxiety and children's behavioral /emotional problems at 4 years: Report from the Avon Longitudinal Study of Parents and Children. *British Journal of Psychiatry*, 180: 502-508.

O'Hara M (1986) Social support, life events and depression during pregnancy. *Archives of General Psychiatry*, 43: 569-573.

O'Hara MW, Swain AM (1996) Rates and risk of postnatal depression - a meta-analysis. *International Journal of Psychiatry*, 8: 37-54.

O'Hara M, Zekoski E (1988) Postpartum depression: a comprehensive review. In: Kumar R, Brockington IF, eds., *Motherhood and mental illness*. London, Butterworth & Co.: 17-63.

O'Hara MW et al. (1991) Controlled prospective study of postpartum mood disorders: psychological, environmental, and hormonal variables. *Journal of Abnormal Psychology*, 100(1): 63-73.

O'Neill T, Murphy P, Greene VT (1990) Postnatal depression - aetiological factors. *Irish Medical Journal*, 83(1): 17-18.

Oppenheim GB (1985) Psychological disorders in pregnancy. In: Priest R, ed., *Psychological disorders in obstetrics and gynaecology*. London, Butterworths: 93-146.

Otterblad Olausson P et al. (2004) Premature death among teenage mothers *BJOG: an International Journal of Obstetrics and Gynaecology*, 111: 793-799.

Paffenberger R (1964) Epidemiological aspects of postpartum mental illness. *British Journal of Social and Preventive Medicine*, 18: 189-195.

Pajulo M et al. (2001) Antenatal depression, substance dependency and social support. *Journal of Affective Disorders*, 65: 9-17.

Parsons LH, Harper MA (1999) Violent maternal deaths in North Carolina. *Obstetrics and Gynaecology*, 94(6): 990-993.

Parvin A, Jones CE, Hull SA (2004) Experiences and understandings of social and emotional distress in the postnatal period among Bangaldeshi women living in Tower Hamlets. *Family Practice*, 21: 254-260.

Patel V (2005) *Gender in mental health research*. Geneva, World Health Organization (Gender and Health Research Series).

Patel V, Andrew G (2001) Gender, sexual abuse and risk behaviours in adolescents: A cross-sectional survey in Goa. *National Medical Journal of India*, 14(5): 263-267.

Patel V, Desouza N, Rodrigues M (2003) Postnatal depression and infant growth and development in low income countries: A cohort study from Goa, India. *Archives of Disease in Childhood*, 88: 34-37.

Patel V, Rodrigues M, Desouza N (2002) Gender, poverty and postnatal depression: a study of new mothers in Goa, India. *American Journal of Psychiatry*, 59: 43-47.

Patel V et al. (2004) Effect of maternal mental health on infant growth in low income countries: new evidence from South Asia. *British Medical Journal*, 328: 820-823.

Paykel E et al. (1980) Life events and social support in puerperal depression. *British Journal of Psychiatry*, 136: 339-346.

Paykel ES (2002) Mood disorders: review of current diagnostic systems. *Psychopathology*, 35(2/3): 94-99.

Pearson V et al. (2002) Attempted suicide among young rural women in the People's Republic of China: possibilities for prevention. *Suicide and Life-Threatening Behaviour*, 32: 359-368.

Perkin M (1999) Cited studies did not show relation between maternal anxiety and birth weight. *British Medical Journal*, 318(7193): 1288-1289.

Petersen R et al. (1997) Violence and adverse pregnancy outcomes: a review of the literature and directions for future research. *American Journal of Preventive Medicine*, 13(5): 366-373.

Pfuhlmann B, Stoeber G, Beckmann H (2002) Postpartum psychoses: prognosis, risk factors, and treatment. *Current Psychiatry Reports*, 4: 185-190.

Phillips MR, Li X, Zhang Y (2002) Suicide rates in China, 1995-99. *Lancet*, 359: 835-840.

Pitt B (1968) "Atypical" depression following childbirth. *British Journal of Psychiatry*, 114: 1325-1335.

Pitt B (1973) Maternity blues. *British Journal of Psychiatry*, 122(569): 431-433.

Pop VJ et al. (1995) Blues and depression during early puerperium: home versus hospital deliveries. *British Journal of Obstetrics and Gynaecology*, 102: 701-706.

Purwar M et al. (1999) Survey of physical abuse during pregnancy GMCH, Nagpur, India. *Journal of Obstetrics and Gynecology Research*, 25(3): 165-171.

Radovanovic Z (1994) Mortality patterns in Kuwait: inferences from death certificate data. *European Journal of Epidemiology*, 10(6): 733-736W.

Rahman A, Hafeez A (2003) Suicidal feelings run high among mothers in refugee camps: a cross-sectional survey. *Acta Psychiatrica Scandinavica*, 108: 392-393.

Rahman A, Iqbal Z, Harrington R (2003) Life events, social support and depression in childbirth: perspectives from a rural community in the developing world. *Psychological Medicine*, 33: 1161-1167.

Rahman A et al. (2003) Mothers' mental health and infant growth: a case-control study from Rawalpindi, Pakistan. *Child: Care, Health and Development*, 30, 21-27.

Ray KL, Hodnett ED (2001) Caregiver support for postpartum depression (Cochrane Review). *The Cochrane Library*, Issue 4, 2002. Oxford: Update Software.

Reardon DC et al. (2002) Deaths associated with pregnancy outcome: a record linkage study of low income women. *Southern Medical Journal*, 95(8): 834-841.

Regmi S et al. (2002) A controlled study of postpartum depression among Nepalese women: validation of the Edinburgh Postpartum Depression Scale in Kathmandu. *Tropical Medicine and International Health*, 7(4): 378-382.

Righetti-Veltema M et al. (1998) Risk factors and predictive signs of postpartum depression. *Journal of Affective Disorders*, 49: 167-180.

Righetti-Veltema M et al. (2002) Postpartum depression and mother-infant relationship at three months old. *Journal of Affective Disorders*, 70: 291-306.

Robinson GE, Stewart DE (1993) Postpartum disorders. In: Stotland N, Stewart D, eds., *Psychological aspects of women's health care: the interface bewteen psychiatry and obstetrics and gynecology*. Washington, DC, American Psychiatric Press.

Rodrigues M et al. (2003) Listening to mothers: qualitative studies on motherhood and depression from Goa, India. *Social Science and Medicine*, 57: 1797-1806.

Romito P (1989) Unhappiness after childbirth. In: Chalmers I, Enkin M, Keirse MJNC, eds., *Effective care in pregnancy and childbirth. Volume 2: Childbirth*. Oxford, Oxford University Press: 1434-1446.

Romito P, Saurel-Cubizolles M, Lelong N (1999) What makes new mothers unhappy: psychological distress one year after birth in Italy and France. *Social Science and Medicine*, 49: 1651-1661.

Rowe-Murray HJ, Fisher J (2001) Operative intervention in delivery is associated with compromised early mother-infant interaction. *BJOG: an international journal of obstetrics and gynaecology*, 108: 1068-1075.

Rowe-Murray H, Fisher J (2002) Baby friendly hospital practices: caesarean section is a persistent barrier to early initiation of breastfeeding. *Birth*, 29(2): 124-130.

Rubertsson C et al. (2005) Depressive symptoms in early pregnancy, two months and one year postpartum: prevalence and psychosocial risk factors in a Swedish sample. *Archives of Women's Mental Health*, 8: 97-104.

Sanson A et al. (1987) The structure of infant temperament: factor analysis of the Revised Temperament Questionnaire. *Infant Behavior and Development*, 10(1): 97-104.

Schweitzer R, Logan G, Strassberg D (1992) The relationship between marital intimacy and postnatal depression. *Australian Journal of Marriage and the Family*, 13(1): 19-23.

Scottish Intercollegiate Guidelines Network (2002) *Postnatal depression and puerperal psychosis. A national clinical guideline.* Edinburgh, Royal College of Physicians.

Sharma V (1997) Effects of pregnancy on suicidal behaviour. *American Journal of Psychiatry*, 154(10): 1479-1480.

Sharp D et al. (1995) The impact of postnatal depression on boys' intellectual development. *Journal of Child Psychology and Psychiatry*, 36: 1315-1336.

Shumway J et al. (1999) Preterm labour, placental abruption, and premature rupture of membranes in relation to maternal violence or verbal abuse. *Journal of Maternal-Fetal Medicine*, 8(3): 76-80.

Silverman JG et al. (2001) Dating violence against adolescent girls and associated substance use, unhealthy weight control, sexual risk behaviour, pregnancy, and suicidality. *Journal of the American Medical Association*, 286(5): 572-579.

Sinclair D, Murray L (1998) Effects of postnatal depression on children's adjustment to schoolteacher's reports. *British Journal of Psychiatry*, 172: 58-63.

Sjostrom K et al. (2002) Maternal anxiety in late pregnancy: effect on fetal movements and fetal heart rate. *Early Human Development*, 67(1-2): 87-100.

Skari H et al. (2002) Comparative levels of psychological distress, stress symptoms, depression and anxiety after childbirth: a prospective population based study of mothers and fathers. *BJOG: an International Journal of Obstetrics and Gynaecology*, 109(10): 1154-1163.

Small R (2000) *An Australian study of Vietnamese, Turkish and Filipino women's experiences of maternity care and of maternal depression after childbirth.* Melbourne, LaTrobe University.

Small R et al. (2000) Randomised controlled trial of midwife led debriefing to reduce maternal depression after operative childbirth. *British Medical Journal*, 321: 1043-1047.

Smith J (1998) Risky choices: the dangers of teens using self-induced abortion attempts. *Journal of Pediatric Health Care*, 12: 147-151.

Stark E, Flitcraft A (1995) Killing the beast within: woman battering and female suicidality. *International Journal of Health Services*, 25(1): 43-64.

Stein G (1982) The maternity blues. In: Kumar R, Brockington IF, eds., *Motherhood and mental illness*, London, Academic Press: 119-153.

Steiner M (1998) Further needs in clinical assessment - perinatal mood disorders: position paper. *Psychopharmacology Bulletin*, 34(3): 301-307.

Stern G, Kruckman L (1983) Multi-disciplinary perspectives on post-partum depression: an anthropological critique. *Social Science and Medicine*, 17: 1027-1041.

Stewart D, Cecutti A (1993) Physical abuse in pregnancy. *Canadian Medical Association Journal*, 149(9): 1257-1263.

Stewart DE, Robinson GE (1996) Violence and women's mental health. *Harvard Review of Psychiatry*, 4(1): 54-57.

Stokoe U (1991) Determinants of maternal mortality in the developing world. *Australian and New Zealand Journal of Obstetrics and Gynaecology*, 31(1): 8-16.

Stowe ZN, Nemeroff CB (1995) Women at risk for postpartum onset major depression. *American Journal of Obstetrics and Gynecology*, 173: 639-645.

Stuart S et al. (1998) Postpartum anxiety and depression: onset and comorbidity in a community sample. *Journal of Nervous and Mental Diseases*, 186(7): 420-424.

Stuchbery M, Matthey S, Barnett B (1998) Postnatal depression and social supports in Vietnamese, Arabic and Anglo-Celtic mothers. *Social Psychiatry and Psychiatric Epidemiology*, 33: 483-490.

Sutter A-L et al. (1997) Post-partum blues and mild depressive symptomatology at days three and five after delivery. A French cross sectional study. *Journal of Affective Disorders*, 44: 1-4.

Tatano Beck C (1998) The effects of postpartum depression on child development: a meta analysis. *Archives of Psychiatric Nursing*, 1: 12-20.

Texiera J, Fisk N, Glover V (1999) Association between maternal anxiety in pregnancy and increased uterine artery resistance index: cohort based study. *British Medical Journal*, 318(7177): 153-157.

Tezcan S, Guciz Dogan B (1990) The extent and causes of mortality among reproductive age women on three districts of Turkey. *Nufusbilim Dergisi*, 12: 31-39.

Thomas T et al. (1996) Psychosocial characteristics of psychiatric inpatients with reproductive losses. *Journal of Health Care for the Poor and Underserved*, 7(1): 15-23.

Thome M (2000) Predictors of postpartum depression in Icelandic women. *Archives of Women's Mental Health*, 3: 7-14.

Thompson JF et al. (2000) Early discharge and postnatal depression: a prospective cohort study. *Medical Journal of Australia*, 172(5 June): 532-536.

Tinker A, Koblinsky M (1993) *Making motherhood safe*. Washington, DC, World Bank.

Viguera AC et al. (2002) Managing bipolar disorder during pregnancy: weighing the risks and benefits. *Canadian Journal of Psychiatry*, 47(5): 426-437.

Warner R et al. (1996) Demographic and obstetric risk factors for postnatal psychiatric morbidity. *British Journal of Psychiatry*, 168(5): 607-611.

Weaver SM et al. (1993) A follow-up study of "successful" IVF / GIFT couples: social-emotional well-being and adjustment to parenthood. *Journal of Psychosomatic Obstetrics and Gynaecology*, 14: 5-16.

Webster J, Chandler J, Battistutta D (1996) Pregnancy outcomes and health care use: Effects of abuse. *American Journal of Obstetrics and Gynaecology*, 174(2): 760-767.

Webster J et al. (2000) Measuring social support in pregnancy: can it be simple *and* meaningful? *Birth: Issues in Perinatal Care*, 27(2): 97-101.

Webster ML et al. (1994) Postnatal depression in a community cohort. *Australian and New Zealand Journal of Psychiatry*, 28(1): 42-49.

Weir J (1984) Suicide during pregnancy in London 1943-1962. In: Kleiner G, Greston W, eds., *Suicide in pregnancy*, Boston, Wright: 40-62.

Wijma K, Soderquist J, Wijma B (1997) Posttraumatic stress disorder after childbirth: a cross sectional study. *Journal of Anxiety Disorders*, 11(6): 587-597.

Wilhelm K, Parker G (1988) The development of a Measure of Intimate Bonds. *Psychological Medicine*, 18: 225-234.

Wilkie G, Shapiro CM (1992) Sleep deprivation and the postnatal blues. *Journal of Psychosomatic Research*, 36(4): 309-316.

Wilson LM et al. (1996) Antenatal psychosocial risk factors associated with adverse postpartum family outcomes. *Canadian Medical Association Journal*, 154(6): 785-799.

Wolke D, Gray P, Meyer R (1994). Excessive infant crying: a controlled study of mothers helping mothers. *Pediatrics,* 94(3): 322-332.

WHO (1992) *International Statistical Classification of Diseases and Related Health Problems*. Tenth Revision. Geneva, World Health Organization.

WHO (2001) *The World Health Report 2001. Mental health: new understanding, new hope*. Geneva: World Health Organization.

WHO (2005) *Proportion of births attended by skilled health personnel. Global regional and subregional estimates - 2005*. Geneva, World Health Organization (http://www.who.int/reproductive-health/global_monitoring/data_regions).

Yalom I et al. (1968) "Postpartum blues" syndrome. A description and related variables. *Archives of General Psychiatry*, 18: 16-27.

Yamashita H et al. (2000) Postnatal depression in Japanese women. Detecting the early onset of postnatal depression by closely monitoring the postpartum mood. *Journal of Affective Disorders,* 58: 145-154.

Yip S-K, Chung TK-H, Lee T-S (1997) Suicide and maternal mortality in Hong Kong. *Lancet*, 350(9084): 1103.

Zelkowitz P, Milet TH (1995) Screening for postpartum depression in a community sample. *Canadian Journal of Psychiatry*, 40: 80-86.

Zuckerman B et al. (1989) Depressive symptoms during pregnancy: relationship to poor health behaviours. *American Journal of Obstetrics and Gynaecology*, 160(5): 1107-1111.

Chapter
3

Psychosocial aspects of fertility regulation

Contraceptive use – Jill Astbury
Elective abortion – Susie Allanson

The availability of safe, reliable, acceptable and affordable contraceptive methods has a profound impact on women's health, including their mental health. It has been estimated that some 123 million women, mostly in developing countries, are not using contraception, despite an expressed wish to space or limit the number of their births (Ross & Winfrey, 2002). At least 350 million couples worldwide do not have access to the full range of modern family planning methods (WHO, 2002).

Contraceptive use interacts with mental health in two main ways. First, the methods themselves may have a direct effect on mood, through biological, biochemical or hormonal pathways. Second, decision-making about the initiation and continuation of contraceptive use may lead to conflict between partners; this, in association with other social determinants, can contribute to depression and anxiety in women. Such decision-making is likely to be influenced by beliefs about gender roles, autonomy and women's reproductive rights. To date, most research in the field has examined the direct effects of contraceptive methods on psychological distress or disorder. The need for increased research on sexuality, gender roles and gender relationships in different cultures, and in particular the effects of discrimination and violence against women, was identified in 1993, as one of the eleven recommendations of the International Symposium on Contraceptive Research and Development for the Year 2000 and Beyond (International Symposium on "Contraceptive Research & Development for the year 2000 and beyond", Mexico City, 1993).

One of the most serious consequences of unintended pregnancy is unsafe abortion. Unsafe abortions, performed by people not trained in medicine and usually carried out in a clandestine manner, contribute significantly to maternal mortality and morbidity in developing regions of the world. It is estimated that 19 million unsafe abortions took place in the year 2000, i.e. approximately one in ten pregnancies ended in an unsafe abortion, giving a ratio of one unsafe abortion to about seven live births. Almost all unsafe abortions take place in developing countries (Ahman & Shah, 2004). Safe abortion, carried out by qualified and trained medical practitioners in a proper medical environment, is a simple and inexpensive procedure (WHO, 2003)

This chapter has two sections. The first summarizes the evidence on the direct effects of various contraceptive methods on women's mental health. The relationship between depression in women and the psychosocial factors that prevent or make it difficult for them to control their fertility are reviewed. Central to this discussion is the question of women's ability to act independently, and how a gender-based lack of power and control can affect their freedom to make contraceptive choices, without duress from their male partners or state reproductive health policies, and can undermine their mental health and emotional well-being. The contraceptive needs of women with severe chronic mental illness are also considered. The second section addresses the psychological aspects of elective abortion.

Contraceptive use and mental health

Effects of contraception on mental health

Methods of contraception can be classified as: modern and reversible (oral contraceptive pills, emergency hormonal contraception, intrauterine devices (IUDs), injectable contraceptives, such as depot medroxyprogesterone acetate (DMPA), levonorgestrel implants (Norplant), and male and female condoms); modern and permanent (male and female sterilization) or traditional (coitus interruptus and abstinence). Different methods have different impacts on rates of psychological disorder and on mood. Hormonal contraceptives have been most thoroughly studied for their possible effect on psychological functioning, followed by sterilization.

A recent survey in five European countries (France, Germany, Italy, Spain and the United Kingdom), of more than 12 000 randomly selected women between 15 and 49 years of age, confirmed that oral contraceptives were the most widely used method of contraception, and were associated with high levels of satisfaction for more than 90% of the women surveyed (Skouby, 2004).

Studies in Malaysia, Nigeria and the West Indies did not find any negative psychological sequelae among women using contraceptive implants, who reported high rates of satisfaction (Arshat et al., 1990; Rattray et al., 1997; Arowojolu & Ladipo, 2003). However, evaluations in the United States have reported cases of major depression and panic disorder developing in women with no prior psychiatric history (Wagner & Berenson, 1994; Wagner, 1996). A study in London, England, which explored acceptability and reasons for discontinuation of implants, found that 5% and 3% of women reported sideeffects of depression and mood swings, respectively, and 6% of the women gave mood swings as the main reason for discontinuing use of the contraceptive (Erskine et al., 2000).

A population-based prospective study of users of DMPA in the United States, which looked specifically at effects on depressive symptoms, found an increased likelihood of reporting depressive symptoms among both DMPA users and discontinuers, in comparison with non-users. Women who had discontinued DMPA use had more severe depressive symptoms prior

to and immediately following discontinuation (Civic et al., 2000). A double-blind, randomized, placebo-controlled trial on the effect of postnatal administration of the long-acting injectable progestogen contraceptive, norethisterone enantate, in a hospital in Johannesburg, South Africa, concluded that women receiving injectable progestogens in the postnatal period are at an increased risk of depression (Lawrie et al., 1998).

Larger systematic investigations have not reached the same conclusion. A prospective cohort study of more than 900 users of contraceptive implants (Westhoff et al., 1998) reported no significant increase in depression scores over 2 years of use. A multicentre study on the relationship between depressive symptoms and two different hormonal contraceptive methods, DMPA and levonorgestrel implants, found no significant increase in such symptoms after one year of DMPA use or two years of implant use (Kaunitz, 1999). Moreover, a five-year follow-up post-marketing surveillance study, conducted in 32 family planning clinics in eight countries (Bangladesh, Chile, China, Colombia, Egypt, Indonesia, Sri Lanka, and Thailand) from 1987 to 1997, came to the conclusion that rates of mood disorders, anxiety and depression were similar in women using levonorgestrel implants and in those using hormonal methods containing estrogen (Fraser et al., 1998). Women are most likely to cease using implants because of concerns about weight gain, headache, raised blood pressure or menstrual problems (Glantz et al., 2000; Arowojolu & Ladipo, 2003).

A placebo-controlled double-blind study in Scotland and the Philippines found that the progestogen-only pill had adverse effects on sexual functioning and was associated with some improvement in well-being in both the centres (Graham et al., 1995). In its review of evidence to determine eligibility criteria for use of hormonal contraceptives, WHO (2000) concluded that there was no evidence to suggest that women with a history of depression should be excluded from using hormonal contraceptives.

Much of the research on the psychological effects of other methods of contraception, including female sterilization and IUDs was carried out in the 1970s and 1980s, and therefore lies outside the timeframe of the current review. Rather more research has been conducted on the psychological effects of voluntary sterilization. In a survey of 1466 German women (Oddens, 1999; den Tonkelaar & Oddens, 2001), 92% of those who had undergone sterilization and 59% of IUD users were satisfied with these forms of contraception, and reported general improvements in their sexual relationships. Negative effects on mood were most usually attributable to lack of confidence in the effectiveness of the method, rather than to side-effects. Khanam, Mullich & Munib (1993) assessed psychiatric symptoms in 100 Bangladeshi women who had been sterilized, and found that 20% were clinically depressed, but that this mood disturbance was more likely to be attributable to coincidental adverse life events, relationship problems and a family history of psychiatric illness than to the procedure. A comprehensive review of studies in Asia, Latin America, North America and Europe (mainly United Kingdom) conducted up to the mid-1980s found that most women do not experience any significant change in sexual activity, and some experience increased sexual enjoyment once the risk of pregnancy is removed (Philliber & Philliber, 1985). Most women reported minimal or negligible change in the quality of the marital relationship after female sterilization and few women regretted being sterilized. However, negative psychological effects were found among certain groups of women, including those who had been coerced into being sterilized, those who did not understand the consequences of sterilization or who experienced health complications after the procedure, those who disagreed with their partner about the sterilization, and those whose marriage was unstable before sterilization (Philliber & Philliber, 1985). Hence, adverse psychological effects were more likely to occur as a consequence of violations of reproductive rights, including the right to accurate health information and the right to give free and informed consent to medical intervention, than to the procedure itself.

More recent research confirms the importance to psychological well-being of women being given adequate information before the procedure, and feeling they have been able to make their own decisions, without pressure from either partners or health care providers (Neuhaus & Bolte, 1995). The timing of the sterilization procedure is also relevant; women who were sterilized immediately after childbirth, Caesarean section or abortion had an increased incidence of psychosomatic complaints and depressive symptoms (Neuhaus & Bolte, 1995). Guidelines for presterilization counselling emphasize the importance of providing accurate information regarding the actual surgical procedure and possible physical health consequences, including failure rates and risk of ectopic pregnancy. They also recommend involving both partners in decision-making, presenting male sterilization as a viable option, and screening for the possibility of poststerilization regret (Association for Voluntary Surgical Contraception, 1996).

Psychosocial determinants of contraceptive use

Reproductive rights and family planning

Contraceptives are crucial to women's ability to exercise their reproductive right to control their fertility and to make decisions about whether, when and how often to become pregnant. Yet, women's ability to exercise this right and to protect themselves against sexually transmitted disease is contingent on their status and position within the family and the broader society. The right to sexual and reproductive health is linked to other important human rights, including economic and social rights and the right to education. Both the International Conference on Population and Development (ICPD) (UNFPA, 1994) and the Fourth World Conference on Women (FWCW) (United Nations, 1995) stressed that the empowerment of women and the provision of comprehensive reproductive health services were critical to the improvement of women's health throughout the world. The concept of reproductive health goes beyond consideration of the biological factors involved in reproduction to encompass the cultural and social context. Government policies determine who has access to health care, including reproductive health care. Social and religious disapproval of sex outside marriage, or of certain forms of contraception, may influence government policy and lead to strict criteria regarding eligibility for government-funded reproductive health care, and restrictions on the types of contraceptive methods available.

Much of the evidence that informs the planning and provision of family planning services is based on data collected from married women aged 15–49 years, who have participated in Demographic and Health Surveys, which have been conducted so far in 70 countries. In many countries, good quality evidence is available only for married women of childbearing age and for the methods of fertility control offered by government or donor-funded family planning programmes. Sexually active unmarried women face the same health risks as their married counterparts, related to pregnancy and sexually transmissible infections. Due to this gap in data collection, many unmarried women who could benefit from the services offered by family planning programmes may not be adequately attended to. However, over the past ten years, the provision of services to women has become less discriminatory in terms of age and marital status. For example, while services to unmarried adolescents were once illegal in many countries (Eschen & Whittaker, 1993), recent recognition of their health needs has led to an increase in the number of adolescent reproductive health services.

Male involvement in the control of women's fertility

Gender inequality persists in most spheres of life (UNDP, 2003), including decision-making around contraceptive use and participation in family planning. Few contraceptive methods are delivered through systems that emphasize the equality and responsibility of both partners (Humble, 1995). The ICPD Programme of Action (UNFPA, 1994) and the Beijing Platform for Action (United Nations, 1995) articulated "the basic right of all couples and individuals to decide freely and responsibly the number and spacing and timing of their children and to have the information and means to do so …".

Historically, reproductive health and family planning programmes have sought to slow down population growth in order to achieve national development objectives. With this goal, women have been the main targets of efforts to promote participation in family planning and to increase uptake of reliable contraceptive methods. While male involvement in family planning programmes is now being increasingly promoted, women remain the predominant users of the contraceptive methods offered. Fertility control therefore presupposes control of women's behaviour in relation to contraceptive use. Male involvement in family planning programmes may serve to increase the level of gender-related control over women's bodies rather than assist in the realization of gender equality in family planning.

For the latter to be achieved, male involvement should not be relied on as a means of increasing female compliance with contraceptive use or of legitimizing (albeit inadvertently) male control over contraceptive decision-making. Moreover, male involvement in family planning, when the male involved is physically, sexually or emotionally violent towards his partner, is dangerous and may exacerbate the woman's risk of violence.

Unmet need, contraceptive intentions and actual behaviour

The relationship between broader situational and interpersonal determinants of contraceptive use, decision-making and the development of emotional distress, depression and other psychological disorders in women has not been adequately investigated. This is puzzling, because there is evidence of the importance of decision-making and control to mental health. Programmes to increase contraceptive use need to be based on an accurate understanding of the multiple determinants involved.

Most research on predictors of contraceptive demand, and the magnitude of and reasons for unmet need for contraception, has been conducted with women. Unmet need has been defined as the number of non-pregnant women who are not currently using contraceptives but who wish to limit family size plus the number of pregnant women who report that the pregnancy was unwanted or untimely. The availability of contraceptive methods may be a necessary condition for their use, but alone is insufficient. Researchers have sought to quantify the extent of unmet need, as well as the disparity between women's stated intention or desire to use contraceptives and their subsequent behaviour, and the reasons for this.

Studies in different contexts (India, Kuwait, Nigeria, Somalia, eastern Turkey) have found that, while a majority of women expressed a desire to use contraception, many did not actually do so. Often, the women gave no explanation for this discrepancy, but those who did cited fear of side-effects, not having a need, not being married, religion and the need for more children. Among some women, religious teachings, their status relative to men, and the impact of an oral tradition in forming attitudes contributed to the low uptake of family planning services. Other women mentioned not having the approval of

The ICPD Programme of Action (UNFPA, 1994) emphasized the importance of male responsibility and participation, stating:

> Men play a key role in bringing about gender equality since, in most societies, they exercise preponderant power in nearly every sphere of life. The objective is to promote gender equality and to encourage and enable men to take responsibility for their sexual and reproductive behaviour and their social and family roles. Governments should promote equal participation of women and men in all areas of family and household responsibilities, including, among others, responsible parenthood, sexual and reproductive behaviour, prevention of sexually transmitted diseases, and shared control in and contribution to family income and children's welfare.

With specific reference to family planning, the Programme of Action states:

> Actions are recommended to help couples and individuals meet their reproductive goals; to prevent unwanted pregnancies and reduce the incidence of high-risk pregnancies and morbidity and mortality; to make quality services affordable, acceptable and accessible to all who need and want them; to improve the quality of advice, information, education, communication, counselling and services; **to increase the participation and sharing of responsibility of men in the actual practice of family planning; …**

The publication, *Selected practice recommendations for contraceptive use* (WHO, 2002), refers to the importance of improving access to high quality care in family planning, and "ensuring that men's and women's rights and perspectives are taken into account in the planning, management and evaluation of services; promoting the widest availability of different contraceptive methods so that people may select what is most appropriate to their needs and circumstances".

the husband or a religious leader, or a belief that family planning was a sin and that use of contraceptives had side-effects. In other studies the negative attitudes of husbands and of the women themselves were critical factors in non-use of contraception (Roy et al., 2003; Orji & Onwudiegwu, 2002; Comerasamy et al., 2003; Sahin & Sahin, 2003; Shah et al., 2003). Erci (2003) investigated decision-making power and perception of status within the family among more than 300 women in Erzurum, Turkey. Women had lower rates of decision-making than men in almost every domain surveyed, except selecting clothes. Men predominated in all decisions related to family planning, including the use of birth control and family size. Women's perception of their position in the family was significantly related to their decision-making status, which was governed by age, educational level and employment status. A low level of education, inadequate income and a large age dif-

ference between husband and wife resulted in women having an ineffective role in decision-making and a low position in the family. Fear of the husband's disapproval is known to be a key reason for discontinuation of use of contraception among women (Jain & Bruce, 1994).

Men's suspicions about the motives of family planning campaigns can also determine whether their wives are allowed to participate in family planning. Hasna (2003) investigated attitudes towards family planning in a Palestinian refugee camp and found that men were more suspicious than women. Men regarded family planning projects as coercive and a mechanism of war, designed to further dispossess and eradicate Palestinians. At the same time, male status was partly related to the exercise of control over family size, wives and children. Another study, in rural Bangladesh, reported that decisions about acceptability of long term contraceptive methods were governed by the number of living male children and by husband's preferences for more children (Nayer et al., 2004).

The beliefs and behaviour of health care providers may also influence contraceptive use. Fears regarding the side-effects and safety of IUDs were expressed by 44% and 69%, respectively, of 107 Navajo Indian health service providers, in response to a question about why they did not recommend this form of contraception to their clients (Espey et al., 2003). While most health care providers in a New Delhi health care facility were familiar with emergency contraception, very few knew about timing of doses or efficacy (Tripathi, Rathore & Sachdeva, 2003). Oral contraceptives are widely used in India, but discontinuation rates are high. A low frequency of field worker visits was found to be strongly associated with discontinuation, and 70% of the women who discontinued did not use any other contraceptive method, despite wishing to avoid pregnancy (Roy et al., 2003).

It is inaccurate to conclude that inconsistencies between intentions to use contraception and actual behaviour indicate that "women failed to adhere to their intention" (Roy et al., 2003). If women's intentions are the only predictors assessed, other influences on their contraceptive behaviour may be overlooked. Service providers and researchers need to recognize the potential impact of gender and gender inequality and to consider whether women possess sufficient independence to make and implement decisions about contraceptive use. It is imperative to determine whether, in reality, women possess sufficient autonomy and decision-making power and resources to formulate and implement their preferences and intentions.

Violence and control of contraceptive decision-making

Sexuality and sexual violence have been largely ignored in family planning programmes (Sundstrom, 2001). Some of the earliest research on the links between contraceptive use and sexual violence was carried out in Latin America. Women reported having little control over their husband's use of contraception and anger when they refused to use it. Some of this was related to "a sense of deep depersonalization, humiliation and physical dissatisfaction" because their husbands mistreated them during sexual rela-

tions (Dixon-Mueller, 1989:147). Various forms of violence, including verbal abuse and sexual coercion, reduce contraceptive use and result in increased rates of unwanted pregnancy and termination of pregnancy (Gazmararian et al., 2000; Jewkes et al., 2001; Rickert et al., 2002; Cabral et al., 2003).

There is substantial evidence that intimate partner violence, including sexual violence, has multiple negative physical, mental and reproductive health effects (Heise & Moreno, 2002; Jewkes, Purna Sen & Garcia-Moreno, 2002; Krug et al., 2002). Multiple mental disorders can result from violence, including depression, anxiety, dysthymia, stress-related syndromes especially post-traumatic stress disorder, phobias, substance use and suicidal ideas (Kilpatrick, Edmunds, & Seymour, 1992; Campbell & Lewandowski, 1997; Resnick, Acierno & Kilpatrick, 1997; Roberts et al., 1998; Campbell & Soeken, 1999; Astbury & Cabral de Mello, 2000). Sexual violence, in particular, carries an increased risk of a range of sexual and reproductive health problems, including unintended pregnancy, abortion, sexually transmissible infection including human papillomavirus and human immunodeficiency virus (HIV) infection, urinary tract infection, chronic pelvic pain, fibroids, vaginal bleeding and cervical dysplasia (Springs & Friedrich, 1992; Lechner et al., 1993; Plichta & Abraham, 1996; Resnick, Acierno, & Kilpatrick, 1997; Letourneau, Holmes & Chasendunn-Roark, 1999; Coker et al., 2000). In addition, sexual violence is associated with decreased use of preventive health care, cervical screening and antenatal care, as well as poorer pregnancy outcomes for both the woman and her offspring (Springs & Friedrich, 1992; Coker et al., 2000; Gazmararian et al., 2000).

The use of coercive control by violent partners is known to extend to areas of behaviour that family planning programmes seek to modify, such as decision-making around contraception. A comparative study in the USA on the sexuality of college students, the circumstances of first intercourse, including the use of contraceptives, and psychological reactions to first intercourse, reported highly significant differences between men and women. Overall, 38.5% of women, but only 8.8% of men said they had felt coerced to have their first sexual encounter ($p \leq 0.0001$); 63.2% of women and 57.4% of men reported that they did not use birth control during first intercourse. Women did not use contraception because the intercourse was unplanned, and men because contraception was not available to them (Darling, Davidson & Passarello, 1992).

In a review of sexual relations among young people in developing countries (WHO, 2001a), many studies highlighted the fact that sexual activity of young women was not always consensual. In the majority of case studies included in the review, between 5% and 15% of young women reported a forced or coercive sexual experience. In several case studies, the figure was higher: 21% among adolescents in Selibe Phikwe, Mahalapye and Kang, Botswana (Kgosidintsi, 1997); 20% among secondary school students in Lima, Cusco and Iquitos, Peru (Alarcon & Gonzales, 2001); and 41% among young women attending night study centres in Lima, Peru (Villanueva, 1992). Among women working in an export zone in the Republic of Korea, 9% reported that their sexual debut had been forced by a factory supervisor or colleague (Kwon, Jin & Cho, 1994). In a case study in Manila, Philippines, 6% of unwed mothers reported that their pregnancy had resulted from rape, and another 7% that it had resulted from sex in exchange for money to support a drug habit (Bautista, 2001). In rural areas of north and north-east Thailand, three of 11 sexually active adolescent females reported that their sexual debut was a result of force or pressure from their partner (Isarabhakdi, 2001). An investigation in South Africa (Jewkes et al., 2001) found that pregnant teenagers were significantly more likely than their non-pregnant counterparts to have experienced forced sexual initiation and to have been beaten, and were less likely to have confronted partners when they discovered they were unfaithful.

Inconsistent use of condoms and prescription contraceptives was associated with verbal abuse of young women, aged between 14 and 26 years, attending family planning clinics in south-east Texas, USA. Clients who had used dual contraception (such as a barrier and a hormonal method) during the last intercourse were less likely to have experienced verbal abuse (Rickert et al., 2002). In a study of 600 American women attending sexual health clinics, personal control in the relationship was predictive of female condom use when male condoms were not used. Male and female condoms were more likely to be used in relationships in which women reported having more control, but both were less likely to be used in relationships characterized by a history of conflict (Cabral et al., 2003).

Contraception and women with serious mental illness, substance use or intellectual disability

Women who are mentally ill or who abuse alcohol or drugs may be unable to consent to sexual activity, are less likely to use contraception effectively, and are at high risk of sexual exploitation (Hankoff & Darney, 1993). They are as likely to be sexually active as women without mental illness (Nimgoankar et al., 1997). Hypomanic behaviour is associated with risky sexual behaviours, including intercourse with multiple partners and rates of unplanned pregnancy are high in women with severe mental illness (Hankoff & Darney, 1993). Compliance with methods that require regular self-administration, particularly oral contraceptives, is lower in women with psychiatric illness. Since some hormonal contraceptives may alter mood and contribute to depression, it is recommended that they are not prescribed to women who are currently depressed (Hankoff & Darney, 1993). However, health professionals are less likely to discuss contraception with women who have serious psychiatric illness (McCandless & Sladen, 2003), and provision of contraception is problematic for groups who do not attend routine medical or reproductive health services.

The reproductive health, rights and contraceptive needs of women with intellectual disabilities have been the subject of extensive legal, ethical and health care deliberations in the United States (Paransky & Zurawin, 2003). The concerns of parents and carers regarding pregnancy and menstrual management have in some cases led to women being surgically sterilized or undergoing hysterectomy (Diekema, 2003). The women's capacity to make autonomous decisions and to care for children is not always clear, and the rights and wishes of the individual women have to be protected as far as possible (Diekema, 2003). Newer medical options, including hormonal implants, permit less invasive and reversible management of fertility and menstruation (Paransky & Zurawin, 2003).

Extensive research on the situations that trigger clinical depression has revealed critical areas of overlap with intimate partner violence. Situations or events that engender depression are typically characterised by a sense of loss, defeat, humiliation and entrapment, diminished self-esteem, and poor coping and decision-making ability. Identical psychological effects are caused by violence (Brown, Harris & Hepworth, 1995; Astbury & Cabral de Mello, 2000). Family planning programmes need to extend their explanatory models for unmet need and non-use or inconsistent use of contraceptives to include the possibility that intimate partner violence may be a major cause of low rates of contraceptive use and several poor reproductive health outcomes.

Women's decision-making latitude, including their control over participation in family planning programmes and use of contraception, is critically linked to their emotional well-being and their status in the family. Support from health professionals for autonomous decision-making is associated with fewer psychosomatic complaints and depressive symptoms.

Mental health and elective abortion

The direct and indirect societal and personal impact of elective abortion varies widely from country to country, because of differences in legal, social, political, religious, cultural and medical restrictions, stigma and practices (Henshaw, Singh and Haas, 1999). In many countries, women cannot access legal, safe, timely or affordable abortion, and they resort to unsafe, clandestine or "backyard" abortions by unqualified practitioners, or to unsafe self-inflicted procedures. Unsafe abortion is one of the major causes of preventable death (WHO, 2005). Safe abortion is a simple and inexpensive procedure (WHO, 2003), with surgical vacuum aspiration the preferred method in the first twelve weeks of gestation and medical abortion (using mifepristone and a prostaglandin) possible in early pregnancy (WHO, 2003). At abortion providing services with medically trained practitioners, women usually simultaneously access contraceptive and other health services, ultimately decreasing the abortion rate and improving their reproductive health (Henshaw, Singh & Haas, 1999).

It is difficult to obtain reliable estimates of abortion rates because there have been few comprehensive epidemiological studies, the terminology used to describe elective abortion is often ambiguous (e.g. induced miscarriage, menstrual regulation), induced abortion may not be distinguished from spontaneous abortion, and

clandestine abortions in both developing and developed countries are likely to be unrecorded (Huntington, Nawar & Abdel-Hady, 1997; Kaye, 2001; Ahman & Shah, 2002; Rossier, 2003). Estimates suggest that 26 million legal abortions and 20 million illegal abortions were performed worldwide in 1995, with one pregnancy termination for every three live births (Henshaw, Singh & Haas, 1999). WHO estimates that 19.7 million unsafe abortions took place in 2003, almost all of which were in the developing world, resulting in approximately 66 500 deaths (WHO, 2007). Some countries, e.g. Ireland and Poland, report near-zero legal abortion rates but these figures say nothing about the number of clandestine abortions and the extent to which women travel to nearby countries for abortion (Henshaw, Singh & Haas, 1999).

The United Nations (1999; 2003) has collected information on the legal status of abortion in countries throughout the world, and has compared the legal grounds on which abortion is permitted in developed and developing countries. The respective percentages of developed and developing countries that permit abortion on specific grounds are as follows: to save a woman's life (96% and 99%); to preserve physical health (88% and 56%); to preserve mental health (85% and 54%); in cases of rape or incest (83% and 32%); in cases of fetal impairment (83% and 27%); for socioeconomic reasons (77% and 19%); on request (67% and 15%). Abortion is totally prohibited in four countries, three in the developing world and one developed country. Laws that permit abortion to protect a woman's health, and more specifically her mental health, suggest recognition of the potential serious adverse impact on women's mental health of having to continue with an unwanted pregnancy. However, such legislation may be implemented leniently, accepting a broad definition of health and mental health, or in a highly restrictive fashion, by requiring that women demonstrate significant physical or psychiatric pathology (Aries, 2002; de Crespingy & Savulescu, 2004; Pinter, 2002; Whittaker, 2002). Legislation may also include gestational limits. Little is known about the incidence of clandestine early abortions (up to twelve weeks' gestation) versus later abortions. In countries with liberal abortion legislation, estimates suggest that more than 90% of legal abortions are early (British Medical Association, 2005; Chan & Sage, 2005).

The following discussion of the mental health aspects of abortion is limited in a number of ways. First, the special cases of late abortion and abortion following a diagnosed fetal abnormality are excluded. Second, the causes of the unintended pregnancy are not examined, notwithstanding the fact that the biopsychosocial context of conception may have an impact on the woman's subsequent decision-making and adjustment to the pregnancy. Variations in women's access to contraceptive methods, contraceptive fallibility, education, economic security, and vulnerability to violence, may all exert independent effects on mental health. Third, there is no detailed examination of the impact on women's mental health of having their requests to abort a pregnancy denied. A rigorous, longitudinal study in the Czech Republic to examine the effects of denied abortion (David et al., 1988; David, Dytrych & Matejcek, 2003; Kubicka et al., 2003) found that women go to great lengths to obtain an abortion when one is initially denied. A significant minority of women who were twice denied abortion in a pregnancy experienced difficulties with long-term adjustment and mother–infant attachment and their children had higher rates of long-term, adverse developmental and emotional consequences than those born to a matched cohort of mothers who desired the pregnancy. Sigal (2004) has made similar observations in a 50-year study of unwanted babies in Quebec, Canada.

Abortion milieu

An ecological model (Krug et al., 2002) suggests that the mental health aspects of abortion may be inextricably linked to the particular "abortion milieu" (Stotland, 1996). Where the abortion milieu is legally restricted, risk is stratified along economic lines, with poor women more likely to resort to unsafe abortion (Whittaker, 2001; Herrera & Zivy, 2002). The medical consequences of unsafe or incomplete abortion can include haemorrhage, sepsis, genital and intra-abdominal injury, pelvic inflammatory disease, toxic reaction, pain, infertility and death (Ba-Thike, 1997; Huntington, Nawar & Abdel-Hady, 1997; Langer et al., 1997; Boonthai & Warakamin, 2001; Whittaker, 2002). Women may also face adverse legal, social and psychological consequences including poverty, shame, social exclusion and imprisonment, and may even be driven to commit suicide (Casas-Becerra, 1997; Herrera & Zivy, 2002).

In Chile, where an estimated 160 000 to 300 000 illegal abortions are performed annually, Casas-Becerra (1997) reported on 40 women prosecuted for performing abortions, 12 prosecuted as accomplices, and 80 prosecuted for having an abortion. Of this last group, eight had sought abortion following rape, many were subsequently imprisoned, all were poor and all underwent high-risk procedures involving the insertion of instruments such as knitting needles and rubber catheters. The majority of women were reported to the authorities by the public hospital where they had sought treatment for abortion-related complications. Casas-Becerra noted that upper- and middle-class women could afford a private, confidential procedure performed by trained doctors. In nineteen other Latin American countries, an estimated 3.4 million abortions are performed annually, the majority of which are clandestine and unsafe. In Mexico, 136 women who went to a public hospital emergency room with post-abortion complications reported punitive, unsympathetic treatment from medical staff, breaches of their privacy and confidentiality, and the withholding of pain relief (Langer et al., 1997).

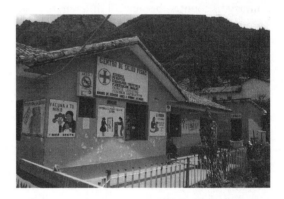

Several countries, including Ethiopia (Gebreselassie & Fetters, 2002) and Kenya (Onyango, Mitchell & Nyaga, 2003) have sought to reduce complications following unsafe abortion by improving the medical response post abortion. Women's health advocates have generally sought reform of restrictive abortion laws (Hessini, 2005).

Maternal mortality and morbidity rates have improved in developing countries that have legalized abortion (Hardy et al., 1997); an associated improvement in mental health may also be expected. Nevertheless, studies in India (Duggal, 2004; Gupte, Bandewar & Pisal, 1997;

Ramachandar & Pelto, 2002), Puerto Rico (Azize-Vargas & Aviles, 1998), Mozambique (Hardy et al., 1997) and elsewhere suggest that "legalisation is an imperfect indicator of the availability of services providing safe abortion" (Hardy et al., 1997:108). Puerto Rico has one of the world's most liberal abortion laws, but a low documented incidence of abortion. In explaining this, Azize-Vargas & Aviles (1998) point to high rates of contraceptive use and sterilization, limited official support, information or services for abortion, and no government subsidy for the cost of abortion. Most women surveyed believed that abortion was illegal. Since abortion was legalized in India in 1972, government-run mobile hospital camps and the private sector provide abortions, but many clandestine abortions continue to be performed annually by unqualified practitioners. Women have complained that the hospital camps lack privacy (initial registration and waiting areas may be in the open air and publicly visible), and women have been verbally abused, coerced into surgical sterilization, or denied abortion on spurious grounds (Ramachander & Pelto, 2002).

In countries with comprehensive health systems and liberal abortion laws, women can attend an accredited medical facility for a medical abortion, or for the ten-minute surgical abortion procedure under general or local anaesthetic. The cost of the abortion may be subsidized by the government. Women can receive emotional support from staff, family and friends, and do not face a threat of death, serious illness or prosecution. An estimated 180 000 pregnancy terminations are performed annually in Great Britain. The Royal College of Obstetricians and Gynaecologists (2000), with support from the National Health Service, regularly updates its evidence-based guidelines on best practice in medical and psychological care of women seeking an elective abortion. In Australia, an estimated 85 000 women terminate a pregnancy each year, although the national data do not distinguish between procedures following missed abortion and elective abortion (Chan & Sage, 2005). Most of the population supports safe, legal abortion services (Kelly & Evans, 2003) and the government subsidizes the cost. However, there is some variation between Australian states in abortion laws, with most requiring demonstration that continuation of the pregnancy is a threat to the woman's mental or physical health. These laws have been criticised for their lack of

clarity and the risks run by both women and abortion providers in terms of potential prosecution and restricted abortion access (de Crespigny & Savulescu, 2004; National Health and Medical Research Council, 1996).

Worldwide, abortion providers and women seeking abortion are under threat from anti-abortion groups (Cavenar, Maltbie & Sullivan, 1978; Woodhouse, 1982; Rizzardo et al., 1991). When accessing abortion providing health clinics, women can face verbal abuse, intimidation and violence from people protesting their opposition to abortion outside abortion-providing clinics (Clapman, 2003; Dean & Allanson, 2004). Approximately one and half million abortions are performed annually in the United States of America. The activities of anti-abortion groups, who believe once a woman is pregnant she must continue the pregnancy no matter what her circumstances, have led to a significant reduction in abortion services, denial of public funding, increased legal restrictions and a well-funded network of Crisis Pregnancy Centres which use a variety of strategies to delay and dissuade women from terminating a problem pregnancy. (Castle & Fisher, 1997; Dean, 2006; Medoff, 2003). United States women who have abortions have been portrayed by anti-abortion groups as "selfish, sexually irresponsible, unfeeling and morally blind individuals who kill their own children for convenience" (Fried, 1997: 41). In this milieu, Fried (1997) has observed American women turning to unsafe abortion practices, including ingestion of poison and violence, either self-inflicted or inflicted by others. In Thailand, anti-abortion rhetoric has labelled women who have an abortion as "morally corrupt" and exemplifying "unrestrained hedonism, vice and temptation" (Whittaker, 2001). During parliamentary debates on abortion in Sri Lanka, women were "variously assumed to be promiscuous and conniving, or vulnerable and needing protection" (Abeyesekera, 1997).

Use of certain words and definitions within the scientific community may also serve to restrict or expand women's reproductive options, and indirectly impact on women's physical and mental health. Definitions and semantics can implicitly and explicitly reflect value judgements. Medical and social assumptions of maternity are embedded in definitions of maternal mortality in relation to abortion (WHO, 2001b). Reflecting on the large number of deaths from unsafe abortions in Bolivia being described as "maternal deaths", Rance (1997) concludes that this "is the price women are expected to pay for having transgressed by refusing maternity", and that "reproductive mortality" (Beral, 1979) or "pregnancy-related deaths" might be a more suitable term. A woman's attitude towards the pregnancy may also be quite distinct from being pregnant (Condon, 1985). To refer to a pregnancy as "unwanted" may suggest fickleness on the part of the woman, while "unplanned" may imply women's contraceptive incompetence or impulsive sexuality. "Problem pregnancy" (Baker, 1985) or "unintended pregnancy" might be preferred where a woman is pregnant in circumstances unfavourable to pregnancy continuation.

Because of the stigma associated with abortion, research in both developing and developed countries has been limited. In developing countries, abortion research on large samples is scarce and primarily focused on the demographic characteristics and contraceptive history of women seeking abortion (Adewole et al., 2002; Angulo & Guendelman, 2002; Perera, de Silva & Gange, 2004). Mental health studies are mostly anecdotal, qualitative and retrospective. Where abortion is illegal, research samples commonly comprise women presenting to public hospitals with serious complications following unsafe abortion. Such research obviously has little to say about women who do not access health facilities, those who do not experience complications requiring medical attention, or those who are wealthy enough to pay for a safe abortion. Accessing abortion research samples can pose dangers to both participants and researchers (Herrera & Zivy, 2002). Research into women's physical health after unsafe abortion has overshadowed research into their mental health. "In trying to understand the traumatic experience they had just survived, their concerns about physical recovery were the most salient, with emotional reactions perhaps being held in suspension" (Huntington, Nawar & Abdel-Hady, 1997).

More is known about women's emotional health in developed countries. However, methodological problems have included ideologically motivated research seeking to demonstrate that abortion is either harmful or benign, and a relative scarcity of rigorously designed studies (Adler, 1992; Dagg, 1991; Major, 2003; Matlin, 2003; McGrath et al., 1990; Stotland, 2004; Turell, Armsworth & Gaa, 1990). Pre-abortion baseline

assessments have been taken from a few hours to two weeks before the procedure, while postoperative assessments have occurred from one hour to two years after the abortion.

Abortion and mental health

The discussion below reflects research on the experiences of women having an unsafe abortion and research from developed countries with relatively liberal abortion laws. Generalizability of the evidence to other abortion milieus is unclear. Where there are gaps in the recent evidence, earlier research is included.

Torres & Forrest (1988) asked 1900 women in American abortion facilities about their reasons for terminating a pregnancy. The most frequent and most important reasons (between 31% and 76% endorsement) were: a concern about life changes if the woman had a baby, inability to afford a baby, relationship problems or a wish to avoid single parenthood, and lack of readiness for the responsibility. Altogether, 31% of respondents mentioned their own immaturity, with 11% indicating this was the most important reason. Only 1% said that the pregnancy was the result of rape or incest, and only 7% gave a health problem as a reason. Studies have not included a specific mental illness category, and such women may or may not fit within the general health category. Despite significant social differences, similar reasons have been found in more recent studies across a variety of cultural contexts, including in developing countries (Tornbom et al., 1994; Adelson, Frommer & Weisberg, 1995; Larsson et al., 2002; Geelhoed et al., 2004; Perera, de Silva & Gange, 2004).

> "A pregnancy may have been planned and intended yet, for a number of reasons, may become unwanted; on the other hand an unplanned pregnancy may become wanted. The term 'unwanted' does not convey the ambivalence felt by many women in categorising a pregnancy in this way" (Royal College of Obstetricians and Gynaecologists, 1991:10).

In a study of 386 American women, Cozzarelli et al. (2000) found that depression scores were significantly lower, and self-esteem scores significantly higher, at two hours, one month and two years after abortion, compared with some hours before the abortion. One month after abortion, mean scores indicated that women felt more relief than positive or negative emotions, and overall more positive emotions than negative emotions. However, 10.8% reported that they felt dissatisfied and had made the wrong decision. At two-year follow-up, the number of women reporting dissatisfaction had increased to 16.3%, and 19% said that the abortion was the wrong decision. Eisen & Zellman (1984) reported similar findings: 80% of 148 adolescents who had an abortion reported satisfaction with the decision six months later.

Major et al. (2000) reported on 418 American women two-years after an early elective pregnancy termination: 20% reported an episode of clinical depression, a rate equal to the national rate of depression; 1% met clinical criteria for post-traumatic stress disorder, which is less than the national rate. This compared with 26% of women reporting clinical depression at some stage prior to the pregnancy. No other psychiatric data were reported. The possibility of mental ill-health being a reason for the abortion, and women's views on whether subsequent mental illness was related to the abortion, were not reported. A pre-pregnancy history of depression was predictive of poorer mental health and more negative abortion-related emotions and evaluations at one hour, one month and two years after the abortion. Though these relationships were statistically significant, the outcome variance explained was quite small (generally less than 10%); most of the variability in women's post-abortion adjustment was unexplained.

Previous psychiatric treatment was not related to scores on a scale measuring the psychological impact of adverse life events, in this case a problem pregnancy and its early termination, three months after the procedure for 96 women in Australia (Allanson, 1999): 31% had sought treatment for emotional problems in the past, with 5% being admitted to hospital. Overall, high psychological distress scores in the days prior to the abortion returned to within normal limits at three months follow-up. The abortion had a very low psychological impact for two-thirds of the sample, while 27% reported some persisting stress symptoms related to the abortion.

Greer et al. (1976) found that, of 216 women who had undergone an early pregnancy termination in London, England, 29% (63) had a history of inpatient or outpatient psychiatric treatment,

and 19% (42) had received psychiatric treatment during the two years following the abortion. Of these 42 women, two-thirds had a pre-abortion psychiatric history, over half (59.5%) reported that the symptoms were unrelated to the abortion, 4 (1.9% of the total sample) reported that their symptoms were related to the abortion, and 13 were unsure. Three months after the abortion, highly significant improvements were observed in measures of depression and guilt (13% reported considerable or moderate guilt compared with 37% before the abortion) and satisfactory sexual adjustment (74% compared with 59%). Satisfaction with the marital relationship did not change from before to after the abortion, but 87% reported improvement in other relationships, while 13% reported deterioration. Some 96% reported resuming normal work activities shortly after the abortion.

In summary, past or current psychiatric illness is apparently rare as a stated reason for elective abortion, and has not been a strong predictor of adjustment to abortion. The stress of facing an unintended pregnancy or unsafe abortion might be expected to increase the risk of onset, or recurrence, of serious mental ill-health, while elective, safe abortion might protect vulnerable women from the long-term stress of pregnancy and parenthood. However, this group of women has attracted negligible research attention. The mental health consequences of unsafe abortion are not known, although qualitative data suggest that unsafe abortion can be traumatic before, during and after the abortion, and is likely to cause psychological harm. Typically, women (including adolescents) experience heightened distress facing a problem pregnancy and prior to safe elective abortion, but show significant improvement on mental health indices afterwards (Mueller & Major, 1989; Cozzarelli, 1993; Major et al., 1997, 2000; Adler, 2000; Barnow et al., 2001; Pope, Adler & Tschann, 2001). Psychiatric sequelae to safe abortion appear to be rare. Approximately 10% of women experience some degree of dissatisfaction with their abortion decision or other psychologically distressing symptoms about their decision to have an abortion, and this can increase to up to 20% within two years after abortion. While unpleasant, such feelings do not necessarily signify clinically significant mental health problems (Major et al., 2000). Evidence-based reviews have consistently concluded that safe, elective, early abortion does not pose a substantial mental health risk and has fewer adverse psychiatric sequelae than childbirth (Adler, 1990; Adler, 1992; Dagg, 1991; Major, 2003; Stotland, 2001; Turell, 1990). Although adverse mental health impacts of safe elective abortion affect a relatively small minority and the number of women experiencing serious adverse impacts appear to be quite small, it appears that the continuing complex biopsychosocial environment of abortion and a desire to optimise women's mental health following safe elective abortion has prompted limited research into risk and protective factors.

Risk and protective factors for mental health after abortion

Pre-abortion optimism about post-abortion adjustment appears to be protective (Cozzarelli, 1993; Cozzarelli, Sumer & Major, 1998). Cozzarelli (1993) investigated 291 American women who had had an abortion, and found that self-efficacy – defined as pre-abortion optimism, perceived personal control and high self-esteem – was strongly associated with better post-abortion adjustment both immediately and three weeks after the procedure. Self-efficacy predicted up to half the variability in post-abortion psychological adjustment. Mueller & Major (1989) randomly assigned 232 women to receive one of three brief verbal presentations before their abortion: (i) to raise expectations of personal coping capacity; (ii) to alter the attributions for unwanted pregnancy; or (iii) a control presentation on a therapeutically neutral topic. Women exposed to one of the experimental interventions had fewer emotional and physical complaints immediately following the termination. The longer-term benefits of the intervention are not known.

Women often involve other people in their decision regarding abortion, but their social networks are not always supportive. Investigations of social support have indicated considerable complexity and contradictions, apparently resulting from subtle differences in the definition of support, the quality of relationships, and the characteristics of study samples (Mueller & Major, 1989; Major et al., 1990; Linn, 1991; Major & Cozzarelli, 1992; Cozzarelli, Sumer & Major, 1998). Major et al. (1997) investigated 617 women's perceptions of support and conflict within three salient relationships: with their partner, mother and friends. Preoperatively,

85% of women had told their partner about the pregnancy and abortion, 69% had told a friend, 25% had told their mother and 17% had told all three. Generally, women viewed all these people as sources of support and reported little conflict, and positive well-being one month after abortion was predicted by support. In identifying factors contributing to less positive adjustment one month post abortion, Major et al noted that women who perceived their mothers and friends as a source of a high level of support as well as conflict were more distressed than if they were just perceived as a source of support. Conflict with the partner, irrespective of his support for her abortion, was related to distress one month after abortion. In a survey of 818 American women presenting for elective abortion, Woo, Fine & Goetzl (2005) found that 17% chose not to disclose the abortion to the partner in the pregnancy. Of these, 45% did not disclose because the relationship had no future, 21% because the partner would oppose the abortion, and 8% because they believed that disclosure would result in their partner physically harming them.

Major & Gramzow (2001) reported on 442 American women followed for two years after abortion. Women who felt that they could not disclose the abortion suppressed more thoughts about it and experienced more intrusive thoughts about it than those in environments in which disclosure was more acceptable. Both suppression and intrusive thoughts were associated with increased psychological distress over time; in contrast, disclosure about the abortion was related to decreased distress.

In-depth interviews with 31 women hospitalized in Egypt with post-abortion complications (Huntington, Nawar & Abdel-Hady, 1997) indicated that practical and emotional support were not forthcoming. The authors surmised that women's predicament was made more difficult by this because women are usually better able to cope with illness and more likely to seek health care when socially supported. The most troubling issues for the women were the need to return immediately to physically demanding work and child care responsibilities, the possibility of people gossiping about them, and criticism, blame and lack of understanding from their husband and his family.

Langer et al. (1997) discuss the apparently compounding, rather than comforting, impact of post-abortion medical attention at a public hospital in Mexico. Almost half the women arrived at the hospital in a highly anxious state and reported fears of dying, infertility and isolation, and constant worry about their children at home. The women found the medical staff rushed and insensitive, and 59% reported more anxiety after the initial examination than before it. In India, women may need to lie about their pregnancy in order to meet legal eligibility requirements for abortion, which include pregnancy resulting from rape for single women, and failed contraception for married women (Gupte, Bandewar & Pisal, 1997).

Women's interpersonal networks can be protective, but social milieus that do not provide support for women's decision about pregnancy may have an adverse impact. "Expressions of disapproval, including attacks on abortion clinics and harassment of women seeking abortions, would be expected to produce negative effects" (McGrath et al., 1999). Empirical research is scarce, but institutionalized "blaming of victims" and withdrawal of social support are likely to have adverse effects on self-regard (Waites, 1993; Cozarelli & Major, 1994; Cozarelli et al., 2000). Taboo and punitive attitudes surrounding abortion prevent women talking about their experiences and may worsen outcomes. The very low abortion rate in the Netherlands (4.0–6.5 per 1000 women aged 15–44 years in 1996, compared with 25.9 per 1000 in the USA) has been linked to the promotion of reproductive options and open discussion and acceptance of sex, contraception and abortion (Henshaw, Singh & Haas, 1999).

Recent research suggests that victimization may play an important role in some women's decision to seek an abortion, and in their abortion-related mental health. It is difficult to draw firm conclusions, however, because of differing definitions of violence, barriers to women's disclosure of violence, and a shortage of research that goes beyond measuring prevalence. A household survey of 2525 women in the USA found that women who reported having an abortion were more likely to report depressive symptoms and lower life satisfaction than those who reported that they had not had an abortion (Russo & Denious, 2001). However, when history of abuse, partner characteristics and background variables were controlled for, abortion was unrelated to poor mental health. In this study, 31% of women who had had an abortion reported violence (including physical or sexual assault during childhood or adulthood and intimate partner violence) compared with 14% of those who reported no abortion.

Prevalence studies in various countries have documented a high incidence of violence against women among those seeking an abortion. In the United States, Glander et al. (1998) found that 40% of 486 women seeking pregnancy termination reported a history of sexual or physical abuse. A United Kingdom survey (Keeling, Birch & Green, 2004) found that 35% of women seeking an abortion reported intimate partner abuse, while a survey of 1127 women attending a hospital abortion service in London (Fisher et al., 2005) found that 20% reported intimate partner physical abuse and 27% reported a history of sexual abuse. Women having a repeat abortion were more likely than first-time abortion seekers to have suffered violence at some time in their life. Leung et al. (2002) found a lifetime prevalence of domestic violence among women seeking abortion in Hong Kong, China, of 27%, compared with 8% for other gynaecology patients and 18% for pregnant women attending antenatal clinics in the same locality. The women seeking abortion had suffered more recent and more serious violence. The authors note, however, that cultural influences probably inhibited the women's reporting of abuse to health professionals. An epidemiological study in Australia (Taft, Watson & Lee, 2004) found that women with previous or recent partner violence were significantly more likely to become pregnant and to report having had an abortion than women without such a history. In a large-sample study in Colombia, Pallitto & O'Campo (2004) documented a moderate relationship between unintended pregnancy and intimate partner violence towards the woman in her current or most recent relationship. The authors estimated that unintended pregnancies in Colombia would decrease by 5% (32 000–45 000 abortions) annually if intimate partner violence were eliminated. A study of women in Uganda reported that 39% of 70 women presenting to a gynaecological emergency ward with complications of induced abortion gave domestic violence as the main reason for inducing the abortion (Kaye, 2001). In a study of 818 American women (Woo et al., 2005), physical abuse, sexual abuse or both within the previous year was twice as common among those who did not disclose their abortion to the partner than among those who did disclose the abortion.

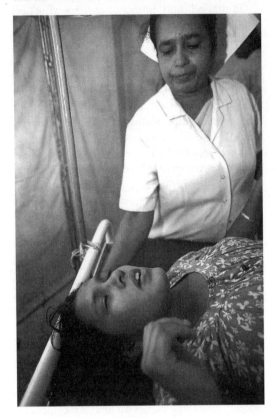

Arguably, violence may interfere with contraceptive use, aggravate relationship instability and undermine a woman's confidence in proceeding with a pregnancy, abortion disclosure, support and women's abortion related mental health. However, research linking abortion, mental health and violence is limited (Bruyn, 2001; Leung, Kung, Lam, Leung and Ho, 2002). Evidence suggests that pregnant women suffering past or current physical and/or sexual violence have worse mental and physical health (Krug, Dahlberg et al., 2002), and among 96 Australian women attending for an early abortion (Allanson and Astbury, 2001), small but statistically significant links were found between these women's experience of violence (40% reported being physically assaulted, 17% sexually assaulted, 9% reported both, and 10% reported violence from the partner in the pregnancy) and poorer mental health outcomes three months post-abortion (Allanson, 1999). Sexual assault history may increase anxiety around childbirth (Jackson, 1997), gynaecological examination (Carlson, 2002) and surgical abortion, with consequent pregnancy ambivalence.

Cultural and social factors that place coercion on women's reproductive health, for example social pressures to have only one child or cultural preferences for sons, may influence mental health after an abortion (Mandal, 2001; Miller, 2001). Based on interviews with 67 women from six villages in India, Gupte et al. (1997) reported that women "who had an abortion after a sex determination test were traumatised compared to those who had an abortion for other reasons". Rothstein (1977a, 1977b) suggests that both subtle and blatant coercion either to continue or terminate a pregnancy is linked to a woman's ambivalence about whether or not to have an abortion. Although ambivalence appears to be a risk factor for post-abortion distress, there has been little clarity in its definition or measurement (Adler et al, 1990; Dagg, 1991; Turrell, Arnmsworth & Gaa, 1990; Allanson & Astbury, 1995). Ambivalence in an abortion decision often has been taken as reflecting a woman's emotional attachment to her pregnancy, leading to grief and a sense of loss if the pregnancy is terminated. Yet, there has been only limited investigation of a woman's relationship with a pregnancy she is considering terminating (Hunter, 1979; Pines, 1990; Allanson & Astbury, 1995), and the discussion above suggests that decision ambivalence may reflect many other facets of a problem pregnancy and abortion. Ambivalence may be a normal part of the psychological process of resolving decisions about abortion, or may be an expression of low self-efficacy. In addition, the relationships between elective abortion and other adverse reproductive experiences, including miscarriage, assisted conception, previous pregnancy complications, and caesarean section have not been investigated, but may influence emotional attachment to a pregnancy or anxieties about pregnancy continuation or termination.

In summary, evidence is emerging about risk and protective factors that are predictive of mental health following an abortion. Post-abortion mental health appears to be enhanced where there is no history of violence, when there is no conflict about the abortion within usually supportive relationships or with the partner, when the abortion is not kept secret from others, and when the woman has high self-efficacy. Research is needed into other possible risk /protective factors, such as history of reproductive trauma, maternal attachment to the pregnancy, and the accessibility of safe reproductive and family planning options. A society's legal, religious, medical and social expectations and infrastructure are likely have an important bearing on all these factors.

Summary

Future research

1. Further participatory research is required to establish accurately needs for contraception.

2. Examination of the disparity between contraceptive intentions and contraceptive use should look beyond women's "failure" to adhere to their intentions.

3. Investigations are needed of the level of coercion and pressure women experience from family planning programmes regarding child-spacing, uptake of contraceptive methods, including sterilization and abortion.

4. With respect to mental health associated with both safe and unsafe abortion, there is a need for methodologically rigorous qualitative and quantitative investigations into women's experiences, needs, biopsychosocial risk and protective factors, and health enhancing interventions.

5. The biopsychosocial aspects of sex-selective abortion are at present unknown and need to be systematically investigated.

6. Research needs to explore the counselling, medical and support needs of women facing an unintended pregnancy and abortion, who may have particular vulnerabilities such as mental illness, violence, reproductive trauma.

Implications for policy

1. Strategies to increase the involvement of men in family planning programmes are essential if the goal of gender equality is to be realized and women's safety protected.

2. Family planning programmes need to give attention to sexual enjoyment as well as fertility control.

3. Strategies to increase women's self-efficacy regarding reproductive options.

Services

1. Women's freedom to make decisions about participation in family planning programmes and fertility control needs to be sensitively ascertained, rather than simply assumed.

2. Sexual violence and coercion, as risk factors for unwanted pregnancy, termination of pregnancy and contraceptive failure, as well as for depression, anxiety and symptoms of traumatic stress, should be ascertained in routine care.

3. Given the high incidence of both safe and unsafe abortion, health professionals need specific training in medical and psychosocial aspects of abortion care.

References

Abeyesekera S (1997) Abortion in Sri Lanka in the context of women's human rights. *Reproductive Health Matters*, 9: 87-95.

Adelson PL, Frommer MS, Weisberg E (1995) A survey of women seeking termination of pregnancy in New South Wales. *Medical Journal of Australia*, 163: 419-422.

Adewole LF et al. (2002) Contraceptive usage among abortion seekers in Nigeria. *West African Journal of Medicine*, 21(2): 112-114.

Adler NE (1992) Unwanted pregnancy and abortion: definitional and research issues. *Journal of Social Issues*, 48(3): 19-35.

Adler NE (2000) Abortion and the null hypothesis. *Archives of General Psychiatry*, 57: 785-786.

Ahman E, Shah I (2002) Unsafe abortion: worldwide estimates for 2000. *Reproductive Health Matters*, 10(19): 13-17.

Ahman E, Shah I (2004) *Unsafe abortion: global and regional estimates of incidence of unsafe abortion and associated mortality in 2000*, 4th ed. Geneva, World Health Organization.

Alarcon I, Gonzales GF (2001) Attitudes towards sexuality, sexual knowledge and behaviour in adolescents in the cities of Lima, Cusco and Iquitos. In: *Sexual relations among young people in developing countries. Evidence from WHO case studies*. Geneva, World Health Organization.

Allanson S (1999) The abortion decision: fantasy, attachment and outcomes. Melbourne, University of Melbourne (unpublished PhD dissertation).

Allanson S, Astbury J (1995) The abortion decision: reasons and ambivalence. *Journal of Psychosomatic Obstetrics & Gynaecology*, 16(3): 123-136.

Allanson S, Astbury J (2001) Attachment style and broken attachments: violence, pregnancy and abortion. *Australian Journal of Psychology*, 53(3): 146-151.

Angulo V, Guendelman S (2002) Crossing the border for abortion services: the Tijuana-San Diego connection. *Health Care for Women International*, 23(6-7): 642-653.

Aries N (2002) The Amercian College of Obstetricians and Gynaecologists and the evolution of abortion policy, 1951-1973: the politics of science. *American Journal of Public Health*, 93(11): 1810-1819.

Arowojolu A, Ladipo O (2003) Nonmenstrual adverse events associated with subdermal contraceptive implants containing normegestrel and levonogestrel. *African Journal of Medicine and Medical Science*, 32(1): 27-31.

Arshat H et al. (1990) A study of the acceptability and effectiveness of Norplant(R) contraceptive implants in Kuala Lumpur, Malaysia. *Malaysian Journal of Reproductive Health*, 8(1): 21-29.

Association for Voluntary Surgical Contraception (1996) Guidelines for pre-sterilization counselling. *Contraceptive Report*, 7: 12-13.

Astbury J, Cabral de Mello M (2000) *Women's mental health: an evidence based review.* Geneva, World Health Organization.

Azize-Vargas Y, Aviles LA (1998) Abortion in Puerto Rico: the limits of a colonial legality. *Puerto Rico Health Sciences Journal,* 17: 27-36.

Baker A (1985) *The complete book of problem pregnancy counselling.* USA: The Hope Clinic For Women.

Barnow S et al. (2001) The influence of psychosocial factors on mental well-being and physical complaints before and after undergoing an in-patient abortion. *Psychotherapie Psychocomatik Medizinisch Psychologie*, 51(9-10): 356-364.

Ba-Thike K (1997) Abortion: a public health problem in Myanmar. *Reproductive Health Matters*, 9: 94-100.

Bautista PF (2001) Young unwed mothers: medical, psychosocial and demographic implications. In: *Sexual relations among young people in developing countries. Evidence from WHO case studies,* Geneva, World Health Organization.

Beral V (1979) Reproductive mortality. *British Medical Journal*, 2: 632-634.

Boonthai N, Warakamin S (2001) Induced abortion: a nationwide survey in Thailand. Paper presented at the *XXV International Congress of the Medical Women's International Association (MWIA) On Women's Health in a Multicultural World*, 19-23 April, Sydney, Australia.

British Medical Association (2005) *Abortion Time Limits: A briefing paper from the BMA* May.

Brown G, Harris T, Hepworth C (1995) Loss, humiliation and entrapment among women developing depression: a patient and non patient comparison. *Psychological Medicine*, 25: 7-21.

Cabral R et al. (2003) Do main partner conflict, power dynamics and control over use of male condom predict subsequent use of the female condom? *Women and Health*, 38: 37-52.

Campbell J, Lewandowski L (1997) Mental and physical health effects of intimate partner violence on women and children. *Psychiatric Clinics of North America*, 20: 353-374.

Campbell J, Soeken K (1999) Forced sex and intimate partner violence: effects on women's health. *Violence Against Women*, 5: 1017-1035.

Carlson K (2002) *Barriers to cervical screening experienced by victims/survivors of sexual assault.* Australia, Centre Against Sexual Assault.

Casas-Becerra L (1997) Women prosecuted and imprisoned for abortion in Chile. *Reproductive Health Matters*, 9: 29-36.

Castle M, Fisher B (1997) Anatomy of a physician education programme. *Reproductive Health Matters*, 9: 46-55.

Cavenar JO Jr, Maltbie AA, Sullivan JL (1978) Aftermath of abortion: anniversary depression and abdominal pain. *Bulletin of the Menninger Clinic*, 42(5): 433-444.

Chan A, Sage LC (2005) Estimating Australian's abortion rates 1985-2003. *Medical Journal of Australia*, 182(9): 447-452.

Chapman K, Gordon G (1999) Reproductive health technologies and gender: is participation the key? *Gender and Development*, 7: 34-44.

Civic D et al. (2000) Depressive symptoms in users and non-users of depot medroxyprogesterone acetate. *Contraception*, 61(6): 385-390.

Clapman A (2003) Privacy rights and abortion outing: a proposal for using common-law torts to protect abortion patients and staff. *Yale Law Journal*, 112(6): 1545-1576.

Coker A et al. (2000) Physical health consequences of physical and psychological intimate partner violence. *Archives of Family Medicine*, 451-457.

Comerasamy H et al. (2003) The acceptability and use of contraception: a prospective study of Somalian women's attitude. *Journal of Obstetrics and Gynaecology*, 23: 412-415.

Cozzarelli C (1993) Personality and self-efficacy as predictors of coping with abortion. *Journal of Personality and Social Psychology*, 65(6): 1124-1236.

Cozarelli C, Major B (1994) The effects of anti-abortion demonstrators and pro-choice escorts on women's psychological responses to abortion. *Journal of Social and Clinical Psychology*, 13: 404-427.

Cozzarelli C, Sumer N, Major B (1998) Mental models of attachment and coping with abortion. *Journal of Personality and Social Psychology*, 74(2): 453-467.

Cozarelli C et al. (2000) Women's experiences with and reactions to anti-abortion picketing. *Journal of Basic and Applied Social Psychology*, 22: 265-275.

Darling C, Davidson JNS, Passarello L (1992) The mystique of first intercourse among college youth. *Journal of Youth and Adolescence,* 21: 97-117.

David H, Dytrych Z, Matejcek Z (2003) Born unwanted: observations for the Prague study. *American Psychologist*, 58(3): 224-229.

David H et al., eds. (1988) *Born unwanted: developmental effects of denied abortion.* New York, Springer.

Dean R, Allanson S (2004) Abortion in Australia: access vs protest. *Journal of Law and Medicine*, 11(4): 510-515.

Dean, R. The erosion of access to abortion in the United States; Lessons for Australia *Deakin Law Review,* 81.

de Bruyn M (2001) *Violence, pregnancy and abortion.* USA: Round Up.

de Crespigny LJ, Savulescu J (2004) Abortion: time to clarify Australia's confusing laws. *Medical Journal of Australia,* 181(4): 201-203.

den Tonkelaar D, Oddens B (2001) Factors influencing women's satisfaction with birth control methods. *European Journal of Reproductive Health Care*, 6(3): 153-158.

Diekema D (2003) Involuntary sterilization of persons with mental retardation: ethical analysis. *Mental Retardation Development and Disability Research Review*, 9(1): 21-26.

Dixon-Mueller R (1989) Psychosocial consequences to women's health of contraceptive use and controlled fertility. In: P. AM, ed., *Contraceptive use and controlled fertility*, Washington, DC, National Academy Press: 140-159.

Duggal R (2004) The political economy of abortion in India: cost and expenditure patterns. *Reproductive Health Matters,* 12(24): 130-137.

Eisen M, Zellman GL (1984) Factors predicting pregnancy resolution decision satisfaction of unmarried adolescents. *Journal of Genetic Psychology*, 143(2): 231-239.

Erci B (2003) Women's efficiency in decision making and their perception of their status in the family. *Public Health Nursing*, 20: 65-70.

Erskine M et al. (2000) Tolerability and reasons for discontinuation of Norplant in an inner city population. *Journal of Obstetrics and Gynaecology*, 20: 180-182.

Eschen A, Whittaker M (1993) Family planning: a base to build on for women's reproductive health services. In: Koblinsky M, Timyam J, Gay J, eds., *The health of women*, Boulder, San Francisco and Oxford, Westview Press: 105-132.

Espey E et al. (2003) IUD-related knowledge, attitudes and practices among Navajo Area Indian Health Service providers. *Perspectives on Sexual and Reproductive Health*, 35: 169-173.

Fisher WA et al. Characteristics of women undergoing repeat induced abortion. *Canadian Medical Association Journal*, 172(5): 637-641.

Fraser I et al. (1998) Norplant consensus statement and background review. *Contraception*, 57: 1-9.

Fried M (1997) Abortion in the US: barriers to access. *Reproductive Health Matters*, 9: 37-45.

Galazios G et al. (2002) Attitudes towards contraceptive pill use in two different populations in Thrace, Greece. *European Journal of Contraception and Reproductive Health Care*, 7: 127-131.

Gazmararian J et al. (2000) Violence and reproductive health: current knowledge and future research directions. *Maternal and Child Health*, 4: 79-84.

Gebreselassie H, Fetters T (2002) *Responding to unsafe abortion in Ethiopia: a facility-based assessment of post-abortion care services facilities in Ethiopia*. Chapel Hill: Ipas.

Geelhoed D et al. (2004) Gender and unwanted pregnancy: a community-based study in rural Ghana. *Journal of Psychosomatic Obstetrics and Gynaecology*, 23(4): 249-255.

Glander S et al. (1998) The prevalence of domestic violence among women seeking abortion. *Obstetrics and Gynecology*, 91(6): 1002-1006.

Glantz S et al. (2000) Norplant (R) use among urban minority women in the United States. *Contraception*, 61(2): 83-90.

Goldberg H et al. (1994) Research on reproduction and women's health. *Demografie*, 36: 30-39.

Graham CA et al. (1995). The effect of steroidal contraceptives on the well-being and sexuality of women: a double-blind, placebo-controlled, two-centre study of combined and progestogen-only methods. *Contraception*, 52: 363-369.

Greer HS et al. (1976) Psychosocial consequences of therapeutic abortion: King's termination study III. *British Journal of Psychiatry*, 128: 74-79.

Gupte M, Bandewar S, Pisal H (1997) Abortion needs of women in India: a case study of rural Maharashtra. *Reproductive Health Matters*, 9: 77-86.

Hankoff L, Darney P (1993) Contraceptive choices for behaviourally disordered women. *American Journal of Obstetrics and Gynaecology*, 168(6S): 1986-1989.

Hardy E et al. (1997) Comparison of women having clandestine and hospital abortions: Maputo, Mozambique. *Reproductive Health Matters*, 9: 108-117.

Harvey S et al. (2003) Sexual decision making and safer sex behaviour among young injection drug users and female partners of IDUs. *Journal of Sex Research*, 40(1): 50-60.

Hasna F (2003) Islam, social traditions and family planning. *Social Policy and Administration*, 37: 181-197.

Heise L, Garcia-Moreno C (2002) Violence by intimate partners. In: Krug EG et al., eds., *World report on violence and health*, Geneva, World Health Organization.

Henshaw S, Singh S, Haas T (1999) Recent trend in abortion rates worldwide. *International Family Planning Perspectives*, 25(1): 44-48.

Herrera AA, Zivy MR (2002) Clandestine abortion in Mexico: a question of mental as well as physical health. *Reproductive Health Matters*, 10(19): 95-102.

Hessini L (2005) Global progress in abortion advocacy and policy: an assessment of the decade since ICPD. *Reproductive Matters*, 13(25): 88-101.

Humble M (1995) Women's perspectives on reproductive health and rights. *Planned Parenthood Challenges*, 2: 26-31.

Hunter EK (1979) *The role of fantasies about the fetus in abortion patients: an adaptive process*. Fresno: California School of Professional Psychology.

Huntington D, Nawar L, Abdel-Hady D (1997) Women's perceptions of abortion in Egypt. *Reproductive Health Matters*, 9: 101-107.

Isarabhakdi P (2001) Determinants of sexual behaviour that influence the risk of pregnancy and disease among rural Thai young adults. In: *Sexual relations among young people in developing countries. Evidence from WHO case studies.* Geneva, World Health Organization.

Jackson C (1997) Carrying more than a baby: women survivors of child abuse. *International Symposium on Contraceptive Research & Development for the year 2000 and beyond, Mexico City, 1993.*

Jain A, Bruce J (1994) A reproductive health approach to the objectives and assessments of family planning programs. In: Sen G, Germain A, Chen L, eds., *Population policies reconsidered: health, empowerment and rights.* Boston, Harvard Centre for Population and Development Studies.

Jewkes R, Purna Sen P, Garcia-Moreno C (2002) Sexual violence. In: Krug EG et al., eds., *World report on violence and health,* Geneva, World Health Organization.

Jewkes R et al. (2001) Relationship dynamics and teenage pregnancy in South Africa. *Social Science and Medicine,* 52: 733-744.

Kaunitz A (1999) Long-acting hormonal contraception: assessing impact on bone density, weight and mood. *International Journal of Fertility and Women's Medicine,* 44: 110-117.

Kaye D. (2001) Domestic violence and induced-abortion: report of three cases, *East African Medical Journal,* 78(10): 555-6.

Kaye D (2005) Domestic violence among women seeking post-abortion care. *International Journal of Gynaecology and Obstetrics,* 75(3): 323-325.

Kelly J, Evans M (2003) Trends in Australian attitudes to abortion 1984-2002. *Australian Social Monitor,* 6: 45-53.

Kgosidintsi N (2001) Sexual behaviour and risk of HIV infection among adolescent females in Botswana. In: *Sexual relations among young people in developing countries. Evidence from WHO case studies.* Geneva, World Health Organization.

Khanam M, Mullich M, Munib A (1993) Pattern of depressive disorder among permanently sterilized women. *Bangladesh Medical Research Council Bulletin,* 19(2): 45-51.

Kilpatrick D, Edmunds C, Seymour A (1992) *Rape in America: a report to the nation.* Arlington, National Victims Centre and Medical University of South Carolina.

Krug E et al., eds (2002) *World report on violence and health.* Geneva, World Health Organization.

Kubicka L et al. (2003) The mental health of adults born of unwanted pregnancies, their siblings, and matched controls: a 35 year follow-up study from Prague, Czech Republic. *Journal of Nervous and Mental Disease,* 190(10): 653-662.

Kwon TH, Jun K, Cho SN (2001) Sexuality, contraception and abortion among unmarried adolescents and young adults: the case of Korea. In: *Sexual relations among young people in developing countries. Evidence from WHO case studies.* Geneva, World Health Organization.

Langer A et al. (1997) Improving post-abortion care in a public hospital in Oaxaca, Mexico. *Reproductive Health Matters,* 9: 20-28.

Larsson M et al. (2002) Reasons for pregnancy termination, contraceptive habits and contraceptive failure among Swedish women requesting an early pregnancy termination. *Acta Obstetrica et Gynecologica Scandinavica,* 81(1): 64-71.

Lawrie T et al. (1998) A double blind randomised placebo controlled trial of postnatal noresthisterone enanthate: the effect on postnatal depression and serum hormones. *British Journal of Obstetrics & Gynaecology,* 105: 1082-1090.

Lechner M et al. (1993) Self-reported medical problems of adult female survivors of childhood sexual abuse. *Journal of Family Practice,* 36: 633-638.

Letourneau E, Holmes M, Chasendunn-Roark J (1999) Gynaecologic health consequences to victims of interpersonal violence. *Women's Health Issues,* 9: 115-120.

Leung WC et al. (2002) Domestic violence and postnatal depression in a Chinese community. *International Journal of Gynecology and Obstetrics,* 79(2): 159-166.

Linn R (1991) Mature unwed mothers in Israel: socio-moral and psychological dilemmas. *Lifestyles: Family & Economic Issues,* 12(2): 145-170.

Mahmood N, Zahid GM (1993) The demand for fertility control in Pakistan. *Pakistan Development Review,* 32: 1097-1104.

Major B (2003) Psychological implications of abortion - highly charged and rife with misleading research. *Canadian Medical Association Journal,* 168(10): 1257-1258.

Major B, Cozzarelli C (1992) Psychosocial predictors of adjustment to abortion. *Journal of Social Issues,* 48(3): 121-142.

Major B, Gramzow R (2001) Abortion as stigma: cognitive and emotional implications of concealment. *Journal of Personality and Social Psychology*, 77(4): 735-745.

Major B et al. (1990) Perceived social support, self-efficacy, and adjustment to abortion. *Journal of Personality and Social Psychology*, 59(3): 452-463.

Major B et al. (1997) Mixed messages: implications of social conflict and social support within close relationships for adjustment to a stressful life event. *Journal of Personality and Social Psychology*, 72(6): 1349-1363.

Major B et al. (2000) Psychological responses of women after first-trimester abortion. *Archives of General Psychiatry*, 57: 777-784.

Mandal S (2001) Modernization and women's status in India: a gender in development perspective on dowry deaths, sex ratios and sex-selective abortion. *Humanities and Social Sciences*, 62(2-A): 797.

McCandless F, Sladen C (2003) Sexual health and women with bipolar disorder. *Journal of Advanced Nursing*, 44(1): 42-48.

McGrath JJ et al. (1999) The fertility and fecundity of patients with psychoses. *Acta Psychiatrica Scandinavica*, 99(6): 441-446.

Medoff MH (2003) The impact of anti-abortion activities on state abortion rates. *Journal of Socio-Economics*, 32(3): 265-282.

Miller BD (2001) Female-selective abortion in Asia: patterns, policies and debates. *American Anthropologist*, 103(4): 1083-1095.

Mueller P, Major B (1989) Self-blame, self-efficacy and adjustment to abortion. *Journal of Personality and Social Psychology*, 57(6): 1059-1068.

Mwakisha J (1996) Female condom study explores role of peer support in sustaining use. *Aidscaptions*, 3: 46-48.

National Health and Medical Research Council (1996) *An information paper on termination of pregnancy in Australia*. Canberra, Commonwealth of Australia.

Nayer I et al. (2004). Acceptance of long-term contraceptive methods and its related factors among the eligible couple in a selected union. *Bangladesh Medical Research Council Bulletin*, 30:31-35.

Neuhaus W, Bolte A (1995) Prognostic factors for preoperative consultation of women desiring sterilization: findings of a retrospective analysis. *Journal of Psychosomatic Obstetrics and Gynaecology*, 16: 45-50.

Nimgoankar V et al. R (1997) Fertility in schizophrenia: results from a contemporary US cohort. *Acta Psychiatrica Scandinavica*, 95(5): 364-369.

Oddens B (1999) Women's satisfaction with birth control: a population survey of physical and psychological effects of oral contraceptives, intrauterine devices, condoms, natural family planning and sterilization among 1466 women. *Contraception*, 59(5): 277-286.

Onyango S, Mitchell M, Nyaga N (2003) *Scaling up access to high-quality post abortion care in Kenya: an assessment of public and private facilities in Western and Nyanza provinces*. Chapel Hill: Ipas.

Orji E, Onwudiegwu U (2002) Prevalence and determinants of contraceptive practice in a defined Nigerian population. *Journal of Obstetrics and Gynaecology*, 22: 540-543.

Pallitto CC, O'Campo P (2004) The relationship between intimate partner violence and unintended pregnancy: Analysis of a national sample from Colombia. *International Family Planning Perspectives*, 30(4): 165-169.

Paransky O, Zurawin R (2003) Management of menstrual problems and contraception in adolescents with mental retardation: a medical, legal and ethical review with new suggested guidelines. *Journal of Pediatric and Adolescent Gynecology*. 16(4): 223-235.

Perera J, de Silva T, Gange H (2004) Knowledge, behaviour and attitudes on induced abortion and family planning among Sri Lankan women seeking termination of pregnancy. *Ceylon Medical Journal*, 49(1): 14-17.

Philliber S, Philliber WW (1985) Social and psychological perspectives on voluntary sterilization: a review. *Studies in Family Planning*, 16: 1-29.

Pines D (1990) Pregnancy, miscarriage and abortion. A psychoanalytic perspective. *International Journal of Psycho-Analysis*, 71: 301-307.

Pinter B (2002) Medico-legal aspects of abortion in Europe. *European Journal of Contraception and Reproductive Health Care,* 7(1):15-19.

Plichta S, Abraham C (1996) Violence and gynaecologic health in women less than 50 years old. *American Journal of Obstetrics and Gynecology*, 174: 903-907.

Pope LM, Adler NE, Tschann JM (2001) Post abortion psychological adjustment: are minors at increased risk? *Journal of Adolescent Health*, 29(1): 2-11.

Ramachandar L, Pelto P (2002) The role of village health nurses in mediating abortions in rural Tamil Nadu, India. *Reproductive Health Matters,* 10(19): 64-75.

Rance S (1997) Safe motherhood, unsafe abortion: A reflection on the impact of discourse. *Reproductive Health Matters*, 9: 10-19.

Rattray C et al. (1997) The Norplant experience at the University Hospital of the West Indies. *Journal of Obstetrics and Gynaecology*, 17(6): 569-572.

Resnick H, Acierno R, Kilpatrick D (1997) Health impact of interpersonal violence. 2: Medical and mental health outcomes. *Behavioral Medicine*, 23: 65-78.

Rickert V et al. (2002) The relationship among demographics, reproductive characteristics and intimate partner violence. *American Journal of Obstetrics and Gynecology*, 187: 1002-1007.

Rizzardo R et al. (1991) Personality and psychological distress in legal abortion, threatened miscarriage and normal pregnancy. *Psychotherapy and Psychosomatics*, 56: 227-234.

Roberts G et al. (1998) How does domestic violence affect women's mental health. *Women and Health*, 28: 117-129.

Ross J, Winfrey WL (2002) Unmet need for contraception in the developing world and the former Soviet Union: an updated estimate. *International Family Planning Perspectives*, 28: 138-143.

Rossier C (2003) Estimated induced abortion rates: a review. *Studies in Family Planning*, 34(2): 87-102.

Rothstein A (1977a) Abortion: a dyadic perspective. *American Journal of Orthopsychiatry*, 47(1): 111-118.

Rothstein A (1977b) Men's reactions to their partners' elective abortions. *American Journal of Obstetrics and Gynecology,* 128: 8.

Roy T et al. (2003) Can women's childbearing and contraceptive intentions predict contraceptive demand? Findings from a longitudinal study in Central India. *International Family Planning Perspectives*, 29: 25-31.

Russo NF, Denious JE (2001) Violence in the lives of women having abortions: implications for practice and public policy. *Professional Psychology Research and Practice*, 32(2): 142-150.

Sahin H, Sahin HG (2003) Reasons for not using family planning methods in Eastern Turkey. *European Journal of Contraception and Reproductive Health Care*, 8: 11-16.

Skouby, S.O. (2004) Contraceptive use and behavior in the 21st century: a comprehensive study across five European countries. *European Journal of Contraception and Reproductive Health Care*. 9(2): 57-68.

Shah M et al. (2003) A profile of contraceptive non use in Kuwait: implication for health and health care. *European Journal of Contraception and Reproductive Health Care*, 8: 99-108.

Sigal JJ (2004) Studies of unwanted babies. *American Psychologist,* 59(3): 183-4.

Springs F, Friedrich W (1992) Health risk behaviours and medical sequelae of childhood sexual abuse. *Mayo Clinic Proceedings*, 67: 527-532.

Stotland NL (1996) Conceptions and misconceptions. Decisions about pregnancy. *General Hospital Psychiatry*, 18(4): 238-243.

Sundstrom K (2001) Reproductive health from an individual and a global perspective. In: Ostlin P et al., eds., *Gender inequalities in health*, Cambridge, MA, Harvard Center for Population and Development Studies: 67-98.

Taft A, Watson L, Lee C (2004) Violence against young women and association with reproductive events: a cross-sectional analysis of a national population sample. *Australian and New Zealand Journal of Public Health*, 28(4): 324-329.

Tornbom M et al. (1994) Evaluation of stated motives for legal abortion. *Journal of Psychosomatic Obstetrics and Gynaecology,* 15: 27-33.

Torres A, Forrest JD (1988) Why do women have abortions? *Family Planning Perspectives*, 20(4): 169-176.

Tripathi R, Rathore A, Sachdeva J (2003) Emergency contraception: knowledge, attitude, and practices among health care providers in North India. *Journal of Obstetrics and Gynaecology Research*, 29(3): 142-146.

UNDP (2003) Human Development Report 2003: *Millennium Development Goals: A compact among nations to end human poverty.* New York, United Nations Development Programme.

UNFPA (1994) *Programme of Action of the International Conference on Population and Development, Cairo, 5-13 September 1994.* New York, United Nations Population Fund.

United Nations (1995) *Fourth World Conference on Women, Beijing, September 1995: Platform for action.* New York www.un.org/womenwatch/daw/beijing/platform/plat1.htm; November 2006.

United Nations (1999) *World abortion policies 1999.* New York, United Nations Population Division (www.un.org/esa/population/ publications/abt/ abt.htm, accessed November 2006).

United Nations Department of Economic and Social Affairs, Population Division(2003) *World Population Policies* 2003, United Nations publication, sales No. E.04. XIII.3.

Villanueva M *Pregnancy and reproductive health in students that attend night school.* Lima, Peru, Cayetano Heredia Peruvian University, Institute for Population Studies (unpublished final report submitted to the Programme in June, 1992).

Wagner KD (1996) Major depression and anxiety disorders associated with Norplant. *Journal of Clinical Psychiatry.* 57(4):152-7.

Wagner K, Berenson AB (1994) Norplant-associated major depression and panic disorder. *Journal of Clinical Psychiatry*, 55: 478-480.

Waites EA (1993) *Trauma and survival: post-traumatic and dissociative disorders in women.* New York, WW Norton & Co.

Webb A (2002) What do women want? Counselling in contraception. *European Journal of Contraception and Reproductive Health Care*, 7: 150-154.

Weber A et al. (2003) High pregnancy rates and reproductive health indicators among female injection-drug users in Vancouver, Canada. *European Journal of Contraceptive and Reproductive Health Care*, 8(1): 52-58.

Westhoff C et al. (1998) Depressive symptoms and Norplant contraceptive implants. *Contraception*, 57: 241-245.

Whittaker A (2001) Conceiving the nation: representations of abortion in Thailand. *Asian Studies Review,* 25(4): 423-451.

Whittaker A (2002) The struggle for abortion law reform in Thailand. *Reproductive Health Matters*, 10(19): 45-53.

Wilmoth GH, de Alteriis M, Bussell D (1992) Prevalence of psychological risks following legal abortion in the U.S.: limits of the evidence. *Journal of Social Issues*, 48(3): 37-66.

Woo J, Fine P, Goetzl L (2005) Abortion disclosure and the association with domestic violence. *Obstetrics and Gynaecology,* 105(6): 1329-1334.

Woodhouse A (1982) Sexuality, femininity and fertility control. *Women's Studies International Forum*, 5(1): 1-15.

WHO (2000) *Improving access to quality care in family planning. Medical eligibility criteria for contraceptive use,* 2nd ed. Geneva, World Health Organization.

WHO (2001a) Sexual relations among young people in developing countries: Evidence from WHO case studies. Geneva, World Health Organization,

WHO (2001b) *Transforming health systems: gender and rights in reproductive health. A training curriculum for health programme managers.* Geneva, World Health Organization.

WHO (2002) *Selected practice recommendations for contraceptive use.* Geneva, World Health Organization.

WHO (2003) *Safe abortion: technical and policy guidance for health systems.* Geneva, World Health Organization.

WHO (2007) *Unsafe abortion: global and regional estimates of incidence of unsafe abortion and associated mortality.* Geneva, World Health Organization. 5th edition.

Yahaya M (2002) Analysis of women's reproductive health situation in Bida Emirate of Niger State, Nigeria. *African Journal of Reproductive Health,* 6: 50-64.

Zellner S (2003) Condom use and the accuracy of AIDS knowledge in Côte d'Ivoire. *International Family Planning Perspectives*, 29: 41-47.

Chapter 4

Spontaneous pregnancy loss

Heather Rowe

It is estimated that 20% of conceptions end spontaneously in miscarriage, most within the first three months of gestation. The actual rate, including those that are not clinically or personally obvious, is estimated to be much higher (Mishell, 1993). In some countries, particularly where legal, safe abortion is unavailable, it is not always possible to make a clear clinical distinction between miscarriage and induced abortion (Vazquez, 2002).

Mental health and spontaneous pregnancy loss

The psychosocial repercussions of miscarriage for individual women are likely to be influenced by culturally specific beliefs and practices surrounding conception, inheritance and ideas of family identity, individual responsibility and attribution of cause. There has been little cross-cultural research on ethnomedical beliefs about pregnancy complications (Asowa-Omorodion, 1997). However, in the available studies the attribution of blame for pregnancy loss to the woman is a common theme. For example, in some societies pregnancy loss is still grounds on which a man may divorce his wife (Vazquez, 2002). This is especially the case where having many children is desirable for social and economic reasons, and where high social status is accorded to fertile and fecund women. Focus groups conducted with Esan women from Edo state in central southern Nigeria revealed that the women believed that attempts to control their fertility would result in pregnancy illness and loss, and that bleeding in pregnancy was a punishment for wrongdoing by the woman. Only if the crime could be established and forgiveness received from the offended party would the bleeding stop (Asowa-Omorodion, 1997).

In developed countries, contemporary discourse emphasizes the desirability of women's autonomy and control of their bodies during pregnancy and childbirth. It is implicit in this that individuals can personally ensure a happy, healthy pregnancy outcome; this can result in self-blame when pregnancy loss does occur (Layne, 2003). Societies differ in the degree to which they permit, or even encourage, discussion of adverse pregnancy events. In contrast to Western social conventions, it is reported that women in some settings, for example Yucatan (Mexico) and Nepal, are able to speak candidly about all kinds of pregnancy loss, which, it is argued, is beneficial (Jordan, 1993; March, 2001). Rice (1999) conducted in-depth interviews and participant observations with Hmong women living in Australia. Her findings revealed that, for these women, miscarriage creates considerable anxiety at both the family and the social level. This is because of a belief that miscarriage may portend the failure of the family to extend its lineage, and because it is seen as a threat to the existence of the clan itself. Religious concerns are focused on the loss of a place within the family for the rebirth of a soul. The reactions of this group of women to miscarriage reflect anxiety about disruption to the harmony between the social and supernatural worlds, which is essential for health.

Responses to miscarriage are shaped by the patterns of socially sanctioned support and mourning behaviour, as well as the time at which pregnancy is publicly acknowledged and the fetus accorded status as a human (Slade, 1994).

Miscarriage is experienced by many women as a significant life crisis (Slade, 1994). Elevated rates of psychological morbidity, in particular depression and anxiety disorders and increased use of psychotropic medication, have been reported after pregnancy loss (Neugebauer, Kline & O'Connor, 1992; Prettyman, Cordle & Cook, 1993; Stirtzinger et al., 1999; Geller, 2001; Garel et al., 1994). Paradoxically, there is also evidence that both health professionals and the lay community tend to minimize the degree of distress, and to assume that women will make a rapid and spontaneous recovery (Layne, 1990; Stirtzinger et al., 1999). It has been argued (Layne, 2003) that, in developed countries, where adverse pregnancy and birth outcomes are rare and the discussion of adverse events is discouraged, women may suffer alone without acknowledgement or support from others. Lack of social acknowledgement of distress about spontaneous pregnancy loss may lead women to experience an invisible bereavement and disenfranchised grief (Cecil & Leslie, 1993). In developing countries, where pregnancy loss of all kinds is more common, it is arguable that miscarriage may be felt as more profound, especially if it represents to the woman the loss of her role as a mother, in a society where alternative roles are limited or nonexistent.

Studies in developed countries have identified a range of emotional reactions to miscarriage, including guilt, sadness, helplessness and anger (Frost & Condon, 1996). The miscarriage itself may be a frightening experience (Prettyman, Cordle & Cook, 1993; Layne, 1997). Nevertheless, not all women in every setting will experience miscarriage as a profound loss, and there appears to be a diversity of reactions, from those requiring psychiatric care at one end of the spectrum, to expressions of ambivalence, relative indifference or relief at the other. This variety is likely to be associated with differences in personal circumstances, as well as familial, social and cultural meanings (Madden, 1994). Women's own descriptions of miscarriages have been interpreted as a process involving the stages of turmoil, adjustment and resolution rather than psychological morbidity (Maker & Ogden, 2003).

Despite a lack of explicit theoretical frameworks in much research on psychological reactions to miscarriage, there is generally an implicit assumption that the bereavement or loss model

is appropriate (Slade, 1994). Psychoanalytical conceptualizations emphasize the normal psychological changes in pregnancy, which include pregnancy as a maturational challenge, when unresolved early conflicts may be re-aroused and an intense narcissistic state may develop. Cognitive modifications may accompany these changes, which are characterized by alterations in primary process thinking. Finally, whether the pregnancy is wanted or not, most women experience some ambivalence towards the fetus, in which the urge to nurture and protect coexists with feelings of being overwhelmed by the irrevocable course of the pregnancy. This conceptualization explains grief reactions to pregnancy loss in terms of an intense narcissistic injury, characterized by feelings of emptiness, shame, helplessness and low self-esteem, which are exacerbated by the absence of an object for which to mourn (Frost & Condon, 1996). Slade (1994) suggests an alternative conceptual framework, which characterizes the experience of pregnancy loss as a stressor, to which individuals will respond according to their individual coping style. However, as yet there has been no empirical investigation of this theoretical position.

> Not all women in every setting will experience miscarriage as a profound loss, and there appears to be a diversity of reactions, from those requiring psychiatric care at one end of the spectrum, to expressions of ambivalence, relative indifference or relief at the other.

Moulder (1994) described two models on which professional care for women having a miscarriage is based. The "medical" model assumes that the miscarriage is a minor mishap, which can be treated, while the "gestational" model recognizes the loss involved, but describes the magnitude of loss in terms of the stage of pregnancy at which it occurred: the later the miscarriage, the greater the loss. Moulder argues that neither of these models accurately explains the diversity of women's responses to pregnancy loss. She proposes a model with greater potential explanatory power, which is based on an understanding of maternal–fetal emotional attachment, loss, and the degree of individual investment in the pregnancy (Moulder, 1994). There has been relatively little research on maternal–fetal emotional attachment in early pregnancy, but the process appears to begin before fetal movements are detected. In addition, a high level of attachment to the fetus can coexist with disenchantment about the pregnancy state itself (Lumley, 1980). The attachment construct is useful in understanding the intensity of emotional reactions to pregnancy loss, but has received little theoretical or empirical attention in the research literature (Condon, 1993).

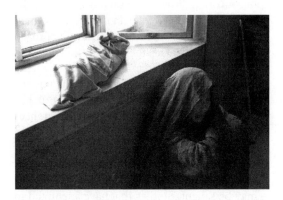

As with other human loss, an understanding of the relationship between grief and depression is essential to understanding the psychological implications of miscarriage (Stirtzinger et al., 1999; Ritsher & Neugebauer, 2002). However, the literature has generally not distinguished between the symptoms of these reactions (Brier, 1999). Grief has been conceptualized as a normal adaptive response to loss, characterized by feelings of sadness, emptiness, angry protest and yearning, which will normally resolve without intervention over time. A pathological grief reaction occurs when symptoms remain intense for a prolonged period, indicating progression to major depression (Beutel et al., 1995). In an attempt to demonstrate empirically the differentiation of grief from depression, Beutel et al. (1995) hypothesized that two kinds of reactions to miscarriage can be distinguished. Grief reactions are preceded by joyful anticipation of motherhood and are of relatively short duration, while depressive reactions are more likely to occur in women with a previous history of depression and elevated distress in pregnancy, and with difficult personal relationships and poor social circumstances. In his study of 125 German women who had recently experienced a miscarriage, those who were categorized on the basis of standard measures to the "depressive reaction" group were twice as likely ($P \leq 0.001$) to have a prior history of depression than those in the "grief only" group, and to have significantly

fewer educational and social resources, more life stressors and greater ambivalence towards the fetus (Beutel et al., 1995).

Despite a lack of consensus regarding the nature and etiology of psychological reactions to miscarriage, there is a body of research describing the incidence and course of psychological symptomatology. Interpretation of these data is hampered by the variety of methodologies employed and of measures used to assess symptoms, but more recent work has generally used standard psychometric measures. In addition, a number of methodological limitations restrict the conclusions that may be drawn from the studies. For example, differences between study and control groups may confound results, and there is variation in the extent to which the study methodology itself may act as a therapeutic intervention. Further, the timing of psychological assessment after miscarriage varies. Meaningful comparisons between these studies are therefore limited (Slade, 1994; Neugebauer, 2003). There is also the question of the potential confounding effect, on the measurement of psychological sequelae of miscarriage, of the provision of psychological care, such as counselling, during or after treatment. It is therefore surprising that very few studies have reported details of any such care that may have been offered to study participants, or whether participants sought or received assistance from professional or lay support groups prior to psychological assessment.

A number of recent, methodologically rigorous studies, using both standardized psychometric measures and comparison groups, have consistently found significantly elevated rates of depressive symptoms in women following miscarriage, in comparison with women with uncomplicated pregnancy, or with women in the community who are not pregnant. Anxiety appears to be less well described than depression (Brier, 1999). Arguably the relevant comparison group is women with uncomplicated pregnancy rather than non-pregnant women; however, similar rates of depressive symptoms have been found in pregnant women and community samples of women of a similar age who are not pregnant (Llewellyn, Stowe & Nemeroff, 1997).

Significantly higher anxiety and depression scores were found in a group of women within 24 hours of surgical treatment for miscarriage compared with a control group of pregnant women;

the difference persisted for six weeks (Thapar & Thapar, 1992). However, the mean gestational age was higher in the pregnant group. Higher levels of psychological symptoms were associated with experience of previous miscarriage, childlessness and an unplanned pregnancy (Thapar & Thapar, 1992; Prettyman, Cordle & Cook, 1993). Symptoms of depression, but not anxiety, persisted for 12 months in a group of women who miscarried (Beutel et al., 1995). In a study conducted in the United States, minor depressive disorder, as assessed by the Diagnostic Interview Schedule (DIS) (Robins et al., 1981), was found in 5.2%, and major depressive disorder in 10.9%, of 229 women, 6 months after miscarriage. Onset of symptoms was within the first month after the loss in 72% of cases. This compared with rates of major and minor depressive disorder of 4.3% and 1%, respectively, in the community cohort (Neugebauer, 1997; Klier, Geller & Neugebauer, 2000). Major depressive disorder, assessed by the Structured Clinical Interview for DSM-III-R (Spitzer et al., 1992) was found in 12% of a group of 150 Chinese women in Hong Kong, China, six weeks after miscarriage (Lee et al., 1997a). Anecdotal reports suggest that a few women will experience miscarriage as a traumatizing event; some of these will meet the criteria for acute stress disorder or post-traumatic stress disorder (PTSD). A different model of care may be warranted for these women (Lee, 1996; Bowles et al., 2000).

A prospective longitudinal study, using a symptom self-reporting scale with 113 women in the Netherlands, found 25% prevalence of PTSD symptoms one month after miscarriage, declining to 7% at four months. In this sample, PTSD symptoms were associated with depression ($P<0.001$) (Engelhard et al., 2001).

Follow-up investigations after pregnancy loss have concluded that symptoms of anxiety and depression resolve spontaneously over time in most women; there is some evidence that anxiety symptoms are more variable and persistent (Prettyman, Cordle & Cook, 1993; Cecil & Leslie, 1993; Janssen et al., 1996). Some women have reported that continuing distress influences the decision to conceive again (Cordle & Prettyman, 1994), and that anxiety recurs in subsequent pregnancies (Statham & Green, 1994).

There is no consistent evidence of a relationship between sociodemographic factors including age, occupation and marital status, pregnancy factors such as gestation and whether the pregnancy was planned or wanted or reproductive history including prior abortion, miscarriage or infertility and the risk of post-miscarriage psychological distress (Lee & Slade, 1996). It has been argued that sociodemographic factors contribute little to the understanding of the meaning of miscarriage to an individual woman (Slade, 1994), and that a more fruitful approach may be to investigate the role of thoughts and cognitions, in particular understanding of the medical explanations of the cause of the miscarriage (Tunaley, Slade & Duncan, 1993). It has also been suggested that individual differences in attributional style – a construct measuring an individual's propensity to locate the cause of an adverse event either internally or with external factors over which he or she has less control – may be salient. Studies that have attempted to investigate the role of cognition in psychological adaptation to miscarriage have produced inconsistent findings (Tunaley, Slade & Duncan, 1993; Robinson et al., 1994). Nevertheless, post-treatment interventions aimed at reducing feelings of self-blame and enhancing self-esteem appear to show promise for improving psychological adaptation to miscarriage (Nikcevic, Kuczmierczyk & Nicolaides, 1998).

More recently, the impact of previous adverse life events on emotional adaptation to pregnancy loss has been investigated. A meticulously conducted study (Neugebauer et al., 1997) of 229 miscarrying women assessed the risk of a first or recurrent episode of major depressive disorder in the six months following loss, and compared it with the risk in a population-based cohort of 230 women drawn from the community. Major depressive disorder was assessed by the Diagnostic Interview Schedule (Robins et al., 1981). The six-month total incidence rates for the miscarrying and the community women were 10.9% and 4.3%, respectively (relative risk, 2.5; 95% confidence interval (CI), 1.2–5.1). The relative risk for depressive disorder in both groups did not differ between women with prior reproductive loss, between younger and older women, by marital status, educational level, or history of elective abortion (Neugebauer, Kline & O'Connor, 1992; Thapar & Thapar, 1992; Prettyman, Cordle & Cook, 1993). In the group of women who had miscarried, neither time of gestation, nor attitude towards the pregnancy, nor length of prior warning of the miscarriage influenced the risk of major depressive disorder. Among women in both groups, the risk of an episode of major depressive disorder was substantially higher among those with a history of major depressive disorder. This finding concurs with those from studies investigating mood disorders at other phases of reproductive life. In particular, in the postpartum period, a personal history of mood disorder or psychiatric diagnosis has been consistently associated with post-pregnancy depression (O'Hara & Swain, 1996; Scottish Intercollegiate Guidelines Network, 2002).

There has been limited discussion in the literature of the factors that contribute to variations in psychological vulnerability among women following miscarriage or perinatal death. However, in a large data-linkage study in the United States (Seng et al., 2001), women who had an ICD-9 code for post-traumatic stress disorder had an odds ratio of 1.9 (95% CI 1.3–2.9) for previous miscarriage, and an odds ratio of 7.4 (95% CI 2.7–20.2) for having been a victim of violence, compared with women without such a diagnosis. This raises the possibility of the causal misattribution of psychopathology to the miscarriage experience itself, when it might more accurately be described in some women as a re-arousal of prior trauma. The interaction between previous adverse life experiences, such as abuse and violence, and the experience of miscarriage warrants specific investigation.

Medical treatment of spontaneous pregnancy loss

Miscarriage, especially late miscarriage, may lead to haemorrhage and infection if pregnancy-related tissue is retained. Appropriate and timely treatment is necessary to effect complete removal of this tissue from the uterus in cases of incomplete miscarriage. Historically, surgical curettage – evacuation of the uterus under general anaesthetic – has been the treatment of choice for miscarriage. The procedure itself carries risks, including cervical trauma and subsequent cervical incompetence, uterine perforation, haemorrhage and intrauterine adhesions (Nanda et al., 2003). There is an international consensus that professional care is needed following miscarriage, but current treatments for miscarriage are not based on randomized controlled studies. The sequelae

of both unsafe induced abortions and surgical treatment of miscarriage consume substantial emergency gynaecological services, especially in developing countries (Hemminki, 1998).

Ultrasound examinations indicate that only a proportion of miscarriages are incomplete, and it is therefore probable that many women have undergone surgical treatment, with its attendant risks, unnecessarily. There is continuing debate about the necessity of routine surgical management (Ballagh, Harris & Demasio, 1998) and practice guidelines now urge conservative attitudes (Lagro-Janssen, 2005). The use of ultrasound could allow active treatment to be restricted to women with an incomplete miscarriage (Vazquez, Hickey & Neilson, 2002). A systematic review of the evidence on the effectiveness and safety of expectant management versus surgical treatment for early pregnancy loss is in preparation (Nanda et al., 2003). Medical treatments for incomplete miscarriage have been developed, and pharmacotherapies are now used with the aim of minimizing morbidity, mortality, and unnecessary surgical intervention (Ashok et al., 1998; Nielsen, Hahlin & Platz-Christensen, 1999; Chung et al., 1999).

> The miscarriage experience including its aftermath are almost universally experienced in the context of clinical care (Hemminki, 1998).

The miscarriage experience and its aftermath are almost universally experienced in the context of clinical care (Hemminki, 1998), and the quality of this care may influence women's emotional recovery. Relevant factors include whether the treatment is medical, surgical or expectant, the attitudes of health care staff, and the availability of counselling, support and other follow-up services. There is debate about the relative efficacy and efficiency of medical and surgical treatments for early miscarriage, and about whether active treatment is needed at all (Henshaw, 1993; Smith, 1993; Nanda et al., 2003). Medical management using a prostaglandin (misoprostol) to promote expulsion of the products of pregnancy is gaining acceptance (Lee et al., 2001). Any evaluation of different treatment regimens would need to investigate the psychological ramifications, which are likely to differ.

There are potential advantages to conservative or expectant management of miscarriage, not the least of which, for women with uncomplicated miscarriage, is the avoidance of hospital admission and separation from family (Smith, 1993). A randomized controlled trial, comparing expectant with medical management for first-trimester miscarriage, found that 76% of 62 women had a complete miscarriage without intervention, compared with 82% of 60 who were given a combination of antiprogesterone and prostaglandin E. Those receiving pharmacological treatment had a longer convalescence time, but there were no differences between the groups in level of pain, bleeding, post-miscarriage complications or satisfaction. Satisfaction was measured on a single, visual, analogue scale, but the fact that it was administered in the treatment setting 14 days after treatment may have limited critical or dissatisfied responses (Nielsen, Hahlin & Platz-Christensen, 1999). It has been argued that the psychological impact of medical management of miscarriage should not be underestimated. Pharmacological treatment may shorten the time to complete miscarriage, but women and health care staff may see the discharged pregnancy-related tissue and find the experience traumatic. Surgical intervention under general anaesthesia, although it carries its own risks, may therefore be the preferred treatment option for some women (Sharma, 1993).

A randomized controlled comparison of medical (misoprostol) versus surgical treatment for early miscarriage, conducted in Hong Kong, China, paid particular attention to psychological and culturally appropriate outcomes for women (Lee et al., 2001). There were no significant differences between the groups in psychological or social functioning, measured two weeks and six months after the procedure. However measures of client satisfaction, made with due care to limit under-reporting of dissatisfaction, showed that the 40% of women who required surgical treatment because of failure of medical treatment were, on several measures, less satisfied than both the surgical treatment group and the group for whom medical treatment was successful. Interestingly, this study investigated the ethnomedical dimension of the treatments for the participants. On measures of the degree to which treatments were seen as having devitalized and damaged the body, women's reports clearly favoured medical treatment. The authors argue that this finding has widespread application, because concern for devitalization of the body is shared by many other cultures. In addition,

misoprostol may prove especially useful in developing countries because it is cheap, stable at room temperature, and has few systemic effects (Vazquez, Hickey & Neilson, 2002) However, its efficacy will need to be improved if its apparent psychological benefits are not to be attenuated by its relatively high failure rate (Lee et al., 2001).

Research into the psychological consequences of miscarriage has been hampered by the problem of potential misattribution of adverse psychological and physical outcomes to the experience of miscarriage itself, rather than to the sequelae of surgical management. Research into the use of medical therapies in miscarriage may help to address this potential flaw.

There is evidence from Australia, the Netherlands, the United Kingdom and the United States that aspects of the primary and hospital care that women receive after miscarriage are consistently regarded by them as unhelpful in their recovery (Cuisinier et al., 1993; Cecil, 1994; Moohan, Ashe & Cecil, 1994; Speraw, 1994; Paton et al., 1999; Harvey, Moyle & Creedy, 2001), and may limit the capacity of primary health care providers to identify psychological morbidity (Wong et al., 2003). Brier (2005) recommends that practitioners should routinely screen for anxiety and depression after miscarriage. Women report insufficient recognition by staff of the magnitude of the experience, insufficient information about why their pregnancy miscarried and the implications for future pregnancies, and deficiencies in psychological or medical follow-up. It has been suggested that unhelpful and insensitive attitudes among staff may reflect their own emotional responses to pregnancy loss (Brier, 1999). When surveyed, 90% of care providers recognized that women were likely to experience emotional distress after miscarriage, which might be ameliorated by discussion of their feelings, but only 20% felt confident that they could do this for women in their care (Prettyman, Cordle & Cook, 1992). It would appear, therefore, that education and training of staff to provide psychologically informed care are needed.

In general, follow-up professional care after miscarriage is not provided, even though women commonly report a desire for it, attend when it is available, and report that it is helpful (Prettyman, Cordle & Cook, 1992; Lee & Slade, 1996; Turner, Flannelly & Wingfield, 1991; Nikcevic, Kuczmierczyk & Nicolaides, 1998). There have been few evaluations of post-treatment interventions, and little description of the form that such follow-up services might take. Given the theoretical conceptualization of miscarriage as significant loss, grief counselling may be appropriate. However, a randomized controlled test of a counselling intervention by nurses found no significant differences in overall mood disturbance one year after miscarriage (Swanson, 1999). The specific features of miscarriage suggest that a broader conceptualization of therapeutic approach is needed. In particular, a combination of explanation of the medical reasons for miscarriage and psychological support may ameliorate the guilt reactions commonly experienced after miscarriage (Nikcevic et al., 1999; Nikcevic, 2003). It is interesting to note, in this context, that two recent prospective longitudinal studies have found no association between miscarriage and psychosocial stress, depression, optimism, spouse abuse (measured by validated psychometric instruments) or biochemical markers of stress and anxiety (Milad et al., 1998; Nelson et al., 2003a; 2003b).

Lee & Slade (1996) proposed a form of post-miscarriage care that acknowledges that miscarriage can potentially precipitate trauma reactions, and that gives attention to post-miscarriage anxiety symptoms. Their proposed model of treatment includes psychological debriefing, a form of crisis intervention used with survivors of trauma (Lee, Slade & Lygo, 1996). This was tested in a small, controlled trial, in which 39 women were randomly assigned to either an hour-long psychological debriefing by a female psychologist in their own home approximately two weeks after the miscarriage, or routine care (no follow-up). The intervention was generally regarded as helpful, but assessments of all trial participants four months after miscarriage revealed no significant differences between the groups in standardized measures of psychological morbidity (Lee, Slade & Lygo, 1996). This is consistent with findings of other trials of psychological debriefing in the context of reproductive loss or trauma (Small et al., 2000; Priest et al., 2003). With the exception of anxiety, which remained above the norm, psychological distress diminished significantly in both groups over time (Lee, Slade & Lygo, 1996). The psychologist who conducted the debriefing in this trial was unable to provide medical information about the possible causes of the miscarriage or about the implications for future reproductive decision-making. It may also be

that the completion of questionnaires as part of the study may itself have had a therapeutic effect, even for women in the control group (Athey & Spielvogel, 2000). The authors suggest that possible adverse effects in some women may have cancelled out beneficial effects, but do not present data to support or refute this interpretation. They further suggest screening using the 30-item General Health Questionnaire, to detect individuals who may benefit from additional psychological assistance (Lee, 1997b). However, such screening does not distinguish women for whom psychological debriefing may be helpful from those for whom it is not, or for whom it could be harmful.

Women's responses to miscarriage are likely to be mediated by the reactions of others, including family members and the broader society in which they live. The extent to which the psychological reactions of the partners of women experiencing miscarriage may limit their capacity to provide emotional support remains under-explored. Men appear to grieve the loss of a pregnancy (Conway & Russell, 2000), but their grief may be less intense and of shorter duration than that of women (Stinson et al., 1992). A small qualitative study revealed that men may experience confusion about how to behave socially, or how to provide appropriate emotional support to their partners, in the presence of their own feelings of loss after miscarriage (Puddifoot & Johnson, 1997). Women who were still depressed six months after spontaneous pregnancy loss were significantly more likely than those who were not depressed to have partners who avoided talking about the loss and who were less supportive (Beutel et al., 1996). In common with other forms of bereavement, support from broader social networks, including local health services, may assist in the adaptation to pregnancy loss (Rajan & Oakley, 1993; Rajan, 1994). In practice, it is unlikely that a single approach to the psychological care of women after spontaneous pregnancy loss will be effective in all settings and for all cultural groups.

There is general agreement in the literature that many women experience miscarriage as highly distressing, and that rates of subsequent psychopathology, including depression and anxiety, are elevated in comparison with community samples. Medical services are routinely involved in preventing the potential complications of miscarriage through active treatment, but are not perceived to provide psychological support at the time of treatment or at follow-up. The particular factors that predispose some women to more intense psychological reactions have not yet been clearly identified, but vulnerability generated by earlier adverse events appears salient and warrants additional investigation. Although psychological reactions to miscarriage resolve spontaneously in most women, there appears to be a role for psychological intervention, immediately after treatment or in the long term. It is not clear whether some or all women would benefit from this type of intervention, or what form it should take, and there has been no evaluation of existing services. However, it is acknowledged that women who use health services after losing a pregnancy may benefit from a more psychologically informed model of care than currently exists in most settings.

Summary

Future research

1. There is a need for research on the impact of prior adverse life experiences, such as abuse and violence, on a woman's predisposition to psychological morbidity after miscarriage, as well as on the form of care that is appropriate for this group.

2. More attention needs to be given to the psychological component of medical care after miscarriage; there is little agreement in the literature about the form that psychological interventions should take, or which would be of most benefit to women.

Policy

Even though it is common, miscarriage should not be regarded as a routine event in women's lives; policies for the assessment and short- and long-term psychological care of women who have experienced miscarriage should be developed.

Services

Health services should ensure that staff are attuned to women's psychological needs following miscarriage, and are trained to respond with empathy and sensitivity.

References

Ashok P et al. (1998) An effective regimen for early medical abortion: a report of 2000 consecutive cases. *Human Reproduction*, 13: 2962-2965.

Asowa-Omorodion FI (1997) Women's perceptions of the complications of pregnancy and childbirth in two Esan communities, Edo State, Nigeria. *Social Science and Medicine*, 44(12): 1817-1824.

Athey J, Spielvogel AM (2000) Risk factors and interventions for psychological sequelae in women after miscarriage. *Primary Care Update: Obstetrics and Gynaecology*, 7(2): 64-69.

Ballagh S, Harris H, Demasio K (1998) Is curettage needed for uncomplicated incomplete spontaneous abortion? *American Journal of Obstetrics and Gynecology*, 179(5): 1279-1282.

Beutel M et al. (1995) Grief and depression after miscarriage: their separation, antecedents, and course. *Psychosomatic Medicine*, 57(6): 517-526.

Beutel M et al. (1996) Similarities and differences in couples' grief reactions following a miscarriage: results from a longitudinal study. *Journal of Psychosomatic Research*, 40(3): 245-253.

Bowles SV et al (2000) Acute and post-traumatic stress disorder after spontaneous abortion. *American Family Physician*, 61(6): 1689-1696.

Brier N (1999) Understanding and managing the emotional reactions to a miscarriage. *Obstetrics and Gynaecology*, 93(1): 151-155.

Brier N (2005) Anxiety after miscarriage: a review of the empirical literature and implications for clinical practice. *Birth*, 31(2): 138-142.

Cecil R (1994) Miscarriage: women's views of care. *Journal of Reproductive and Infant Psychology*, 12: 21-29.

Cecil R, Leslie JC (1993) Early miscarriage: preliminary results form a study in Northern Ireland. *Journal of Reproductive and Infant Psychology*, 11: 89-95.

Chung T et al. (1999) Spontaneous abortion: a randomized controlled trial comparing surgical evacuation with conservative management using misoprostol. *Fertility and Sterility*, 71(6): 1054-1059.

Condon JT (1993) The assessment of antenatal emotional attachment; development of a questionnaire instrument. *British Journal of Medical Psychology*. 66: 167-183.

Conway K, Russell G (2000) Couples' grief and experience of support in the aftermath of miscarriage. *British Journal of Medical Psychology*, 73: 531-545.

Cordle C, Prettyman R (1994) A 2-year follow-up of women who have experienced early miscarriage. *Journal of Reproductive and Infant Psychology*, 12: 37-43.

Cuisinier MC et al. (1993) Miscarriage and stillbirth: time since the loss, grief intensity and satisfaction with care. *European Journal of Obstetrics, Gynaecology and Reproductive Biology*, 52(3): 163-168.

Engelhard I et al. (2001) Post-traumatic stress disorder after pregnancy loss. *General Hospital Psychiatry*, 23: 62-66.

Frost M, Condon JT (1996) The psychological sequelae of miscarriage: a critical review of the literature. *Australian and New Zealand Journal of Psychiatry*, 30: 54-62.

Garel M et al. (1994) Long-term consequences of miscarriage: the depressive disorders and the following pregnancy. *Journal of Reproductive and Infant Psychology*, 12: 233-240.

Geller PA et al. (2001) Anxiety disorders following miscarriage. *Journal of Clinical Psychiatry*, 62(6): 432-438.

Harvey J, Moyle W, Creedy D (2001) Women's experience of early miscarriage: a phenomenological study. *Australian Journal of Advanced Nursing*, 19(1): 8-14.

Hemminki E (1998) Treatment of miscarriage: current practice and rationale. *Obstetrics and Gynecology*, 91(2): 247-253.

Henshaw R et al. (1993) Medical management of miscarriage: non-surgical uterine evacuation of incomplete and inevitable spontaneous abortion. *British Medical Journal*, 306: 894-895.

Janssen HJEM et al. (1996) Controlled prospective study on the mental health of women following pregnancy loss. *American Journal of Psychiatry*, 153(2): 226-230.

Jordan B (1993) *Birth in four cultures. A crosscultural investigation of childbirth in Yucatan, Holland, Sweden, and the United States. Revised and expanded by Robbie Davis-Floyd.* Illinois, Waveland Press.

Klier CM, Geller PA, Neugebauer R (2000) Minor depressive disorder in the context of miscarriage. *Journal of Affective Disorders*, 59: 13-21.

Lagro-Janssen AL (2005) The practice guideline 'Miscarriage' (second revision) from the Dutch College of General Practitioners; a response from the perspective of general practice. *Nederlands Tijdschrift voor Geneeskunde,* 149(6): 278-280.

Layne L (1990) Motherhood lost: cultural dimensions of miscarriage and still birth in America. *Women and Health,* 16: 69-98.

Layne L (1997) Breaking the silence: an agenda for a feminist discourse of pregnancy loss. *Feminist Studies,* 23(2): 289-315.

Layne L (2003) Unhappy endings: a feminist reappraisal of the women's health movement from the vantage of pregnancy loss. *Social Science and Medicine,* 56: 1881-1891.

Lee C, Slade P (1996) Miscarriage as a traumatic event: a review of the literature and new implications for intervention. *Journal of Psychosomatic Research,* 40: 235-244.

Lee C, Slade P, Lygo V (1996) The influence of psychological debriefing on emotional adaptation in women following early miscarriage: a preliminary study. *British Journal of Medical Psychology,* 69(1): 47-58.

Lee D et al. (1997a) Psychiatric morbidity following miscarriage: a prevalence study of Chinese women in Hong Kong. *Journal of Affective Disorders,* 43: 63-68.

Lee DT et al. (1997b) Screening psychiatric morbidity after miscarriage: application of the 30-item General Health Questionnaire and the Edinburgh Postnatal Depression Scale. *Psychosomatic Medicine,* 59(2): 207-210.

Lee DTS et al. (2001) A comparison of the psychological impact and client satisfaction of surgical treatment with medical treatment of spontaneous abortion: A randomized controlled trial. *American Journal of Obstetrics and Gynecology,* 185(4): 953-958.

Llewellyn AM, Stowe ZM, Nemeroff CB (1997) Depression during pregnancy and the puerperium. *Journal of Clinical Psychiatry,* 58(15): 26-32.

Lumley J (1980) The image of the fetus in the first trimester. *Birth and the Family Journal,* 7: 5.

Madden ME (1994) The variety of emotional reactions to miscarriage. *Women and Health,* 21(2/3): 85-104.

Maker C, Ogden J (2003) The miscarriage experience: more than just a trigger to psychological morbidity? *Psychology and Health,* 18(3): 403-415.

March K (2001) Childbirth with fear. In: Chase S, Rogers M, eds., *Mothers and children: feminist analyses and personal narratives.* New Brunswick, NJ, Rutgers University Press: 168-173.

Milad MP et al. (1998) Stress and anxiety do not result in pregnancy wastage. *Human Reproduction,* 13: 2296-3200.

Mishell D (1993) Recurrent abortion. *Journal of Reproductive Medicine,* 38(4): 250-259.

Moohan J, Ashe R, Cecil R (1994) The management of miscarriage: results from a survey at one hospital. *Journal of Reproductive and Infant Psychology,* 12: 17-19.

Moulder C (1994) Towards a preliminary framework for understanding pregnancy loss. *Journal of Reproductive and Infant Psychology,* 12: 65-67.

Nanda L et al. (2003) Expectant care versus surgical treatment for miscarriage (Protocol for a Cochrane Review). In: *The Cochrane Library,* Issue 3, Oxford Update Software.

Nelson D et al. (2003) Does stress influence early pregnancy loss? *Annals of Epidemiology,* 13: 223-229.

Nelson D et al. (2003) The effect of depressive symptoms and optimism on the risk of spontaneous abortion among inner city women. *Journal of Women's Health,* 12(6): 569-576.

Neugebauer R (2003) Depressive symptoms at two months after miscarriage: interpreting study findings from an epidemiological versus clinical perspective. *Depression and Anxiety,* 17: 152-161.

Neugebauer R, Kline J, O'Connor P (1992) Determinants of depressive symptoms in the early weeks after miscarriage. *American Journal of Public Health,* 82: 1332-1339.

Neugebauer R et al. (1997) Major depressive disorder in the 6 months after miscarriage. *Journal of the American Medical Association,* 277(5): 383-388.

Nielsen S, Hahlin M, Platz-Christensen J (1999) Randomised trial comparing expectant with medical management for first trimester miscarriages. *British Journal of Obstetrics and Gynaecology,* 106: 804-807.

Nikcevic A (2003) Development and evaluation of a miscarriage follow-up clinic. *Journal of Reproductive and Infant Psychology,* 21(3): 207-217.

Nikcevic AV, Kuczmierczyk AR, Nicolaides KH (1998) Personal coping resources, responsibility, anxiety and depression after early pregnancy loss. *Journal of Psychosomatic Obstetrics and Gynaecology,* 19(3): 145-154.

Nikcevic AV, Tunkel SA, Nicolaides KH (1998) Psychological outcomes following missed abortions and provision of follow-up care. *Ultrasound in Obstetrics and Gynaecology,* 11: 123-128.

Nikcevic AV et al. (1999) Investigation of the cause of miscarriage and its influence on women's psychological distress. *British Journal of Obstetrics and Gynaecology,* 106(8): 808-813.

O'Hara MW, Swain AM (1996) Rates and risk of postnatal depression - a meta-analysis. *International Journal of Psychiatry,* 8: 37-54.

Paton F et al. (1999) Grief in miscarriage patients and satisfaction with care in a London hospital. *Journal of Reproductive and Infant Psychology,* 17(3): 301-315.

Prettyman RJ, Cordle CJ (1992) Psychological aspects of miscarriage: attitudes of the primary health care team. *British Journal of General Practice,* 42(356): 97-99.

Prettyman RJ, Cordle CJ, Cook GD (1993) A three-month follow-up of psychological morbidity after early miscarriage. *British Journal of Medical Psychology,* 66(4): 363-372.

Priest S et al. (2003) Stress debriefing after childbirth: a randomised controlled trial. *Medical Journal of Australia,* 178(2 June): 542-545.

Puddifoot J, Johnson M (1997) The legitimacy of grieving: the partner's experience at miscarriage. *Social Science and Medicine,* 45(6): 837-845.

Rajan L (1994) Social isolation and support in pregnancy loss. *Health Visitor,* 67(3): 97-101.

Rajan L, Oakley A (1993) No pills for heartache: the importance of social support for women who suffer pregnancy loss. *Journal of Reproductive and Infant Psychology,* 11: 75-87.

Rice PL (1999) When the baby falls!: The cultural construction of miscarriage among Hmong women in Australia. *Women and Health,* 30(1): 85-103.

Ritsher J, Neugebauer R (2002) Perinatal bereavement grief scale. Distinguishing grief from depression following miscarriage. *Assessment,* 9(1): 31-40.

Robins L et al. (1981) National Institute of Mental Health Diagnostic Interview Schedule: its history, characteristics and validity. *Archives of General Psychiatry,* 38: 381-389.

Robinson GE et al. (1994) Psychological reactions in women followed for 1 year after miscarriage. *Journal of Reproductive and Infant Psychology,* 12: 31-36.

Scottish Intercollegiate Guidelines Network (2002) *Postnatal depression and puerperal psychosis. A national clinical guideline.* Edinburgh, Royal College of Physicians.

Seng JS et al. (2001) Posttraumatic stress disorder and pregnancy complications. *Obstetrics and Gynaecology,* 97(1): 17-22.

Sharma J (1993) Medical management of miscarriage. *British Medical Journal,* 306: 1540.

Slade P (1994) Predicting the psychological impact of miscarriage. *Journal of Reproductive and Infant Psychology,* 12: 5-16.

Slade P, Cecil R (1994) Understanding the experience and emotional consequences of miscarriage - editorial. *Journal of Reproductive and Infant Psychology,* 12: 1-3.

Small R et al. (2000) Randomised controlled trial of midwife led debriefing to reduce maternal depression after operative childbirth. *British Medical Journal,* 321(7268): 1043-1047.

Smith LF (1993) Should we intervene in uncomplicated miscarriage? *British Medical Journal,* 306(5 June): 1540-1541.

Speraw SR (1994) The experience of miscarriage: how couples define quality in health care delivery. *Journal of Perinatology,* 14(3): 208-215.

Spitzer RL et al. (1992). The Structured Clinical Interview for DSM-III-R (SCID): I. History, rationale, and description. *Archives of General Psychiatry,* 49: 624-629.

Statham H, Green J (1994) The effects of miscarriage and other "unsuccessful" pregnancies on feelings early in a subsequent pregnancy. *Journal of Reproductive and Infant Psychology,* 12: 45-54.

Stinson K et al. (1992) Parents' grief following pregnancy loss: a comparison of mothers and fathers. *Family Relations,* 41: 218-223.

Stirtzinger RM et al. (1999) Parameters of grieving in spontaneous abortion. *International Journal of Psychiatry and Medicine,* 29(2): 235-249.

Swanson KM (1999) Effects of caring, measurement, and time on miscarriage impact and women's well-being. *Nursing Research*, 48(6): 288-298.

Thapar AK, Thapar A (1992) Psychological sequelae of miscarriage: a controlled study using the general health questionnaire and the hospital anxiety and depression scale. *British Journal of General Practice*, 42(356): 94-96.

Tunaley J, Slade P, Duncan S (1993) Cognitive processes in psychological adaptation to miscarriage: a preliminary report. *Psychology and Health*, 8: 369-381.

Turner M, Flannelly G, Wingfield M (1991) The miscarriage clinic: an audit of the first year. *British Journal of Obstetrics and Gynaecology*, 98: 306-308.

Vazquez JC, Hickey M, Neilson JP (2002) Medical management for miscarriage (Protocol for a Cochrane Review). In: *The Cochrane Library*, Issue 4. Oxford, Update Software.

Wong MKY et al. (2003) A qualitative investigation into women's experiences after a miscarriage: implications for the primary healthcare team. *British Journal of General Practice*, 53: 697-702.

Chapter

5

Menopause

Jill Astbury

Between 1980 and 1998, global average life expectancy increased from 61 to 67 years. The increase, however, was not evenly distributed. For example, high rates of human immunodeficiency virus (HIV) infection in sub-Saharan Africa caused life expectancy to fall to 47 years on average; life expectancy has fallen in 34 countries since 1990 (UNDP, 2003).

In high-income countries, women outlive men by 5–8 years. However, in low-income countries, the differential is reduced to 0–3 years (World Bank, 2006), and in three countries – Nepal, Pakistan and Zimbabwe – women's life expectancy is lower than men's (UNDP, 2003).

In six African countries, women's life expectancy is less than 40 years. These are Malawi (39.1 years), Rwanda (38.7 years), Sierra Leone (35.8 years), Swaziland (39.9 years), Zambia (33.4 years) and Zimbabwe (35.4 years). In high-income developed countries, women's average life expectancy is more than 80 years. These countries include Australia (81.9 years), France (82.6 years), Japan (84.7 years), Spain (82.6 years), Sweden (82.4 years) and Switzerland (82.2 years).

As life expectancy increases, more women are living to the age of menopause and beyond. Even in countries with low average life expectancy, such as those in sub-Saharan Africa, the majority of women not infected by HIV live to menopause and beyond. The marked differences in life expectancy underline the fact that the priority of menopause and its mental health dimensions, as a reproductive health problem, will vary considerably between countries.

Mental health and the perimenopausal period

Menopause is defined retrospectively as the end of menstruation. During the perimenopausal period, women gradually stop menstruating and become unable to conceive and bear children without assisted reproductive technology. In high-income countries, the average age at menopause is around 50 years for nonsmokers. Women who smoke tend to reach menopause approximately 18 months earlier. A low socioeconomic position over the lifetime is also associated with an earlier age at menopause (McKinlay, Brambilla & Posner, 1992; Luoto, Kaprio & Uutela, 1994; Shinberg, 1998; Wise et al., 2002). In low-income countries, an overall earlier age at menopause has been reported. Menopause is earliest among women who have suffered from malnutrition (Khaw, 1992; Leidy, 1994).

Menopause is characterized by simultaneous physical, hormonal, and psychosocial changes. Physically, health status may decline and chronic diseases associated with ageing may appear for the first time. Hormonally, the perimenopausal transition is characterized by declining ovarian follicular activity and hormonal fluctuations that result in vasomotor instability. Symptoms include hot flushes, vaginal dryness and sleep problems.

Dominant views on fertility, ageing and female roles help shape women's expectations of and attitudes towards menopause, and influence the social status accorded to women in midlife. These views inform women's expectations and subjective experiences, and the meanings they attach to menopause (Lock, 1994; McMaster, Pitts &

Poyah, 1997; Boulet et al., 1994). Cultural conceptions of menopause can vary, from its being perceived as a normal and unproblematic part of human development and the female life course to its being seen as a hormone-deficiency disease that gives rise to severe, disabling physical and psychological symptoms requiring medical treatment and surveillance.

A comprehensive review of cross-cultural and comparative research concluded that the majority of women do not find menopause a difficult experience (Lock, 2002). Similar findings on women's attitudes towards natural menopause have been reported in the USA (Avis & McKinlay, 1995). In the longitudinal Massachusetts Women's Health study, the majority of participants did not seek medical help for menopause, and held primarily positive or neutral attitudes towards it (Avis & McKinlay, 1995). Again, few women in the Seattle Midlife Women's Health Survey (Woods & Mitchell, 1997) defined menopause as a time when increased symptoms, disease risk or medical care should be expected. Most women viewed menopause as a normal developmental process.

The prevalence of menopausal symptoms varies considerably, even within countries. For example, Bosworth et al. (2001), in a study of perimenopausal American women (aged 45–54 years) in North Carolina, found high rates of hot flushes (65%), night sweats (56%), difficulty sleeping (45%), mood swings (49%) and memory problems (44%). Conversely, Woods & Mitchell (1997) reported much lower rates of symptoms for women participating in the Seattle Midlife Women's Health Study. In this study only 17% reported hot flushes and night sweats. In contrast, a longitudinal study of Australian women reported an increase in vasomotor symptoms, such as hot flushes, night sweats, breast tenderness and vaginal dryness over the perimenopausal transition (Dennerstein et al., 2000).

Cross-cultural studies have found significant variations between women in different countries in the level and type of menopausal symptoms experienced and the degree of physical and psychological distress associated with them (Punyahotra & Dennerstein, 1997; Fu, Anderson & Courtney, 2003). Women in Japan (Lock, 1994) and other Asian countries, including China (Hong Kong SAR, and Province of Taiwan), Indonesia, Republic of Korea, Malaysia,

the Philippines, and Singapore, tend to report fewer menopausal symptoms than those in the United States (Boulet et al., 1994). Lock (2002) cautions against dismissing reports of fewer symptoms in these societies simply as learned cultural expectations.

Psychosocially, the perimenopausal transition takes place in a context that may be marked by significant life changes and upheavals. Family composition may change through death or divorce, children may leave or return home, and parents may become more dependent. In addition, work status and level of participation in paid work may decline.

While there is a large literature on hormonal treatments for menopause and the effect of such treatments on breast cancer, heart disease, osteoporosis, dementia and depression, this research is not the focus of the current review. First, results from the Women's Health Initiative, the world's largest randomized controlled trial involving more than 16 000 women in the USA, indicated that the combination of estrogen and progestogen, given for treatment of menopause, was associated with significant health risks. This study, begun in 1997, was initially intended to be completed in 2005, but was terminated three years early, because analysis revealed significantly increased health risks. These included increased risks of breast cancer (Chlebowski et al., 2003), heart disease (Pradhan et al., 2002), stroke (Wassertheil-Smoller et al., 2003) and poor cognitive functioning (Rapp et al., 2003). Second, menopause research has been criticized for being carried out primarily in middle- and high-income countries on samples of middle class white women (Standing & Glazer, 1992). Treating menopause in low-income countries carries a high cost and has low public health relevance. Where there are high rates of HIV infection, high maternal mortality rates and low life expectancy for women, other reproductive and mental health issues are of more concern, and require more urgent attention, than treatments for menopause.

This chapter focuses on the relationship between menopause and psychological distress in midlife. It will consider the factors that have been identified as playing a significant role in women's emotional health and well-being at this time, especially those associated with increased rates of depression. The relative contributions of physical, hormonal and psychosocial changes to depression have received considerable attention from researchers, and evidence on the relationships will be reviewed. Most research has been carried out in high-income countries and the validity of these findings for women in resource-poor settings is largely unknown. Caution in extrapolating findings from high-income countries is especially warranted with regard to studies from the USA, where rates of gynaecological surgery (hysterectomy) and hormone replacement therapy are high, and hence natural menopause is by no means a universal experience.

Menopause: a time of increased risk for poor mental health?

Evidence from national surveys permits comparison of population-based rates of depression over the lifespan. Throughout their reproductive years, women experience significantly higher rates of depression than men, with female:male ratios approximately 2:1 (Astbury & Cabral de Mello, 2000). This difference first emerges in puberty (Wade, Cairney & Pevalin, 2002; Kessler, 2003) and declines from midlife onwards, although evidence on the age when the sex difference ceases to be important varies from one study and one country to another. For Australian women aged between 45 and 54 years, the rate of depression was 7%, considerably lower than that for women aged 18–24 years (11%) (Andrews et al., 1999). Two national surveys in the USA have indicated a U-shaped relationship between age and depression, with the lowest rates occurring in the age group 45–49 years (Kessler et al., 1992). The United Kingdom National Survey of Psychiatric Morbidity found that the sex difference in the prevalence of depression disappeared after the age of 55 years (Bebbington et al., 2003).

Despite the fact that the gender difference in depression is most marked during the reproductive years, experiences related to changes in sex hormones, such as pregnancy, the use of oral contraceptives, hormone replacement therapy and menopause, do not appear to account for this difference (Stephens & Ross, 2002; Kessler, 2003). Large-scale epidemiological surveys of mental health have found no substantial increase in rates of depression among women in midlife. Yet researchers remain interested in identifying the factors that distinguish between women who do

and do not experience depression at this time. These include the role of hormonal changes, menopausal status and menopausal symptoms, such as hot flushes and disturbed sleep, psychosocial, socioeconomic and physical health factors, and a history of depression (Bosworth et al., 2001).

In order to investigate whether menopause has a direct or an indirect effect on depression, it is necessary to clarify through prospective, longitudinal research whether depression is a cause or consequence of high levels of symptoms, including hot flushes, insomnia and vaginal dryness. Over the past decade or so, an increasing number of such studies have been carried out in high-income countries, including Australia, Canada, the United Kingdom, and the United States (Woods & Mitchell, 1997; Avis et al., 2001; Glazer et al., 2002; Kaufert, Gilbert & Tate, 1992; Kuh, Wadsworth & Hardy, 1997; Dennerstein, Lehert & Guthrie, 2002). Most longitudinal studies have used multidimensional models to investigate why some, but not all, women experience depression during the menopausal transition. These have been designed to assess the contributions of sociocultural factors, attitudes towards and expectations of menopause, health status and health behaviours, and history of depression, as well as the impact of age, menopausal status, and symptoms.

> Do women with negative expectations of menopause have more frequent symptoms and rate these symptoms more negatively than women who hold positive expectations and in turn do such women have more negative experiences of menopause and higher rates of depression?

A stress model of depression is congruent with a multidimensional approach to understanding the pathways to depression in midlife (Woods & Mitchell, 1997). Stress, as a highly important mediating factor linked to depression, may arise from a number of different sources: from the menopausal transition itself, because of changes in menstrual patterns and the appearance and persistence of vasomotor symptoms; from the woman's life context, which can have a direct impact on mood but is also influenced by negative socialization experiences and attitudes to menopause and poor health; and from acute or

Three main hypotheses have been proposed regarding the relationship between menopause and depression for women in midlife:

Hypothesis 1. Direct effect

There is a close relationship between hormones and mood, and menopausal change in hormonal status will have direct effects on depression. The specific questions arising from this view include whether lower estrogen levels are associated with increased rates of depression and whether decreases in estrogen bring about neurochemical changes that lead to depression.

Hypothesis 2. Indirect effect

Depression is a consequence of menopausal symptoms (the "domino" hypothesis). The main question related to this hypothesis is whether high rates of menopausal symptoms predict increased depression and reduced emotional well-being.

Hypothesis 3. No effect

Menopause and its associated hormonal changes are largely irrelevant in explaining depression among women in midlife. Depression during menopause can be primarily accounted for by the classical determinants of depression over the life course, and menopausal status and symptoms make no meaningful additional contribution. Implicit in this view is a criticism of other research on menopause that does not include all the previously identified predictors of depression.

The central question is: to what extent do classical determinants of depression, such as low socio-economic status, lack of social support and a confiding relationship with a partner, unemployment, previous history of depression, negative life events and high levels of past or current stress account for depression in midlife?

chronic health conditions and thus the physical and psychological health status and history.

Using this multidimensional framework, researchers have investigated the different contributions of various stressors to depression and troublesome menopausal symptoms. The stressors have included menopausal status, age, life context factors such as psychosocial adversity, negative life events, negative socialization and attitudes towards menopause, as well as general physical health status and health behaviours.

Overall, there is little evidence that menopausal or hormonal status exerts a strong or direct effect on depression. Rather, the evidence supports a "domino" hypothesis that an increased level of distressing symptoms is a cause of depression. Avis et al. (2001), in a longitudinal study, found that depression was positively associated with

symptoms such as hot flushes, night sweats and difficulty sleeping, but not with menopausal status or change in estradiol levels. Estradiol had no direct effect on depression independent of symptoms. Glazer et al. (2002), in the longitudinal Ohio Midlife Women's Study, also found that menopausal status did not significantly predict depression in midlife. Loss of resources and low level of education – both classical determinants of depression – were, however, strongly predictive of depression in this cohort. Anxiety was also predicted by loss of resources but the effectiveness of women's coping strategies and education were important too. The researchers concluded that stress, as indicated by loss of resources, was a better predictor of poor health outcomes than menopausal status.

Bosworth et al. (2001) conducted a cross-sectional study of a random sample of women aged

45–54 years residing in Durham County, North Carolina. Variables included depression (measured by the abbreviated Centre for Epidemiologic Studies –Depression Scale (CES-D), perceived menopausal stage, climacteric symptoms, health behaviour and markers of socioeconomic status. Overall 164 women (28%) were using hormone replacement therapy (HRT), and 236 (41%) reported ever using HRT. Almost one-third (29%) of women in the sample had CES-D scores indicating significant depressive symptoms, but there was no significant difference in menopausal status between depressed and non-depressed women. Depressed women had higher rates of night sweats, hot flushes, insomnia, memory loss/forgetfulness and mood swings. Maartens, Knottnerus & Pop (2002) found that stage of menopausal transition in Dutch women was significantly and independently related to depression, after other risk factors were taken into account. Rates of depression, as measured by the Edinburgh Depression Scale, significantly increased from pre- to perimenopause, and again from peri- to postmenopause. However, other risk factors significantly associated with depression in this study included unemployment, inability to work, financial problems, death of a partner or child, and a previous episode of depression, all of which had higher odds ratios than any stage of the menopausal transition. Two of these – unemployment and the death of a child – conferred particularly high risks of depression in midlife. On the other hand, Dennerstein, Lehert & Guthrie (2002) found that menopausal symptoms exerted no demonstrable effect on women's well-being over time; rather, there was an improvement in well-being from early to late phases of the menopausal transition. Psychosocial variables were most significant in determining this, particularly when a woman formed a new marriage or partnership and experienced increased satisfaction in work.

In population-based longitudinal studies in Massachussetts, USA (Avis et al., 1994) and Manitoba, Canada (Kaufert, Gilbert & Tate, 1992), stressful life events and circumstances were found to be strongly associated with depression persisting or occurring for the first time in midlife. Sources of stress included marital and relationship problems, difficulties with children, and demands from friends and family. Similarly, Woods & Mitchell (1997) reported that a stressful life context and poor health status had significant direct effects on depressed mood. Stressful life context was significantly associated with having more severe vasomotor symptoms. Women who experienced more menopausal changes tended to have more negative expectations for midlife and poorer health status.

The major explanatory role assigned to attitudes and expectations of menopause in the development of depression presupposes that the majority of women formed these attitudes earlier in life. Avis & McKinlay (1991), in a longitudinal study, found that negative attitudes towards menopause predicted both subsequent symptom reporting during menopause and depression. However, in an interview-based study of more than 500 premenopausal women with a median age of 41 years, participating in the Seattle Midlife Women's Health Study, Woods & Mitchell (1997) found that most were uncertain about their expectations of their own menopause.

Another possible risk factor for depression during menopause is sexual functioning and changes in the frequency of sex or in the level of sexual pleasure and satisfaction. Some studies have reported a decrease in sexual functioning with age, which becomes more marked in midlife (Palacios et al., 1995; Avis, 2000; Dennerstein, Dudley & Burger, 2001). An obvious difficulty for research in this area is separating the effect of increasing age from menopausal status. One longitudinal Swedish study disentangled the effects of these two factors and reported that menopausal status, rather than age, was the important factor for explaining decreased sexual functioning (Hallstrom & Samuelsson, 1990). In addition to age and menopausal status, risk factors for decreased sexual desire included lack of a sexual partner, a poor, non-confiding relationship with the sexual partner, insufficient support, alcohol dependence and the partner's own sexual difficulties. Stressors, employment, negative attitudes towards menopause, previous level of sexual functioning, and poor physical or psychological health also contribute to decreased sexual desire and functioning in midlife (Hallstrom & Samuelsson, 1990; Avis, 2000; Dennerstein, Dudley & Burger, 2001). These factors are also predictive of depression. Difficulties or dissatisfaction with sexual functioning can add to stress during the menopausal transition.

Well-being in midlife and the importance of the life course

In addition to investigating the predictors of depression in midlife, a number of researchers have sought to identify and understand the determinants of positive health and general well-being during this period. Dennerstein, Dudley & Guthrie (2003) noted a small decline in self-rated health with increasing age, but this was not attributable to the effect of the menopausal transition. A decline in self-rated health eight years after enrolment, among women who had initially rated their health as better than average, was associated with only two variables following multivariate analysis: a change in weight and a change in libido and feelings for the partner. Women who reported a decline in self-rated health and were in paid employment were significantly more likely than other women to have had an operation or procedure in the previous year. Kuh, Wadsworth & Hardy (1997) also found that women who were obese had the highest rates of psychological symptoms, while women who were of normal weight had lower levels of self-reported symptoms than women who were under- or overweight.

As these studies illustrate, factors preceding menopause can exert a strong influence on the likelihood of poor mental health at the time of menopause. In general, longitudinal studies of menopause recruit women who are approaching or are already experiencing the perimenopausal transition. This means that potentially important risk factors for depression that have occurred earlier in the life course can only be assessed retrospectively and are therefore susceptible to recall bias. A notable exception is the study by Kuh, Wadsworth & Hardy (1997), who investigated the links between earlier experiences (in childhood, adolescence or earlier adult life) and mental health in midlife. Participants in this research were part of the larger Medical Research Council National Survey of Health and Development (MRCNSHD), a prospective cohort study of a representative sample of the British population born in 1946 and assessed repeatedly over subsequent decades. Data on midlife were collected over a 6-year period when participants were aged between 47 and 52 years. Data were collected on anxiety, depression, irritability, tearfulness and feelings of panic. From these data, researchers calculated an overall psychological score (range 0–12). Risk factors were grouped in six clusters: family background, characteristics of the child, adult health, adult socioeconomic circumstances, social support, lifestyle and current life stress. Pathways through which risk factors determined psychological distress in midlife included cumulative losses, social adversity, and negative events and experiences over the course of the women's lives. The importance of negative life events, such as adverse changes in family and work life, for mental health was confirmed in this study. No variation was found in psychological symptoms in midlife according to menopausal stage, in keeping with the results of most other studies.

Following multivariate analysis, three significant associations remained between family background variables and symptoms of psychological distress. Women who were psychologically distressed were more likely to have lived in council housing, had parents who divorced, and had mothers who had high scores on a measure of neuroticism. Certain characteristics of the women during childhood and adolescence were significantly associated with adult psychological symptom scores. These included level of neuroticism and antisocial behaviour in adolescence. Women with higher psychological symptom scores in midlife were significantly more likely to have had health problems earlier in adult life. Of particular note were psychological illness between 15 and 32 years, anxiety and depression at 36 years, reported health problems at 36 years and physical disability at 43 years. This study, like many others, found significant relationships between adult circumstances, social relationships, health behaviour and current life stress and high psychological symptom scores.

A significant inverse relationship was found between social class, educational qualifications and psychological symptoms. Women living in households where the income was earned by manual labour, or who were themselves on a low income, had higher symptom scores than those from non-manual-labour households or with higher income. Similarly, divorced or separated women had a higher symptom score than those who were married or single. Although the number of children exercised no effect on symptom scores, the scores were worse in women whose children were teenagers or younger. Higher social support, including emotional support, good social networks and access to help in a crisis were associated with low symptom scores. However, after simultaneous adjustment of all risk factors, social networks were no longer independently associated with midlife symptoms. Some health risks, such as smoking and weight, were related to symptom scores in midlife. Smokers had the highest symptom scores, lifelong non-smokers the lowest and ex-smokers had intermediate scores. Women of normal weight had lower scores than women who were under- or overweight, while obese women had the highest scores. Alcohol intake and past physical activity were not systematically related to symptom scores.

The researchers concluded that markedly different life course trajectories were associated with psychological distress in midlife, and argued that the relationship between the woman's parents may be even more important than their findings on parental divorce suggested. No measures of parental conflict, parental indifference, or physical, sexual or psychological abuse were included in their study. They commented further that a retrospective question, asked when the women were 42 years old, identified a small number who may have suffered abuse or serious neglect of some kind in childhood. This limited measure of parental maltreatment was strongly associated with midlife psychological distress after adjusting for all other early experiences, and was mediated by mental health status in adult life.

Other research has confirmed the importance of different forms of adversity in childhood, including sexual abuse, for multiple health outcomes in adult life (Felitti et al., 1998). In addition, there is a well documented link between childhood sexual abuse and intimate partner violence in adult life and increased rates of a number of adverse mental health outcomes, including depression, anxiety and post-traumatic stress disorder (Astbury & Cabral de Mello, 2000). Women in the sixth year of follow-up for the Melbourne Women's Midlife Health Project completed a questionnaire on lifetime experience of violence: 28.5% (101/362) reported having experienced some form of domestic violence – physical, sexual or emotional – during their lifetime.

Research into the relationship between depression in midlife and possible risk factors, including menopausal and hormonal status and symptoms, faces a number of methodological challenges. While prospective studies minimize reliance on recall for contemporary events and experiences, bias remains a problem for more distant events and past experiences. Only the life course prospective study by Kuh, Wadsworth & Hardy (1997) avoided recall bias altogether, but such longitudinal studies are extremely costly to run. As a result, the comparison of findings across studies is limited by differences in methodological approach, ranging from the research design, the method of sample selection, differences in recruitment strategies, and choice of instruments for measuring risk factors and outcome variables. Studies also vary in the choice of methods for defining, detecting and measuring outcome variables, such as depression. Some studies have measured symptoms of depression, some have used standardized measures that permit diagnostic criteria to be applied, and others have used non-standardized self-report measures. There are differences in the age groups of women recruited to the studies, not all important covariables are taken into consideration, and most studies do not consider the impact of cultural factors. The sample in a longitudinal study is not necessarily representative of the general population, especially if there is a low response rate to the initial invitation to participate. For example, the response rate to the invitation to participate in the Melbourne Women's Midlife Health Project was only 56% (Dennerstein, Lehert & Guthrie, 2002). As further attrition in prospective samples occurs with time, sample bias is compounded. It may be that those participating in a cross-sectional study, where only one attempt to recruit participants is needed, are more similar to the general population than those who remain in a longitudinal study. However, cross-sectional studies cannot disentangle cause from effect or capture temporal changes. Prospective studies are needed to document time-related changes in indicators of health, including recent hormonal, social and psychological changes. All of these may influence and help to explain variations in menopausal symptoms and depressive symptoms between individual women. In addition, significant social and cultural changes can occur over a single generation. Changes in social organization and gender roles, including increased rates of divorce, decreased fertility rates and increased participation by women in paid work, raise new issues that can affect women's sense of well-being in midlife. Recent cohorts of women might differ from earlier cohorts in the significance they assign to work and personal achievement in their lives (Woods & Mitchell, 1997).

Overall, therefore, multidimensional models are needed to explain depression in midlife. Depression is more likely to be a consequence of distressing menopausal symptoms than a cause of them. The classical social and contextual determinants of depression, such as unemployment, socioeconomic adversity, negative life events, lack of social support, loss of partner through bereavement or separation, or lack of a confiding relationship with a partner, continue to exercise a powerful influence during menopause. Obesity, smoking and depression in midlife are related. Health promotion programmes that seek to reduce these high-risk behaviours among women in midlife will be successful only if they simultaneously address the causes of depression

Summary

Further research

While there is considerable anthropological literature on the cultural construction of menopause in low- and middle-income countries, and on women's expectations and experiences of it, data on the links between mental health and menopause are more limited. Research on this relationship is needed to provide culturally specific data for decision-making at programme, policy and service-provision levels. In particular, the following questions should be addressed:

1. Are the factors identified in high-income countries as critical to women's mental life in midlife equally important for the mental health and well-being of women in low- and middle-income countries?

2. If not, what other socioeconomic, cultural or interpersonal factors play a significant role?

3. What sources of assistance do women in low- and middle-income countries have for health problems and physically or psychologically distressing symptoms related to menopause?

4. How satisfied are women with these sources? What additional sources of assistance or services would they like to have? Do they think such services should be integrated in existing reproductive health services or stand alone?

Policy

Answers to the above questions are essential to provide data for the development of evidence-based policies on women's health, including their mental health in midlife.

Services

Research to date has the following implications for services and health care providers:

1. It is necessary to look beyond menopausal status, hormone levels and menopausal symptoms to adequately explain depressed mood in women at midlife.

2. A life-course, rather than a cross-sectional, approach is necessary to understand emotional distress in midlife.

3. The "classical" social determinants of depression, as well as the presence of distressing somatic symptoms and decreased sexual functioning and pleasure, are likely to contribute to dysphoria and depression.

4. A history of depression and high levels of psychosocial adversity may be more important than menopausal status in explaining current levels of emotional distress, and should be taken into account.

5. It is important to evaluate the sources and impact of stress, and of social support, on women's emotional well-being. This may include stressful demands from family and friends, who can function as conduits of stress as well as sources of positive social support.

References

Andrews G et al. (1999) *The mental health of Australia.* Canberra, Commonwealth Department of Health and Aged Care.

Astbury J, Cabral de Mello M (2000) *Women's mental health: an evidence based review.* Geneva, World Health Organization.

Avis NE (2000) Sexual function and aging in men and women: community and population-based studies. *Journal of Gender-Specific Medicine,* 3(2): 37-41.

Avis NE, McKinlay SM (1991) A longitudinal analysis of women's attitudes toward the menopause: results from the Massachusetts Women's Health Study. *Maturitas,* 13(1): 65-79.

Avis NE, McKinlay SM (1995) The Massachusetts Women's Health Study: an epidemiologic investigation of the menopause. *Journal of the American Medical Women's Association,* 50: 45-49.

Avis NE et al. (1994) A longitudinal analysis of the association between menopause and depression. *Annals of Epidemiology,* 4: 214-220.

Avis NE et al. (2001) Longitudinal study of hormone levels and depression among women transitioning through menopause. *Climacteric,* 4: 243-249.

Bebbington P et al. (2003) The influence of age and sex on the prevalence of depressive conditions: report from the National Survey of Psychiatric Morbidity. *International Review of Psychiatry,* 15: 74-83.

Bosworth HB et al. (2001) Depressive symptoms, menopausal status, and climacteric symptoms in women at midlife. *Psychosomatic Medicine,* 63: 603-608.

Boulet MJ et al. (1994) Climacteric and menopause in seven south east Asian countries. *Maturitas,* 19: 157-176.

Chlebowski RT et al. (2003) Influence of estrogen plus progestin on breast cancer and mammography in health postmenopausal women. *Journal of the American Medical Association,* 289:3243-3253.

Dennerstein L, Dudley E, Burger H (2001) Are changes in sexual functioning during midlife due to aging or menopause? *Fertility and Sterility,* 76: 456-460.

Dennerstein L, Dudley E, Guthrie J (2003) Predictors of declining self rated health during the transition to menopause. *Journal of Psychosomatic Research,* 54: 147-153.

Dennerstein L, Lehert P, Guthrie J (2002) The effects of the menopausal transition and biopsychoscial factors on well being. *Archives of Women's Mental Health,* 5: 15-22.

Dennerstein L et al. (1999) Mood and the menopausal transition. *Journal of Nervous and Mental Disease,* 1187: 685-691.

Dennerstein L et al. (2000) Life satisfaction, symptoms, and the menopausal transition. *Medscape Women's Health,* 5(4): E4.

Felitti VJ et al. (1998) Relationship of childhood abuse and household dysfunction to many of the leading causes of death in adults. The Adverse Childhood Experiences (ACE) Study. *American Journal of Preventive Medicine,* 14: 245-258.

Fu SY, Anderson D, Courtney M (2003) Cross-cultural menopausal experience: comparison of Australian and Taiwanese women. *Nursing and Health Sciences,* 5: 77-84.

Glazer G et al. (2002) The Ohio Midlife Women's Study. *Health Care for Women International,* 23: 612-630.

Hallstrom T, Samuelsson S (1990) Changes in women's sexual desire in middle life: the longitudinal study of women in Gothenburg. *Archives of Sexual Behaviour,* 19: 259-268.

Kaufert PA, Gilbert P, Tate R (1992) The Manitoba Project: a re-examination of the link between menopause and depression. *Maturitas,* 14(2): 157-160.

Kessler RC (2003) Epidemiology of women and depression. *Journal of Affective Disorders,* 74: 5-13.

Kessler RC et al. (1992) The relationship between age and depressive symptoms in 2 national surveys. *The Psychology of Ageing,* 7: 119-126.

Khaw HT (1992) Epidemiology of the menopause. *British Medical Bulletin,* 48: 249-261.

Kuh D et al. (2002) Lifetime risk factors for women's psychological distress in midlife. *Social Science and Medicine,* 55: 1957-1973.

Kuh DL, Wadsworth M, Hardy R (1997) Women's health in midlife: the influence of the menopause, social factors and health in earlier life. *British Journal of Obstetrics and Gynaecology,* 104(8): 923-933.

Leidy LE (1994) Biological aspects of menopause across the lifespan. *Annual Review of Anthropology,* 23: 231-253.

Lock M (1994) Menopause in cultural context. *Experimental Gerontology,* 29: 307-317.

Lock M (2002) Symptom reporting at menopause: a review of cross cultural findings. *Journal of the British Menopause Society,* 8: 132-136.

Luoto R, Kaprio J, Uutela A (1994) Age at menopause and sociodemographic status in Finland. *American Journal of Epidemiology,* 139: 64-76.

Maartens LW, Knottnerus JA, Pop VJ (2002) Menopausal transition and increased depressive symptomataology: a community based prospective study. *Maturitas,* 42: 195-200.

Mazza D et al. (2001) The physical, sexual and emotional violence history of middle aged women: a community based prevalence study. *Medical Journal of Australia,* 175: 199-201.

McKinlay SM, Brambilla DJ, Posner GJ (1992) The normal menopause transition. *Maturitas,* 14(2): 103-115.

McMaster J, Pitts M, Poyah G (1997) The menopausal experiences of women in a developing country: there is a time for everything, to be a teenager, a mother and granny. *Women and Health,* 26: 1-13.

Palacios S et al. (1995) Changes in sex behaviour after menopause: effects of tibolone. *Maturitas,* 22 (2): 155-161.

Pradhan AD et al. (2002) Inflammatory biomarkers, hormone replacement therapy, and incident coronary heart disease. *Journal of the American Medical Association,* 288: 980-987.

Punyahotra S, Dennerstein L (1997) Menopausal experiences of Thai women. Part 2: The cultural context. *Maturitas,* 26: 9-14.

Rapp SR et al. (2003) Effect of estrogen plus progestin on global cognitive function in postmenopausal women. The Women's Health Initiative Memory Study: A randomized controlled trial. *Journal of the American Medical Association,* 289: 2663-2672.

Shinberg D (1998) An event history of age at last menstrual period: Correlates of natural and surgical menopause among midlife Wisconsin women. *Social Science and Medicine,* 46: 1381-1396.

Standing TS, Glazer G (1992) Attitudes of low income clinic patients toward menopause. *Health Care for Women International,* 13: 271-280.

Stephens C, Ross N (2002) The relationship between hormone replacement therapy use and psychological symptoms: no effects found in a New Zealand sample. *Health Care for Women International,* 23: 408-414.

UNDP (2003) *Human Development Report 2003. Millennium Development Goals: A compact among nations to end human poverty.* New York, Oxford, Oxford University Press.

Wade TJ, Cairney J, Pevalin DJ (2002) Emergence of gender differences in depression during adolescence: national panel results from three countries. *Journal of the American Academy for Child and Adolescent Psychiatry,* 41: 190-198.

Wassertheil-Smoller S et al. (2003) Effect of estrogen plus progestin on stroke in postmenopausal women. *Journal of the American Medical Association,* 289: 2673-2684.

Wise LA et al. (2002) Lifetime socioeconomic position in relation to onset of perimenopause. *Journal of Epidemiology and Community Health,* 56: 851-860.

Woods NF, Mitchell ES (1997) Pathways to depressed mood for midlife women: observations from the Seattle Midlife Women's Health Study. *Research in Nursing and Health,* 20: 119-129.

Woods NF, Mariella A, Mitchell ES (2002) Patterns of depressed mood across the menopausal transition: approaches to studying patterns in longitudinal data. *Acta Obstetrica Scandanavica,* 81: 623-632.

World Bank (2006) Women in development. In: *2006 World Development Indicators,* Washington, DC: 34-37.

Chapter
6

Gynaecological conditions

Non-infectious gynaecological conditions – Heather Rowe
Infectious gynaecological conditions – Lenore Manderson & Narelle Warren
Malignant conditions – Lenore Manderson & Narelle Warren

One of the most important aspects of women's health care is the prevention of maternal mortality and the after-effects of injury sustained in pregnancy and childbirth (Wall, 1999). The main focus in this area has, understandably, been on maternal mortality, despite the fact that maternal injury affects substantial numbers of women globally. For every woman who dies from pregnancy-related causes, approximately 30 others incur injury, infection or disability, which, for the most part, remains untreated (Adamson, 1996). Many more women experience other, non-pregnancy-related gynaecological health problems.

Non-infectious gynaecological conditions

The causes of much obstetric and gynaecological morbidity stem from the neglect and abuse associated with the low social position accorded to females in many societies. Malnutrition in childhood and early adulthood, early age at marriage and first pregnancy, and lack of access to obstetric services result in high rates of obstetric morbidity. Myths associated with sex and reproduction result in many women feeling ashamed of their reproductive functions and being blamed for gynaecological infections, injuries and consequent infertility (Adamson, 1996; Miller & Rosenfield, 1996; Wall, 1998). The physical dimensions of these conditions have received little attention, and the mental health implications even less.

The International Conference on Population and Development (ICPD) in 1994 recognized

sexual and reproductive health and rights as fundamental to human rights and development. The ICPD Programme of Action aimed to increase the availability of good quality reproductive health services in developing countries. Too often, such services are of poor quality, with inadequately trained staff and no counselling services. Appropriate provider–patient interactions may be adversely affected by local social hierarchies (Mayhew, 2000), and women have reported disrespectful and abusive treatment by health care providers (Petchesky, 1998). Services are often designed with scant regard for the needs of women with respect to the timing of clinics and the availability of female doctors (Jaswal, 2001). In addition, an emphasis on family planning, and particularly discrimination and coercion in various population programmes, may discourage women from attending. Services should respond to the needs of a wider clientele than is represented in the "unmet need for family planning", which is narrowly defined as the 100–150 million married women who wish to space or limit births, but are not using contraceptives. Women value services staffed by trusted providers, who are respectful of local beliefs and practices (Toussaint, Mark & Straton, 1998; Hunt & Geia, 2002). Monitoring of progress should include indicators that are of importance to women (Germain, 2000).

Barriers to attendance at reproductive health services are commonly linked to cultural factors. Decisions about seeking treatment, for example, are often in the hands of husbands and mothers-in-law. Other structural factors also inhibit women's use of health services. The low level of literacy and formal education of women in many countries, their limited opportunities for employment and therefore lack of economic independence, and the poor development of other sectors, such as transport and communication, all inhibit women's access to services and have a negative effect on women's reproductive health (Aoyama, 2001). In addition, policies and services have often been based on the assumption that addressing barriers to physical health is sufficient and that, once this is attained, mental health will follow (Gulcur, 2000).

Studies continue to report high rates of gynaecological health problems in developing countries (Bhatia & Cleland, 2000). Prevalence studies in communities and clinical settings have used a variety of methods of measurement, including interviews to obtain self-reports of symptoms, clinical examinations, and laboratory analysis of specimens. Data derived from representative community-based samples are more generalizable than those from clinic-based studies, as women frequently do not seek treatment for these conditions because of financial and cultural constraints. However, data collected in community settings often underestimate health problems, both because women under-report the conditions and because of the lack of reliable and qualified personnel willing to travel to remote places in adverse conditions to collect information. Women are often reluctant to agree to clinical examination or blood collection, which further undermines the feasibility of community-based epidemiological studies (Bonetti, Erpalding & Pathak, 2002).

There is little consistency in the results of the different studies. Women's own reports, in particular, are influenced by the context of the interview (Bhatia & Cleland, 2000). Frequently, self-reported symptoms do not correspond to medically diagnosed morbidities, although there is no clear evidence-based explanation of the differences (WHO, 2001a). Difficulties in transporting equipment and samples, and the cost of the studies, further limit the evidence base (Bonetti, Erpalding & Pathak, 2002). Finally, very few research studies have addressed the mental health implications of gynaecological or obstetric health problems.

Obstetric fistula

An obstetric fistula is a tract between the bladder and the vagina, or the rectum and the vagina, which causes urinary or faecal incontinence or both. It is a devastating morbidity of pregnancy, which is prevalent in resource-poor countries. It primarily affects young, poor women with little education and limited social roles, who do not have access to adequate obstetric care (Muleta, 2004). A combination of malnutrition in childhood (which causes growth retardation), early marriage, and pregnancy before pelvic growth is complete results

> While the physical consequences of fistula are disabling, so too are the social consequences: stigmatization, isolation and loss of social support, divorce or separation, worsening poverty, malnutrition and suffering, and ultimately premature death (UNFPA, 2001).

in cephalopelvic disproportion and obstructed labour – "days of futile contractions repeatedly grinding down the skull of an already asphyxiated baby onto the soft tissues of a pelvis that is just too small" (Adamson, 1996). Prolonged obstructed labour in the absence of emergency obstetric services results in maternal death or, in many of those who survive, "obstructed labour injury complex" – obstetric fistula.

A woman with fistula suffers from constant vaginal wetness, which causes genital ulcerations, frequent infections and terrible odour. Long-term health consequences include skeletal injuries, and a combination of cervical injury, amenorrhoea, vaginal scarring and stenosis, leading to secondary infertility (Wall, 1999). Approximately 20% of women who are in obstructed labour for long enough to develop fistula also develop neurological injuries, including a condition known as "foot drop" which makes walking difficult (Wall, 1999). Most such labours in developing countries end in stillbirth; the typical patient is small and short (less than 44 kg in weight and under 150 cm tall) and married early (average age at marriage, 15.5 years) (Wall et al., 2004).

The fetal death rate in obstructed labour is over 90% (Wall, 1999). Most cases of obstructed labour occur in women having their first baby, who have a high probability of remaining childless thereafter. Amenorrhoea following fistula is common. In a society where childbearing is central to women's status, the loss of both a child and the role of motherhood is especially harsh, and many of these women face stigma. The rate of suicide in such women is unknown, but thought to be notable (Adamson, 1996). Social isolation confirms the woman's belief that she is to blame and has brought shame on her family. A study of women with fistula attending a clinic in the United Republic of Tanzania revealed that half of them were not living with their husband; three-quarters of these said that the reason for the separation was the fistula (Bangser, Gumodoka & Berege, 1999).

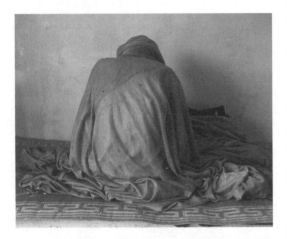

Women with untreated fistula face a lifetime of disability, pain, humiliation, abandonment, poverty, and malnutrition, often ending in premature death. Because of the shame associated with the condition, it is often hidden. Despite the undoubted psychological consequences of the physical and social burdens endured by women with fistula, there have been no systematic investigations. There are no reliable data on prevalence, but between 500 000 and two million women are estimated to be living with the condition (Adamson, 1996; Donnay & Weil, 2004; UNFPA, 2001). It is thought that, every year, between 50 000 and 100 000 women develop fistula. In sub-Saharan Africa the number of new cases annually is around 33 000 (Vangeenderhuysen, Prual & Ould el Joud, 2001). Most of these go untreated. Lack of services for safe childbirth and timely repair of fistula violates women's internationally recognized human right to reproductive health care (Cook, Dickens & Syed, 2004). There are anecdotal reports that some women with fistula can continue to live a dignified, productive life, but the determinants of apparent individual differences remain uninvestigated (Hilton & Ward, 1998).

Fistula is almost unknown in developed countries, where there is both universal access to high quality obstetric services and lower rates of teenage pregnancy. Unlike in developing countries, where 90% of fistulae result from obstetric injury, in the United Kingdom over 70% of fistulae follow pelvic surgery (Hilton, 2001). Obstetric fistula is almost entirely preventable and nearly always curable, although repairs can break down and require repeat surgery. Success rates of surgical repair are above 90% among trained surgeons (Bazeed et al., 1995; UNFPA, 2002). Most affected women and girls in developing countries are unable to afford the cost of fistula repair (UNFPA, 2001). However, when the Bugando Medical Centre Project on fistula opened in the United Republic of Tanzania in 1997, with assistance from personnel from the Addis Ababa Fistula Hospital in Ethiopia, women overcame enormous obstacles to attend in large numbers (Bangser, Gumodoka & Berege, 1999).

Timely access to skilled antenatal and intrapartum services is the key to preventing injury in childbirth (Donnay & Weil, 2004). However, in order to reduce the incidence of obstructed labour, two social changes are also needed: girls' nutrition must be improved, to ensure adequate growth of the pelvis; and the average age at first birth must increase. Gender discrimination in household food allocation is common in societies where females are accorded low social status, and is associated with poor access to health care (Messer, 1997). The pelvis continues to grow after menarche and full adult height have been reached, i.e. after the age at which pregnancy can occur (Moerman, 1982). Micronutrient and protein deficiencies in girls and young women compromise this growth and development (Messer, 1997). In Nigeria, maternal and child health education is being introduced into the Koranic school curriculum, with the aim of helping to ensure that young women are better able to have a safe pregnancy and obtain appropriate health care (Ibrahim, Sadiq & Daniel, 2000).

Social changes that promote the value of girls and delay marriage and first birth are potentially powerful agents for reducing the incidence of fistula and other obstetric injuries.

Pelvic organ prolapse

Pelvic organ prolapse is a significant descent of the uterus and vagina, which may protrude partly or completely beyond the vulva. It causes disturbing symptoms, such as pelvic fullness, back pain, incontinence, vaginal discharge, and bleeding (Aoyama, 2001).

The global prevalence of pelvic organ prolapse is estimated to be between 2% and 20% among women under 45 years (Bonetti, Erpalding & Pathak, 2002). Estimates in developing countries vary widely, from 3.4% in South India (Bhatia et al., 1997) to as high as 56% in Egypt (Younis et al., 1993). Even in developed countries, data on pelvic organ prolapse are inadequate, and there is little agreement on prevalence (Bump & Norton, 1998; Luber, Boero & Choe, 2001). The prevalence is higher in postmenopausal women because of hormonally mediated increases in tissue laxity. In developed countries, pelvic organ prolapse is associated with mature age (Luber, 2001), but in developing countries it occurs in a younger population.

The causes of prolapse are believed to be multifactorial. Multiparity is considered to be the primary predisposing factor, although in one study in Nepal, most women with prolapse had only one child (Bonetti, Erpalding & Pathak, 2002). Chronic health problems that increase abdominal pressure, such as obesity, constipation, chronic coughing and poor nutrition, may contribute to the condition. Heavy manual labour, including lifting and carrying of heavy objects, such as water and wood for cooking, is also a risk factor (Bonetti, Erpalding & Pathak, 2002). Women themselves explain prolapse in terms of difficult first delivery, first birth at a young age, gynaecological surgery, and miscarriage. In turn, women with pelvic organ prolapse are reported to be at a much greater risk of reproductive tract infections (Younis et al., 1993). Symptoms reported by women with prolapse, such as itching and foul-smelling discharge, may in fact be symptoms of other conditions.

Poor medical history-taking appears to result in underdiagnosis of the condition. However, of 227 women with self-reported prolapse in a household survey conducted in north India, 57% had not sought treatment. The majority of those who did seek care consulted a traditional birth attendant, not a doctor. Women reported shyness, lack of cooperation of the husband, and lack of time or money as reasons for not consulting a doctor. Of those who were offered surgery, few took it up (Kumari, Walia & Singh, 2000).

In developed countries, surgery is the principal treatment and over 390 000 repairs are performed annually in the United States of America (Norton et al., 1995). It is estimated that in the USA more than 10% of women will undergo a surgical procedure for symptoms of pelvic organ prolapse, including urinary incontinence, by the age of 80 years (Olsen, 1997), despite the fact that many women with incontinence do not seek medical help (Walters, 2004). There have been few evaluations of the success of surgical treatment, and women and clinicians may disagree on whether surgery has been successful (Hullfish et al., 2002).

Strategies to prevent urinary incontinence, including pelvic floor exercises, are included in antenatal and postnatal education programmes in developed country settings (Mason, 2001). These strategies may also help prevent pelvic organ prolapse. However, they do not address the risk factors for pelvic organ prolapse, such as heavy manual labour.

Little attention has been paid to psychosocial effects and quality of life measures among women with prolapse. Recently validated condition-specific instruments to assess the quality of life of women with pelvic organ prolapse include questions on distress caused by symptoms and their general impact, but there has been no validated assessment of psychological functioning for use pre- or post-surgery (Barber et al., 2001). The impact on women's mental health of progressive, long-term pelvic floor dysfunction remains underinvestigated. In a prospective study conducted in the USA, the pre-surgery goals of a group of 33 predominantly white women were elicited. At 6 and 12 weeks post-surgery, prior to the physician visit, the women were asked about their perceptions of the outcome of surgery. At 6 weeks, women agreed that most of their goals in relation to activity, symptoms, health and appearance had been met, but only by 12 weeks had their goals relating to social interaction and self-image been achieved (Hullfish et al., 2002).

Infectious gynaecological conditions

Reproductive tract infections (RTIs) include all infections of the genital tract in both men and women; some of these, but not all, are sexually transmitted. Environmental conditions, poor general health status and poor personal hygiene can lead to higher rates of reproductive tract infections that are not sexually transmitted (Whittaker 2002). These infections may have an impact on women's mental health. Research in India highlighted the association between reproductive tract infections and psychological distress (Prasad, Abraham et al. 2003), and demonstrated that presence of a symptom for more than one month – most commonly vaginal discharge – and a history of similar symptoms over the past year were risk factors for the development of common mental disorders, including depression, anxiety and somatization disorders.

Unexplained vaginal discharge

Some reproductive tract infections in women are caused by overgrowth of organisms that are normally present. Itching, irritation, and abnormal but non-bloody vaginal discharge can be distressing, but diagnosis is frequently difficult (Younis et al., 1993; Bhatia & Cleland, 1995; Zurayk et al., 1995; Koenig et al., 1998). Symptoms related to the reproductive tract are extremely common among low-income women, in both developing and developed countries (Jaswal, 2001; Dekker et al., 1993). The prevalence of unexplained vaginal symptoms is difficult to determine, since estimates tend to be based on clinical presentation and laboratory analysis of specimens. There is, however, a low correlation between vaginal discharge and laboratory evidence of infection (Wathne et al., 1994; Zurayk et al., 1995; Patel & Oomman, 1999; Bhatia & Cleland, 2000), and rates of self-reported symptoms are not accurate estimates of the prevalence of gynaecological morbidity (Koenig et al., 1998). In Nepal, for example, laboratory diagnosis indicates low rates of infection in symptomatic women, supporting a cautious approach to symptomatic treatment for RTIs (Bonetti, Erpalding & Pathak, 2002). Similarly, a survey in general practice in the Netherlands found that, in 25% of women presenting with vaginal symptoms, no microbial infection could be diagnosed (Dekker et al., 1993). However, Karaca et al. (2005), in a systematic comparison of microbiological laboratory testing and clinical examination of pregnant women, found that reproductive tract infections were underdiagnosed in settings where laboratory facilities were limited.

Epidemiological data may indicate that reproductive tract infections are not a cause for public health concern. However, women report that the symptoms have a profound effect on their life.

In Asian societies, there is a widespread belief that vaginal discharge is abnormal, depletes vital energy, and causes weakness, fatigue and aches and pains (Chaturvedi et al., 1993; Whittaker, 2002). Women may fear that the symptoms indicate or will lead to serious disease, such as cancer. In other cases, women may be reluctant to seek medical advice because they believe that these conditions are sexually transmitted. Strong cultural taboos and shame may prevent women from seeking professional treatment; they may, instead, try to treat themselves, which in turn may endanger their health (Jaswal, 2001; Boonmongkon, Nichter & Pylypa, 2001; Guo, Wang & Yan, 2002; Whittaker, 2002). In many cultures, women endure vaginal symptoms as an "inevitable" part of womanhood.

The experience of gynaecological symptoms is associated with psychological distress, particularly when no genital tract pathology is diagnosed (Stewart et al., 1990; Patel & Oomman, 1999). The impact on women's mental health of chronic, distressing symptoms, which have no medical explanation and remain unresolved – and by implication, undervalued – has not been fully examined. The symptoms can have deep cultural meanings (Dekker et al., 1993; Trollope-Kumar, 1999), and may in themselves be somatic expression of depression and psychosocial distress (Patel & Oomman, 1999).

Candidiasis

Candidiasis (vaginal thrush or monilia) is one of the most common causes of vaginal discharge and discomfort. Distress is related both to the symptoms and to misunderstanding of their cause. *Candida* yeast is always present in the body. Candidiasis arises when, under certain conditions, the yeast multiplies, leading to an infection characterized by a thick, clumped discharge. The infection can be very debilitating, causing vulval and vaginal itching, discomfort or irritation, redness and/or swelling of the vagina and vulva, and a stinging or burning sensation when urine is passed. The pain, itchiness and general discomfort associated with recurrent candidiasis can cause considerable distress.

The most common causes of candidal overgrowth are antibiotic treatment, oral contraceptives, pregnancy, diabetes, immune system disorders and general illness. Cleaning the anus by wiping towards the vagina can also spread yeast from the digestive tract. Contemporary products, such as some soaps, antiseptic douches, perfumed sprays, and tight-fitting and synthetic underwear, can also change the local environment in the vagina and may result in overgrowth of yeast. Candidiasis is rarely sexually transmitted. All women are exposed at some time to at least some of the biological factors associated with thrush, and 75% of all women will experience the infection during their life (CDC 2005). Candidiasis is treated as a minor infection and its impact is rarely studied. Because it is often associated with menstruation, pregnancy and the use of oral contraceptives, it is frequently considered trivial by women and their health care providers. However, urination and intercourse during infection can be extremely painful, and lesions may occur as a result of friction with swollen tissue, increasing the woman's risk of acquiring other infections, including human immunodeficiency virus (HIV).

Treatment is usually with an antifungal cream or suppositories, such as miconazole or clotrimazole, although such treatments are rarely available and affordable for women in poor countries. Women may also experiment with natural therapies (e.g. by including yoghurt in their diet) and by applying various herbs topically, but few studies have reported on women's perceptions and self-management of this condition, or on its effects on their mental and emotional health (Bechart 1996).

In a small cross-sectional study of women with chronic vaginal candidiasis, the women reported that recurrent infection seriously interfered with their sexual and emotional relationships (Irving, Miller et al. 1998). The women were significantly more likely than controls to suffer from clinical depression, to be dissatisfied with life, to have low self-esteem, and to perceive their lives as stressful. Similarly, in a small study in the United Kingdom, women reported that thrush had a major adverse impact on their life, making them feel miserable, unable to work, embarrassed, and even stigmatized (Chapple, Hassell et al. 2000). Women of south Asian descent drew attention to the physical discomfort, personal distress and embarrassment, and the impact that infection had on their personal and professional lives; they reported feeling "dirty", embarrassed, depressed and stigmatized (Chapple 2001).

Bacterial vaginosis

Bacterial vaginosis is caused by overgrowth of anaerobic bacteria, and is characterized by vaginal inflammation and discharge. It has serious adverse consequences, in particular an increased risk of premature birth, pelvic inflammatory disease and sexually transmitted infection, including HIV and herpes simplex 2 (Harville, Hatch & Zhang, 2005; Uma et al., 2005). It is thought to be more common in women who have reduced immunity as a result of chronic stress. Ehrstrom et al. (2005) found higher levels of stress hormones in women with recurrent bacterial vaginosis than in age-matched healthy controls. However, Harville, Hatch & Zhang (2005) found that rates of bacterial vaginosis infection were no higher in a sample of 411 African American women with high self-reported life stress than in those without.

Bacterial vaginosis may be more likely to occur in women living in chronic adversity, whose general health status is low. Poor women attending an outpatient clinic in Hyderabad, India, who were seriously undernourished, were more likely to have bacterial vaginosis than those who were adequately fed (Yasodhara et al., 2006). Sex workers are at increased risk of concurrent infection with bacterial vaginosis and sexually transmitted infections (STIs), and it is thought that bacterial vaginosis may increase vulnerability to STI (Kim et al., 2005; Uma et al., 2005).

Sexually transmitted infections of the reproductive tract

Sexually transmitted infections are a major cause of morbidity, disability, psychological suffering and death worldwide. In addition to their direct effects, they can make people more vulnerable to infection with the human immunodeficiency virus and cause infertility.

In both industrialized and poor countries, the prevalence and incidence of sexually transmitted bacterial and viral infections have increased since 1995 (WHO 2001b). In 1999, an estimated 340 million new cases of sexually transmitted bacterial infections (syphilis, gonorrhoea, chlamydial infections and trichomoniasis) occurred in men and women aged 15–49 years; this number has continued to rise (WHO 2001; 2006). Precise global surveillance data on the prevalence and incidence of sexually transmitted viral infections (other than HIV) are difficult to find, but indicators suggest that 630 million, or two-thirds of people who have ever been sexually active, are infected with a human papillomavirus (Baseman and Koutsky 2005; Pagliusi and Vaccine Research and Development [2001] 2003). The prevalence of genital herpes (herpes simplex virus type 2 (HSV2) and, to a lesser extent, type 1 (HSV1)) varies widely, from 4% in the United Kingdom to up to 80% in sub-Saharan Africa (Paz-Bailey, Ramaswamy et al. 2007). In addition to the primary symptoms, HSV infection increases the likelihood of developing other sexually transmitted infections, such as genital ulcer disease (GUD) and HIV infection (Paz-Bailey, Ramaswamy et al. 2007).

Poverty, low income, urbanization, unemployment and migration are all associated with the incidence and continued transmission of STIs (Holtgrave and Crosby 2003), in particular when condoms are unaffordable or unavailable (Duncan, Tibaux et al. 1997). STI epidemics have been reported from the emerging states of Eastern Europe and other countries experiencing rapid structural, political and social change (Purevdawa, Moon et al. 1997; Axmann 1998; Aral, Lawrence et al. 2003). Marginalized communities are also highly vulnerable. In Australia, for example, indigenous communities have extremely high rates of sexually transmitted infections of all kinds, as well as high rates of sexual violence, and non-sexual physical and mental health problems. In one descriptive study among indigenous Australians, over a quarter of women aged 20–43 years were infertile. Nearly 50% of women in rural northern Australia had been infected with genital chlamydia and there were high rates of previous pelvic inflammatory disease (PID), gonorrhoea and syphilis (Kildea and Bowden 2000). Effective public health interventions are hindered by a history of dispossession, violence and racism, as much as by structural, social and economic barriers to service (Kirk et al., 1998).

Sexually transmitted infections can result in pelvic inflammatory disease, tubal occlusion and consequent infertility, ectopic pregnancy, adverse pregnancy outcomes, genital neoplasia, and neurological complications. Although these infections cause pain, disability and reduced functioning, little research has been conducted into their psychological séquelae, in either developed or developing country settings. In relative terms, more evidence is available on specific infections for North America and Western Europe.

Diagnosis is universally described as stressful. Being diagnosed with an STI is stigmatizing (1997; Duncan, Hart et al. 2001; Donovan 2004), and carries an implication of one's own or the partner's infidelity. In addition, infection may have implications for reproductive health in the long term; establishing or maintaining a sexual relationship may become problematic; and there may be concerns about preventing recurrence of disease. These psychosocial responses may be exacerbated or compounded if clinic staff have negative attitudes (Connell, McKevitt et al. 2004). Universally, the research literature draws attention to the short- and long-term psychological responses of individuals to STI diagnoses and recurrent infections, the particular emotional, social and mental health costs of these for women, and the lack of systematic responses to meet the mental health needs (Prasad, Abraham et al. 2003).

> Lack of information on reproductive health problems means that women are often unaware that conditions are treatable, and that without treatment many conditions have serious long-term implications.

Infertility in women, as a result of untreated sexually transmitted reproductive tract infections, causes particular distress and hardship, with social and emotional consequences for both men and women, and social stigmatization, particularly of women (Papreen, Sharma et al. 2000).

Various factors impede diagnosis and treatment and contribute to a substantial global underestimate of reproductive tract infections of all kinds. Most women in developing countries have poor access to appropriate, acceptable, gender-sensitive health services. Rural women, in particular, are unfamiliar with reproductive tract infections, confuse sexually and non-sexually transmitted infections, and perceive and experience considerable social stigma on diagnosis (Guo 1999; Go, Quan et al. 2002; 2002). Reproductive tract and sexually transmitted infections are typically associated with sexual freedom, and in much of the world, women's sexuality is tightly controlled. Any symptom of infection may be taken as evidence of infidelity, and this may have serious consequences for women and their children in terms of personal safety and security.

For women whose quality of life is tied to their fertility, reproductive tract and sexually transmitted infections cause short- and long-term problems that affect their economic and domestic life (Walraven, Scherf et al. 2001). Women who are vulnerable and who fear informing their partner about an infection may not accept that they have been infected, because of profound feelings of shame and stigma, as well as fears of intimate partner violence. In Morocco, for example, STIs are viewed as women's illnesses (Manhart, Dialmy et al. 2000); a diagnosis of STI can lead to victimization and stigmatization, by both the male partner and family members. As a result of gender discrimination in sexual health services, women may remain untreated and vulnerable to sequelae of the infection. In Zimbabwe, women's psychological reactions to repeated multiple STIs highlight their lack of power to negotiate safe sex within marriage, their lack of choice in terms of conditions of marriage, and the lack of social support networks for infected women (Pitts, Bowman et al. 1995). Women reported fear or worry about the risk of HIV/AIDS, yet highlighted their feelings of shame, social isolation and stigma; they also related their infections to being unable to trust their husband's sexual behaviours. This finding was supported by data collected from men, most of whom indicated they were unlikely to change their sexual practices (multiple partners, not using condoms) despite the infection. Research in Uganda has also illustrated that psychosocial factors, including gender relations and types of sexual partner, as well as poor quality of health care, discourage women from referring their sexual partner for treatment (Nuwaha, Faxelid et al. 2000). Limited financial resources and a perception that symptoms are not severe discourage women from seeking care. A study in Nairobi, Kenya, demonstrated that women waited longer than men before seeking reproductive and sexual health care (Voeten, O'Hara et al. 2004).

Few studies have documented the social and cultural aspects that lie behind recognition, diagnosis and treatment of reproductive health problems in women. Ethnographic research in north-eastern Thailand highlighted how family life and sexual relations are disrupted by fears of gynae-cological problems, regardless of the diagnosis. This influences the extent to which women treat themselves, and their concerns about the seriousness of recurrent ailments (Boonmongkon, Nichter et al. 2001; Boonmongkon, Nichter et al. 2002). Women typically minimize their concerns about their gynaecological problems and employ self-management strategies rather than seek medical advice. As the gynaecological problem therefore remains unresolved, these factors result in substantial suffering. Elsewhere in south-east and south Asia, women find reproductive tract symptoms stressful, leading a number of authors to suggest that women over-report vaginal discharge for reasons that are unclear but may be culturally constructed (Bang and Bang 1994; Ramasubban and Rishyasringa 2001; Ross, Laston et al. 2002). Such research highlights how discharge is commonly culturally constructed and therefore perceived by women as being unrelated to sexual contact (Bhatti and Fikree 2002), regardless of its cause. These findings suggest that, while not all discharge is indicative of reproductive tract infection, women may over-report some symptoms and under-report others, because of confusion about their origin. In particular, women who fear the social repercussions of sexually transmitted infections may report somatic symptoms, such as dizziness, backache and weakness, rather than discharge (Trollope-Kumar 2001). As a further complication, women seeking treatment for reproductive tract symptoms may receive unnecessary treatment, especially in areas of high STI prevalence, and may experience fungal infections (candidiasis) as a side-effect of the overprescription of antibiotics (Hawkes, Morison et al.), which compounds rather than reduces their distress.

Sexually transmitted infections are prevalent among women who have experienced sexual violence, compounding effects on their mental health, sexual functioning and social relationships (Holmes 1999; Jewkes 2000; Firestein 2001; Brokaw, Fullerton-Gleason et al. 2002; Upchurch and Kusunoki. 2004). Gender-based violence is associated with STI infection; both are associated with other physical and mental health problems, including mood changes, sleep disturbances, self-harm, and psychosomatic symptoms (Suris, Resnick et al. 1996; Kawsar, Anfield et al. 2004; Plazaola-Castano and Perez 2004).

Young people are at high risk for STIs, because of various social, economic, environmental, psychosocial and behavioural factors (Bishop Townsend 1996). In addition, young women are physiologically at greater risk of lesions during sexual activity, whether intercourse is forced or not. Adolescents may be asymptomatic or unaware of the significance of their symptoms, and not attend for investigation; as a result, STIs may remain undetected and untreated. Risk is higher among young women with multiple partners, or whose partners have multiple partners, who use condoms inconsistently. In many countries, access to condoms and relevant information is limited and they may be completely unavailable to those who are unmarried. Young women typically lack the skills to negotiate with partners regarding the occurrence of sex and the use of condoms.

In various settings other factors may complicate the effect of gender-related variables (Boyer, Shafer et al. 2000). In a study among young people in Lima, Peru, 18% had a history of STI symptoms or diagnosis, but only 11% of those who were heterosexually active reported consistent use of condoms. Those with a history of STI were more likely than others to associate condom use with casual sex, and to report a history of sexual coercion or of having paid or been paid for sex. For women, sex at a young age was a risk factor for STI and unplanned pregnancy (Caceres, Marin et al. 1997). Mental health problems, including depression and low self-esteem, appear to be significantly associated with risky sexual behaviour among young people. In the United States, depressive symptoms are associated with an increased probability of not having used a condom during the last sexual intercourse; for girls, they are associated with a history of STI (Shrier, Harris et al. 2001). Rosenthal & Biro (Rosenthal and Biro 1991) draw attention also to the presence of intrusive or avoidant thoughts in young women following infection, and argue for the need to explore the coping mechanisms of young people with sexually transmitted infections.

Syphilis

Syphilis is highly infectious and was epidemic until the early twentieth century (De Schryver and Meheus 1990; WHO 2001b). Efforts to control it had some success in the 1960s, but prevalence increased in the mid-1980s coincident with a general increase in STIs. Specific targeted programmes aimed at high-risk populations in some parts of southern Africa have been successful in reducing incidence rates (for example, in Botswana: Creek, Thuku et al. 2005), as have programmes in the Caribbean (Jamaica: Figueroa 2004) and South America (Argentina: Pajaro, Barberis et al. 2001). These declines, largely in developing countries, have contributed to an overall decrease in the global incidence of syphilis (De Schryver and Meheus 1990; Piot and Islam 1994; Gerbase, Rowley et al. 1998; WHO 2001b). Nevertheless, focal epidemics continue to occur in most parts of the world (Finelli, Levine et al. 2001), particularly in rapidly developing and developed countries. Data from South Africa demonstrate that the prevalence of syphilis has increased since 2003 (Department of Health (South Africa) Directorate 2006); similar trends have been observed elsewhere, including central America (Nicaragua: Hoekstra, Riedijk et al. 2006) and Asia (Thirumoorthy 1990; Reynolds, Risbud et al. 2006; Chen, Zhang et al. 2007). Syphilis prevalence has increased to critical levels in some populations across Western Europe (Cowan, 2004; Cronin et al., 2004; Marcus, Bremer & Hamouda, 2004; Righarts et al., 2004; Sasse, Defraye & Ducoffre, 2004; Defraye & Sasse, 2005; Lautenschlager, 2005; Oliver & Christensen, 2005; Payne et al., 2005; Simms et al., 2005; Wallace, Winter & Goldberg, 2005; Del Giudice et al., 2006), Eastern Europe (Tichonova, Borisenko et al. 1997; Uuskula, Silm et al. 1997; Ciment 1999; Dencheva, Spirov et al. 2000; Grgic-Vitek, Klavs et al. 2002; Karapetyan, Sokolovsky et al. 2002; Zakoucka, Polanecky et al. 2004; Resl and Kumpova 2005; Yakubovsky, Sokolovsky et al. 2006), the United States (CDC 2006; Kerani, Handsfield et al. 2006) and the Pacific region (Thirumoorthy 1990; Mak, Johnson et al. 2004; Azariah 2005; Johnston, Fernando et al. 2005). Prevalence rates are different in men and women; surveillance data from Serbia suggest that the incidence of syphilis has remained fairly stable in women since the mid-1980s, despite significant fluctuations – with a recent surge – in men (Bjekic, Vlajinac et al. 2001). Recent increases, globally, have been attributed to substantial increases in incidence among men who have sex with men (Cowan 2004; Fairley, Hocking et al. 2005; Fenton and Imrie 2005; Wade, Kane et al. 2005; Kerani, Handsfield et al. 2006) and female sex workers (Hernandez-Giron, Cruz-Valdez et al. 1998; Smacchia, Parolin et al. 1998; Uribe-

Salas, Conde-Glez et al. 2003; Nigro, Larocca et al. 2006).

The disease is caused by a bacterium (spirochaete), and can be diagnosed by a blood test. The first symptoms, usually a painless, often isolated ulcer at the site of inoculation, generally appear 10–90 days after infection. Secondary infection can occur in any part of the body, from 6–8 weeks after infection. Symptoms may include fever, a flat red body rash, hair loss, various cutaneous eruptions on the genitals and anus, myalgia, arthralgia and depression. Secondary syphilis is highly contagious, both sexually and transplacentally. Fetuses of infected women may suffer from extreme developmental disorders and often die *in utero* or at birth (Brockmeyer and Reimann 1998). An untreated infected individual can infect others through sexual contact for up to two years. There is then a latency period of 2–10 years followed, in about one-third of untreated individuals, by the development of skin, mucocutaneous and long bone disorders. In some cases, severe complications of the brain and spinal cord may result in progressive paralysis.

Gonorrhoea

Gonorrhoea is a bacterial infection, caused by *Neisseria gonorrhoeae*, the gonococcus. It is usually diagnosed through laboratory testing. In men, infection can cause a burning sensation on passing urine and a yellow discharge from the penis. In women, it is mostly asymptomatic, although some women may have a yellow vaginal discharge, low abdominal pain, or irregular menstrual bleeding. Gonorrhoea is relatively rare in industrialized countries, except in poor groups. In Australia, its prevalence among indigenous Australians is 78 times greater than in the rest of the population (Roche 2001). Gonorrhoea can be treated effectively; if left untreated, the infection can spread to the reproductive organs, causing pelvic inflammatory disease and infertility; it can thus have a major impact on women's quality of life. Psychosocial research related to gonorrhoea has focused on issues relevant to disease control, including barriers to partner referral (Nuwaha, Faxelid et al. 2000; Fortenberry, Brizendine et al. 2002).

There has been virtually no consideration of the mental health factors associated with diagnosis or outcomes of either of these conditions.

Human papillomavirus (HPV) infection

There are a number of human papillomaviruses (HPV), some of which are transmitted through sexual contact. Sexually transmitted HPV infection is common in women, particularly young women. Prevalence rates vary by population group and country of residence: HPV infection has been found in 16% of women in China (Li, Dai et al. 2006), 11–38% in Australia (O'Keefe, Gardner et al. 2006; Posner, Boyle et al. 2006), 51% of women in the United States (Kahn, Slap et al. 2005) and 58% in Brazil (Oliveira, Rosa et al. 2006). Genital HPV infection may be asymptomatic, or may cause genital warts, or genital or cervical intraepithelial neoplasia (often diagnosed by cervical smear tests Tinkle 1990; Stoler 1996; often diagnosed by cervical smear tests Wiley and Masongsong 2006). The association of cervical intraepithelial neoplasia and cervical cancer with HPV has led to increasing interest in testing for HPV during screening for cervical abnormalities. It has also stimulated the development of vaccines against two types of HPV involved in the development of cervical cancer (Frazer and Cox 2006; Leggatt and Frazer 2007); (Wiley and Masongsong 2006). Epidemiological data indicate that genital warts and cervical intraepithelial neoplasia are caused by different HPV types. Thus, the presence of warts does not indicate that a smear test will be abnormal (Ault 2006; Dalstein, Briolat et al. 2006; Wiley and Masongsong 2006). Women's knowledge about the association between HPV, cervical screening and cancer remains limited; in all but one Australian study (Giles and Garland 2006), most women were unaware of any association (Andersson-Ellstrom & Milsom, 2002; Pitts & Clarke, 2002; Gudmundsdottir et al., 2003; Kahn et al., 2005; Klug, Hetzer & Blettner, 2005; McMullin et al., 2005; Philips, Avis & Whynes, 2005).

Diagnosis of HPV infection has a significant psychological impact (Conaglen, Hughes et al. 2001), yet little research has been conducted on the mental health effects of HPV. For a small proportion of women (~3% in an Indian study: Singh, Sehgal et al. 1995), the physical manifestation of HPV is cauliflower-like warts on the labia and in the vagina (due to two specific strains of HPV: Handsfield 1997). Genital warts can provoke a sense of shame, depression, and anxiety (Linnehan and Groce 2000; Cox, Petry et al. 2004; Philips, Avis et al. 2005;

McCaffery, Waller et al. 2006; Friedman and Shepeard 2007), affecting the woman's health behaviour, including her sexual practices and attendance for cervical screening (Ault 2006); this may have consequences subsequently for her physical health. In one of the few studies exploring women's responses to a diagnosis of HPV infection, McCaffery et al. (McCaffery, Waller et al. 2006) argued that it is the diagnosis itself that prompts a range of negative psychosocial responses, which need to be addressed. Specifically, they noted that women often felt distressed, anxious or upset following diagnosis – which often occurred in the context of limited knowledge about HPV – and expressed concerns about their future health, fertility, and cancer risk. In addition, women viewed HPV as a highly stigmatizing condition, which left them feeling "unclean", "dirty", or "infectious"; they felt guilty and responsible for the infection, which had significant implications in terms of their sexual relationships (McCaffery, Waller et al. 2006). Such findings suggest that greater attention should be given to psychosocial issues associated with cervical screening and HPV diagnosis (Miller, Mischel et al. 1996; Waller, McCaffery et al. 2004).

Genital herpes

Genital infection with herpes simplex virus type 2 (HSV2) is one of the most common sexually transmitted viral infections in the world. It is incurable and can cause recurrent painful outbreaks. Infants may become infected during birth, and develop serious illness. Infection with HSV2 increases the risk of infection with HIV. Control of HSV2 is a key factor in reducing transmission of HIV in settings where HIV is widespread (del Mar Pujades Rodriguez et al., 2003; Kamali et al., 2003).

Diagnosis of HSV2 infection is associated with a range of psychological responses, including anguish, anger, lowered self-esteem, and hostility towards the person believed to be the source of the infection. Distress may be associated with the diagnosis itself, the adjustment to the infection, the type of social supports available to the person, and the need to decide whether to tell other people (Fraley 2002). Melville et al. (Melville, Sniffen et al. 2003) reported strong emotional and psychosocial responses to a diagnosis of herpes infection, including denial, confusion, distress, disappointment, relief, fear of

telling sexual partners, anger at the source partner, guilt about acquiring or transmitting the infection, and concern about transmitting it to future offspring. Dalkvist et al. (Dalkvist, Wahlin et al. 1995) and Cohen et al. (Cohen, Kemeny et al. 1999) found that persistent stress and anxiety were particularly predictive of recurrence of symptoms, but not transient changes in mood, short-term stressors, life change events, or phase of the menstrual cycle. Chronic elevated stress may result in recurrence of symptoms and, in a cyclical fashion, further worsen mental health and quality of life (Rein 2000; Judlin 2002; Pereira, Antoni et al. 2003). Women experiencing chronic social and economic adversity may therefore be especially likely to experience recurrent outbreaks of herpes.

Depression is common among people diagnosed with genital herpes; it appears to be more severe in women than in men (Mindel 1996; Dibble and Swanson 2000) and in those with a first episode of genital herpes. Ongoing responses include fear of telling future partners, continued concern about transmission, and feeling sexually undesirable and socially stigmatized. Continuing psychological problems include interference with sexual relationships, a sense of despair and low quality of life. People with genital herpes have also been found to use health services more often (Spencer, Leplege et al. 1999; Taboulet, Halioua et al. 1999; Melville, Sniffen et al. 2003).

Despite its global prevalence, little work has been conducted on the mental health impact of herpes outside North America and Western Europe. Psychosocial considerations are important in the management of recurrent genital herpes (Longo and Koehn 1993). Cognitive coping strategies and support from a partner appear to help with adjustment (Mindel 1996). Women with herpes tend to have a more negative self-view and more confusion and stress symptoms than infected men. Gender-specific interventions for young adults with genital herpes have therefore been advocated (Lewis, Rosenthal et al. 1999; Dibble and Swanson 2000).

Overall, herpes infection results in significant psychological stress and psychosexual morbidity, and has a marked negative impact on quality of life (Wild, Patrick et al. 1995; Mindel 1996; Brentjens, Yeung-Yue et al. 2003).

Chlamydia

Chlamydial infection is caused by the bacterium *Chlamydia trachomatis*. It is diagnosed by laboratory testing of swabs collected from the cervix in women or the urethra in men. It can be treated with antibiotics. Untreated chlamydia may spread through the uterus to the fallopian tubes, causing salpingitis, a painful condition, which may result in pelvic inflammatory disease, infertility or ectopic pregnancy. In men, chlamydia can result in infertility through inflammation around the testes. Chlamydial infection is very common, often occurring in young adults, and can be passed from mother to child during birth, causing conjunctivitis or pneumonia.

Most people with chlamydia do not have symptoms and remain unaware of infection. Symptoms in men may include urethritis. In women, infection often starts in the cervix, and symptoms may include vaginal discharge, burning on urination, lower abdominal pain, or pain during sexual intercourse, causing considerable suffering. Little work has been conducted on the mental health effects of the diagnosis, the disease itself, or its long-term effects (France, Thomas et al. 2001). According to one small study in Glasgow, most infected women had not considered that they were at risk of STI; this negatively affected their reactions to diagnosis, and produced anxiety about disclosing their infection to others and about the possible effects on their future reproductive health (Duncan, Hart et al. 2001). Risk factors, other than behavioural factors such as non-use of condoms, are unclear (Williams, Wingood et al. 2002), and there appears to be a complex interaction between geographical location, age, ethnic group, social deprivation and multiple simultaneous sexual partnerships (Potterat, Zimmerman-Rogers et al. 1999; Winter, Sriskandabalan et al. 2000; Connell, McKevitt et al. 2004). While better population-based data are needed, street youth, sex workers, and individuals with social problems appear to be at high risk of infection in all settings (Paris, Gotuzzo et al. 1999).

Other psychological, behavioural and social factors have yet to be linked to chlamydia (Claman, Toye et al. 1995), but it is often diagnosed in women who have experienced sexual violence (Martin, Matza et al. 1999). The prevalence of chlamydia associated with sexual violence in young people points to the need for services to appropriately assess and respond to their mental health needs (Kawsar, Anfield et al. 2004). There is evidence from the USA that young people diagnosed with conditions such as chlamydia subsequently felt less comfortable during sex, had negative feelings about themselves, and felt angry after sex (Whitten, Rein et al. 2003). This points to the emotional costs of such diagnoses and the need for readily available mental health services and interventions targeted to specific subgroups, particularly young people or women who have experienced sexual violence.

Malignant conditions

Cervical cancer

Cervical cancer is associated with infection with human papillomavirus, a sexually transmitted virus. It is the second most common cancer in women after breast cancer (Lambley, 1993; (Parkin, Bray et al. 2005), accounting for approximately 15% of all cancers in women. Its incidence is increasing: each year, worldwide, approximately 500 000 new cases of cervical cancer are diagnosed and some 270 000 women die of the disease (WHO, 2004(Parkin, Bray et al. 2005). The incidence of cervical cancer is higher in developing than in developed countries, and 78% of all new cases occur in developing countries (Parkin 1994; Parkin, Bray et al. 2005). In developing countries, the burden of disease from cervical cancer is higher than that from breast cancer; approximately 80% of women who die from the disease are in these countries (Parkin, Pisani et al. 1999); Rohan et al., 2003; WHO, 2004). The highest incidence rates – over 30 per 100 000 women per year – occur in Melanesia, Central and South America, and eastern and southern Africa (WHO, 2004). The lowest incidences are found in Europe, North America, east Asia and the western Pacific (Parkin, Pisani et al. 1999). Cervical cancer rates are higher in countries in which there is a general lack of awareness of the disease, lack of recognition of premalignant cervical changes, lack of screening programmes, and limited treatment services (WHO, 2004). Death rates from cervical cancer are highest among women aged over 50 years, who may be less likely than women of reproductive age to attend gynaecological services (WHO, 2004).

The difference in incidence and mortality rates between developing and developed countries reflects differences in both stage of disease at diagnosis and availability of effective treatment. The Papanicolaou cytological test (Pap smear), which can detect premalignant changes in cervical cells, is recommended by WHO for population screening. Early intervention among those found positive can reduce cervical cancer mortality by at least 80% (Van Til, MacQuarrie & Herbert, 2003; WHO, 2004). Effective screening, however, places high demands on resources, and is not common in poor countries, where visual inspection of the cervix is often the only method available to detect cervical dysplasia (WHO, 2004). In developing countries, diagnosis of cervical cancer typically occurs at an advanced stage, and the 5-year survival rate is around 48% (ranging from 41% in Eastern Europe to 49% across the African continent) ((Parkin, Pisani et al. 1999). The only treatments for cervical cancer are radiotherapy and surgery, which are costly and often unavailable to women in developing countries. Prevention therefore offers the most effective strategy for controlling the disease (WHO, 2004).

Individual, social, cultural, logistic, practical, and economic factors associated with participation in cervical screening services have been investigated, in particular to learn about barriers to accessing screening, with the ultimate aim of encouraging women to attend these services. Screening programmes in developed countries have led to improved survival rates, but there are still groups of women who are not adequately screened, and are diagnosed when disease is advanced (IARC, 2004). Members of minority ethnic groups and immigrants are less likely to present for screening than other women and subsequently experience higher cervical cancer incidence and mortality rates. Women may be reluctant to attend for screening because it involves an intimate vaginal examination, especially if they have inadequate knowledge about the causes and development of cervical cancer.

Relatively little research has been conducted outside the United States on the mental health aspects of cervical cancer and knowledge of the wider psychological and social factors associated with it is limited. Studies in the USA have found that: women with disabilities have low utilization rates of cervical screening services (Havercamp, Scandlin & Roth, 2004); African-American women are more likely to be diagnosed with late stage cervical cancer than other women born

in the USA (Schwartz et al., 2003); and Asian immigrants have higher rates of cervical cancer mortality (Singh & Miller, 2004). American-born and immigrant Vietnamese women are five times more likely to be diagnosed with the disease than white women born in the USA (Taylor et al., 2004), and cervical cancer incidence and mortality rates in Latin American immigrants are more than double those of white women (Scarinci et al., 2003). These authors interpret the findings as indicating that poor, marginalized and immigrant women in the USA have a poor understanding of cervical cancer etiology, prevention, and symptoms, and therefore do not attend existing services (Perez-Stable et al., 1992; Suarez et al., 1997a; 1997b; Phipps et al., 1999).

In Canada, women of low socioeconomic status are less compliant with screening recommendations and more likely to be identified when precancerous tissue is already present (Gupta et al., 2003). Screening rates are low in Hong Kong, China, which has been found to be related to cost, low knowledge about risk factors, lack of education about the importance of early detection, cultural values related to modesty, and embarrassment. Consequently the incidence of cervical cancer is relatively high (Holyroyd, Twinn & Adab, 2004). Women with a history of sexual abuse are also less likely to attend for screening, and these women appear also to be at higher risk of developing cervical cancer (Coker et al., 2000; Farley, Golding & Minkoff, 2002).

Many women experience anxiety and uncertainty when attending for screening. Ambivalence is generated by the tension between the reassurance potentially offered by screening and the possibility of diagnosing an abnormality. Uncertainty may also derive from a lack of knowledge about whether screening involves a Pap smear, colposcopy or visual examination. Although it is promoted as a preventive measure, many women see screening as a way of detecting cancer (Howson, 2001). Intimate screening examinations are invasive, may be physically uncomfortable and can arouse anxiety. Even when women present for cervical screening, they may doubt that there is an effective treatment for any abnormalities detected (Gregg & Curry, 1994; Temple-Smith et al., 1995; Kirk et al., 1998; Manderson, Kirk & Hoban, 2001). The situation is more complicated in developing countries. Women in one Thai province understood the Pap smear as a way of diagnosing all gynaecological problems, rather than a way of screening for precancer (Boonmongkon et al., 2002). Thai women are familiar with some risk factors for cervical cancer, such as a history of sexually transmitted infections or multiple sexual partners, but attributed its occurrence also to poor vaginal and perineal hygiene, fertility control and *karma* (the negative effects of past action) (Boonmongkon, Nichter & Pylypa, 2001; Jirojwong & Manderson, 2001; Boonmongkon et al., 2002).

Testing blood for the presence of HPV antibodies has been suggested as an additional or alternative screening technique to the Pap smear. It is less invasive than other screening methods, would reduce demands on resources and is likely to improve access for older women and hard-to-reach populations (Rohan, Burk & France, 2003). Maissi et al. (2005) compared groups of women with normal or abnormal Pap smear results, who had or had not been tested for HPV infection. While there were no differences in mood or quality of life between the four groups six months after the test, specific anxiety about abnormal test results remained and was highest in the group not tested for HPV. Among the HPV-positive women in this study, those who were younger, perceived themselves to be at high risk of cancer, and who had difficulty understanding the test results were most distressed (Maissi et al., 2004).

However, the association of HPV infection and cervical cell abnormalities can discourage women from attending for screening. Kavanagh & Broom (1998) found that women who had an abnormal Pap smear result rejected the explanation that their own sexual behaviour could have caused their condition, and indicated that they were afraid that their personal morality would be judged. McCaffrey et al. (2004) surveyed 428 adult women following routine cervical screening in London, England, and found that those who were HPV-positive were more anxious than those who tested negative; the women were especially concerned about the impact on future sexual relationships. Indigenous Australian and South African women also associate cervical cancer with promiscuity, linking sexuality, dirt and disease (Wood, Jewkes & Abrahams, 1997; Manderson, Kirk & Hoban, 2001).

For some women, any gynaecological symptoms are alarming indicators of possible cervical can-

cer. Kavanagh & Broom (1997, 1998) and Karasz, McKee & Roybal (2003) found that women believed that vaginal itching and discharge could be indicators of cervical cancer and lead to an abnormal smear result. Women in north-east Thailand, with recurrent symptoms of abdominal or lower back pain, and vaginal discharge, itching or odours, also believed that these could develop into cervical cancer (Boonmongkon et al., 2002). Misunderstandings about risk generate high levels of fear. In Thailand, women's fear and worry about their cervical cancer risk led to psychological symptoms, including anxiety, insomnia, and increased stress (Boonmongkon et al., 2002).

Women who have dysplasia (abnormal cervical cell changes) or cervical cancer may have no symptoms and generally feel well. Signs of cervical cancer include irregular vaginal bleeding, unusual vaginal discharge, postcoital discomfort or bleeding, pelvic pain, excessive fatigue, swollen legs and backache. However, these signs may also indicate other conditions. Lack of knowledge about the implications of an abnormal smear test often exacerbates women's confusion, fear and anxiety following a positive result (Kavanagh & Broom, 1997; Karasz, McKee & Roybal, 2003). Limited knowledge about the natural history of cervical cancer may also contribute to women's confusion regarding medical responses to a cervical abnormality (Karasz, McKee & Roybal,. 2003). The detailed physical investigations that follow an abnormal screening result are sometimes unexpected and can be emotionally disruptive; they have been described as intense and traumatic (Howson, 2001) and as having an adverse impact on day-to-day psychological functioning (Forss et al., 2004).

Relatively little is known about women's mental health once cervical cancer has been diagnosed. Studies have tended to focus on women's need for support, with less attention being paid to other aspects of psychological functioning. In general, women of low socioeconomic status and members of minority ethnic groups have been found to be more pessimistic about their prognosis than other women. While this may be realistic, because the disease is detected at a more advanced stage, it is also a result of misinformation and poor education about the progression and implications of the condition (Rodney et al., 2002). Diagnoses of cancer commonly arouse fears of illness, infirmity and death, and are often associated in the short term with elevated rates of anxiety and depression.

Women's reactions to the diagnosis, treatment and prognosis of cervical cancer have been described in general terms and include: difficulty adjusting to side-effects of treatment, including nausea, loss of weight, and hair loss; concern about the impact on relationships; and fear of recurrence of cancer after treatment. These reactions affect confidence, self-esteem and general quality of life. Some studies have indicated that women who survive cervical cancer may experience anger and frustration that they can no longer have children (Basen-Engquist et al., 2003). Others have found reduced sexual interest and higher levels of sexual dysfunction than among survivors of other cancers, including problems with arousal, genital pain and altered sexual self-concept (Lagana et al., 2001; Jensen et al., 2004). A recent study with poor Latin American immigrants in the United States identified high levels of self-reported depression related to having cancer (Meyerowitz et al., 2000). Zulu women patients in South Africa also had high levels of psychiatric morbidity (Nair, 2000). In the long term, cervical cancer has a more severe adverse effect than other chronic conditions on women's quality of life; psychologically informed cancer support services are needed by all (Lalos & Eisemann, 1999; Li, Samsioe & Iosif, 1999; Klee, Thranov & Machin, 2000).

Ovarian, endometrial and other gynaecological cancers

Globally, ovarian cancer is most common among older, socioeconomically advantaged women in highly industrialized countries. Among American women, it is the fifth most common cancer and the leading cause of death from all gynaecological cancers. Although the cause is as yet unknown, the risk of developing ovarian cancer is increased in women who carry mutations of the BRCA1 and BRCA2 genes. Endometrial cancer appears to be associated with early age at menarche, late age of menopause and nulliparity, as well as infertility, obesity, diabetes and hypertension. However, many cases occur in women without any known risk factors (Holschneider & Berek, 2000; Loman et al., 2001; Purdie & Green, 2001; Runnebaum & Stickeler, 2001). Mental health research has focused on effective communication regarding familial risk and decision-making about prophylactic oophorectomy.

Mutations in BRCA genes can now be identified through DNA testing, which is available in most rich countries. The psychological impact of this testing is complex and has been examined in survey and interview studies. In a twelve-month post-investigation comparison of tested women who were and were not found to carry the mutation, those carrying mutations and who had not undergone prophylactic oophorectomy were the most distressed. Non-clinical distress, specific to cancer, was apparent in all carriers (Claes et al., 2005). Anxieties related to development of disease were persistent in carriers of genetic mutations (Watson et al., 2004), but there was a general reduction in distress after screening (Tiffen, Sharp & O'Toole, 2005). The alternative to prophylactic oophorectomy is regular gynaecological screening and women using one or other of these approaches were compared prospectively by Madalinska et al. (2005). Women who had surgery had fewer cancer-specific anxieties and a more optimistic view of the future, but worse sexual functioning and more menopausal symptoms. The authors concluded that these risks need to be weighed against the benefits of surgery in the clinical care of individual women. In a systematic review, Nelson et al. (2005) found that cancer risk assessment and genetic testing did not have adverse psychological sequelae, but that counselling and expert advice were needed to help women interpret the risk assessment. While professional support is beneficial for all those who screen positive (Hopwood, 2005), individual reactions are influenced by personality factors, in particular whether the person has an active or avoidant coping style; counselling needs to take this into account (Aziz et al., 2005; Hopkins et al., 2005).

In common with all those diagnosed as having cancer, women with ovarian cancer often try to make sense of their illness by seeking a cause. Unfortunately, with ovarian cancer, no direct cause can usually be identified. In Canada, women with ovarian cancer believed they had developed the disease because of a wide variety of factors, including stress, genetic factors, environmental pollution, hormones, sexual practices and smoking (Stewart et al., 2001). Awareness of cancer is generally related to age, access to information and economic status (Perez-Stable et al., 1992; Dyck, 1995; Suarez et al., 1997a; DiGiacomo, 1999; Phipps et al., 1999).

Ovarian cancer commonly presents with non-specific abdominal symptoms. Accurate diagnosis may be delayed, and women report considerable frustration regarding their experiences in seeking help, as doctors dismiss complaints such as back pain and discomfort (Markovic, Manderson et al. 2006). In women who are members of minority groups, disease is usually detected at a more advanced stage, because of delays in seeking treatment; as a result, these women have higher mortality and morbidity rates. Delays in diagnosis influence both survival and mental health status.

Length of survival depends on age at diagnosis, cancer stage and the type of tumour. The physical effects of surgery and adjuvant treatment affect quality of life and emotional well-being. Depression can occur in response to both the disease and its treatment, including to post-surgical pain, nausea, hair loss, weight loss, uncertain prognosis and the prospect of premature death. Delays in diagnosis, the high mortality rate and lack of curative treatments have an adverse impact on mental health, which should always be taken into account in routine care. Many women with ovarian cancer experience a pervasive diminution in quality of life, with preoccupation about risk of recurrence and life purpose, and gradual social withdrawal (Ferrell et al., 2005). Distress is worse in those who are younger and poor, and have a personal history of cancer or a family history of breast or ovarian cancer (Halbert et al., 2005; Geirdal et al., 2005). Social support assists adjustment following chemotherapy for ovarian cancer (Hipkins et al., 2004), but there is significant psychological morbidity during treatment and more than one-third of patients have clinically significant depression and anxiety.

Other gynaecological cancers, including vulval and vaginal cancers and teratomas, are rare. As a result, women who develop these diseases often feel isolated and distressed, linked to an inadequate general understanding of their disease and inaccurate beliefs about their causes. Treatment may involve surgical excision of the vulva, which is deeply traumatic and adversely affects body image, self-esteem, social confidence and sexual life. Its impact on mood and interpersonal relationships has not yet been systematically investigated (Andersen & Vanderdoes, 1994; Andersen, 1999a, 1999b; Barton, 2003).

Overall, poor gynaecological health has direct effects on women's mental health and psychological functioning, which need to be considered during routine health care.

Summary

Future research

1. The psychosocial consequences of obstetric injury, reproductive tract morbidity and cancers in women need to be considered and included in all research into these conditions.
2. Primary prevention programmes for gynaecological morbidity need to be designed and evaluated.
3. The specific needs of women in culturally diverse settings for advice, support and counselling during treatment and rehabilitation for gynaecological conditions should be systematically ascertained.

Policy

1. Policy and service delivery need to address both prevention and treatment of obstetric injury and gynaecological morbidity.
2. Where women's access to health services is constrained by social and cultural factors, strategies to reduce obstetric injury and gynaecological morbidity should be accompanied by efforts to improve women's social position.
3. Obstetric injuries and consequent gynaecological morbidity can be reduced by: encouraging social changes that promote the value of girls and delay marriage and first birth; ensuring rapid access to trained personnel during labour and childbirth; and ensuring that women do not return to hard manual labour shortly after childbirth.

Services

1. Gynaecological and obstetric health services need to be accessible, affordable and appropriate to women's needs.

2. The staff of such services should be trained to manage sensitively gynaecological morbidity and obstetric injury; they should try to change cultural practices that reduce women's self-determination and to identify psychological distress and anxiety.

3. Health service staff should offer non-judgemental, empathic care, which encourages women to talk about their reproductive health concerns. They should also be capable of providing support to minimize the mental health impact associated with treatment and care.

4. Gynaecological and cancer screening services should recognize that women may be fearful, embarrassed or ashamed of tests, treatment and possible disease, and should ensure that they understand the nature of screening.

References

Adamson P (1996) Commentary: a failure of imagination. In: *The progress of nations 1996.* New York, UNICEF (http://www.unicef.org/pon96/womfail.htm).

Andersen BL (1999a) Sexual self concept (schema) and adjustment following cancer. *Psychosomatic Medicine*, 61(1): 130.

Andersen BL (1999b) Surviving cancer: the importance of sexual self-concept. *Medical and Pediatric Oncology*, 33(1): 15-23.

Andersen BL, Vanderdoes J (1994) Surviving gynecologic cancer and coping with sexual morbidity – an international problem. *International Journal of Gynecological Cancer*, 4(4): 225-240.

Aoyama A (2001) *Reproductive health in the Middle East and North Africa: well-being for all.* Washington, World Bank.

Aral SO et al. (2003) The social organization of commercial sex work in Moscow, Russia. *Sexually Transmitted Diseases* 30(1): 39-45.

Ault KA (2006). Epidemiology and natural history of human papillomavirus infections in the female genital tract. *Infectious Diseases in Obstetrics Gynecology* 14(1): 40470.

Axmann A (1998) Eastern Europe and community of independent states. *International Migration*, 36 (4): 587-607.

Azariah S (2005) Is syphilis resurgent in New Zealand in the 21st century? A case series of infectious syphilis presenting to the Auckland Sexual Health Service. *New Zealand Medical Journal* 118(1211): U1349.

Bang R, Bang A (1994) Women's perceptions of white vaginal discharge: Ethnographic data from rural Maharashtra. *Listening to Women Talk About their Health: Issues and Evidence from India*. Gittlesohn J, Bentley ME, Pelto PJ et al. New Dehli, Ford Foundation, Har-Anand Publishers.

Bangser M, Gumodoka B, Berege Z (1999) A comprehensive approach to vesico-vaginal fistula: a project in Mwanza, Tanzania. In: Berer M, Sundari Ravindran T, eds., *Safe motherhood: critical issues*, London, Blackwell Science: 157-165.

Barber M et al. (2001) Psychometric evaluation of two comprehensive condition-specific quality of life instruments for women with pelvic floor disorders. *American Journal of Obstetrics and Gynecology*, 185: 1388-1395.

Baseman JG, LA Koutsky (2005) The epidemiology of human papillomavirus infections. *Journal of Clinical Virology* 32 Suppl 1: S16-24.

Bazeed M et al. (1995) Urovaginal fistulae: 20 years' experience. *European Urology,* 27(1): 34-38.

Bechart E (1996) Recurrent vaginal candidiasis. Reflections of a psychosomatic gynecologist. *Contraception, Fertilite, Sexualite* 24(3): 233-7.

Bhatti LI, Fikree FF (2002) Health-seeking behavior of Karachi women with reproductive tract infections. *Social Science & Medicine* 54(1): 105-117.

Bhatia J, Cleland J (1995) Self-reported symptoms of gynecological morbidity and their treatment in South India. *Studies in Family Planning,* 26(4): 203-216.

Bhatia J, Cleland J (2000) Methodological issues in community-based studies of gynecological morbidity. *Studies in Family Planning,* 31(4): 267-277.

Bhatia J et al. (1997) Levels and determinants of gynecological morbidity in a district of South India. *Studies in Family Planning,* 28(2): 95-103.

Bishop Townsend V (1996) STDs: Screening, therapy, and long-term implications for the adolescent patient. *International Journal of Fertility and Menopausal Studies* 41(2): 109-114.

Bjekic M, Vlajinac H et al. (2001) Trends of gonorrhoea and early syphilis in Belgrade, 1985-99. *Sexually Transmitted Infections* 77: 387-389.

Bonetti T, Erpelding A, Pathak L (2002) *Reproductive morbidity – a neglected issue? A report of a clinic-based study held in Far-Western Nepal.* Kathmandu, Nepal Ministry of Health, GTZ, UNFPA.

Boonmongkon PM, Nichter et al. (2001) Mot Luuk problems in northeast Thailand: why women's own health concerns matter as much as disease rates. *Social Science & Medicine* 53(8): 1095-1112.

Boonmongkon P, Nichter M et al. (2002) Women's health in northeast Thailand: Working at the interface between the local and the global. *Women & Health* 35(4): 59-80.

Boyer CB, Shafer MA et al. (2000) Associations of sociodemographic, psychosocial, and behavioral factors with sexual risk and sexually transmitted diseases in teen clinic patients. *Journal of Adolescent Health* 27(2): 102-111.

Brentjens MH, Yeung-Yue KA et al. (2003) Recurrent genital herpes treatments and their impact on quality of life. *Pharmacoeconomics* 21(12): 853-863.

Brockmeyer NH, Reimann G (1998) Syphilis - clinical aspects, diagnosis and therapy. Part 1 - clinical aspects. *Medizinische Welt* 49(12): 618-623.

Brokaw J, Fullerton-Gleason L et al. (2002) Health status and intimate partner violence: A cross-sectional study. *Annals of Emergency Medicine* 39(1): 31-38.

Bump R, Norton P (1998) Epidemiology and natural history of pelvic floor dysfunction. *Obstetrics and Gynecology Clinics of North America,* 25: 723-746.

Caceres CF, Marin BV et al. (1997) Young people and the structure of sexual risks in Lima. *AIDS* 11: S67-S77.

CDC, C. f. D. C. a. P. (2005) Genital Candidiasis (Vulvovaginal Candidiasis (VVC), vaginal yeast infections). *Candidiasis.* D. o. B. a. M. D. Coordinating Center for Infectious Diseases. Atlanta, GA, CDC. 2007.

CDC, C. f. D. C. a. P. (2006) Primary and secondary syphilis--United States, 2003-2004. *Morbidity and Mortality Weekly Report* 55(10): 269-73.

Chapple A (2001) Vaginal thrush: perceptions and experiences of women of south Asian descent. *Health Education and Research* 16(1): 9-19.

Chapple A, Hassell K et al. (2000) You don't really feel you can function normally: women's perceptions and personal management of vaginal thrush. *Journal of Reproductive and Infant Psychology* 18(4): 309-319.

Chaturvedi S et al. (1993) Somatization misattributed to non-pathological vaginal discharge. *Journal of Psychosomatic Research,* 37(6): 575-579.

Chen ZQ, Zhang GC, et al. (2007) Syphilis in China: results of a national surveillance programme. *Lancet* 369(9556): 132-8.

Ciment J (1999) Health situation in former communist bloc is dire, says Unicef. *BMJ* 319(7221): 1324.

Claman P, Toye B et al. (1995) Serologic Evidence of Chlamydia-Trachomatis Infection and Risk of Preterm Birth. *Canadian Medical Association Journal* 153(3): 259-262.

Cohen F, Kemeny ME, et al. (1999) Persistent stress as a predictor of genital herpes recurrence. *Archives of Internal Medicine* 159(20): 2430-2436.

Conaglen HM, Hughes R et al. (2001) A prospective study of the psychological impact on patients of first diagnosis of human papillomavirus. *International Journal of STD & AIDS* 12(10): 651-658.

Connell P, McKevitt C et al. (2004) Investigating ethnic differences in sexual health: focus groups with young people. *Sexually Transmitted Infections* 80(4): 300-305.

Cook RJ, Dickens BM, Syed S (2004) Obstetric fistula: the challenge to human rights. *International Journal of Gynaecology & Obstetrics*, 87(1):72-77.

Cowan S (2004) Syphilis in Denmark-Outbreak among MSM in Copenhagen, 2003-2004. *European Surveillance* 9(12): 25-7.

Cox JT, Petry KU et al. (2004) Using imiquimod for genital warts in female patients. *Journal of Womens Health* 13(3): 265-271.

Creek TL, Thuku H et al. (2005) Declining syphilis prevalence among pregnant women in northern Botswana: an encouraging sign for the HIV epidemic? *Sexually Transmitted Infections* 81(6): 453-455.

Dalkvist J, Wahlin TBR et al. (1995) Herpes-Simplex and Mood - a Prospective-Study. *Psychosomatic Medicine* 57(2): 127-137.

Dalstein V, Briolat J et al. (2006) The epidemiology of genital human papillomavirus infections. *Review of Practice* 56(17): 1877-81.

De Schryver A, Meheus A (1990) Epidemiology of sexually transmitted diseases: the global picture. *Bulletin of the World Health Organization* 68(5): 639-54.

Dekker JH et al. (1993) Vaginal symptoms of unknown aetiology: a study in Dutch general practice. *British Journal of General Practice*, 43(371): 239-244.

Dencheva R, Spirov G et al. (2000) Epidemiology of syphilis in Bulgaria, 1990-1998. *International Journal of STD and AIDS* 11(12): 819-22.

Department of Health (South Africa) Directorate, E. a. S. (2006) *National HIV and syphilis antenatal sero-prevalence survey in South Africa, 2005*. Pretoria, National Department of Health: 20.

Dibble SL, Swanson JM (2000) Gender differences for the predictors of depression in young adults with genital herpes. *Public Health Nursing* 17(3): 187-194.

Donnay F, Weil L (2004) Obstetric fistula: the international response. *Lancet*, 363(9402): 71-72.

Donovan B (2004) Sexually Transmitted infections other than HIV. *Lancet* 363(9408): 545-556.

Duncan B, Hart G et al. (2001) Qualitative analysis of psychosocial impact of diagnosis of Chlamydia trachomatis: implications for screening. *British Medical Journal* 322(7280): 195-199.

Duncan ME, Tibaux G et al. (1997) STDs in women attending family planning clinics: A case study in Addis Ababa. *Social Science & Medicine* 44(4): 441-454.

Dyck I (1995) Hidden geographies: the changing lifeworlds of women with multiple sclerosis. *Social Science & Medicine*, 40(3): 307-320

Fairley CK, Hocking JS et al. (2005) Syphilis: back on the rise, but not unstoppable. *Medical Journal of Australia* 183(4): 172-173.

Fenton KA, Imrie J (2005) Increasing rates of sexually transmitted diseases in homosexual men in Western europe and the United States: why? *Infectious Diseases Clinics of North America* 19(2): 311-31.

Figueroa JP (2004). An overview of HIV/AIDS in Jamaica: strengthening the response. *West Indian Medical Journal* 53(5): 277-82.

Finelli L, Levine WC et al. (2001) Syphilis outbreak assessment. *Sexually Transmitted Diseases* 28 (3): 131-135.

Firestein BA (2001) Beyond STD prevention: Implications of the new view of women's sexual problems. *Women & Therapy* 24(1-2): 27-31.

Fortenberry JD, Brizendine E et al. (2002) The role of self-efficacy and relationship quality in partner notification by adolescents with sexually transmitted infections. *Archives of Pediatrics & Adolescent Medicine* 156(11): 1133-1137.

Fraley SS (2002) Psychosocial outcomes in individuals living with genital herpes. *Journal of Obstetric Gynecologic and Neonatal Nursing* 31 (5): 508-513.

France C, Thomas K et al. (2001) Psychosocial impacts of chlamydia testing are important. *British Medical Journal* 322(7296): 1245.

Frazer IH, Cox J (2006) Finding a vaccine for human papillomavirus. *Lancet* 367(9528): 2058-9.

Friedman AL, Shepeard H (2007) Exploring the Knowledge, Attitudes, Beliefs, and Communication Preferences of the General Public Regarding HPV: Findings from CDC Focus Group Research and Implications for Practice. *Health Education and Behaviour*.

Gerbase AC, Rowley JT et al. (1998) Global prevalence and incidence estimates of selected curable STDs. *Sexually Transmitted Infections* 74 Suppl 1: S12-6.

Germain A (2000) Population and reproductive health: where do we go next? *American Journal of Public Health*, 90(12): 1845-1847.

Giles M, Garland S (2006) A study of women's knowledge regarding human papillomavirus infection, cervical cancer and human papillomavirus vaccines. *Australian and New Zealand Journal of Obstetrics and Gynaecology* 46(4): 311-5.

Go VF, Quan VM et al. (2002) Barriers to reproductive tract infection (RTI) care among Vietnamese women - Implications for RTI control programs. *Sexually Transmitted Diseases* 29(4): 201-206.

Grgic-Vitek M, Klavs I et al. (2002) Syphilis epidemic in Slovenia influenced by syphilis epidemic in the Russian Federation and other newly independent states. *International Journal of STD and AIDS* 13 Suppl 2: 2-4.

Gulcur L (2000) Evaluating the role of gender inequalities and rights violations in women's mental health. *Health and Human Rights*, 5(1): 46-66.

Gupta S et al. (2003) Delivering equitable care: comparing preventive services in Manitoba. *American Journal of Public Health*, 93(12): 2086-2092.

Guo SF (1999) Cultural and personal behavioral factors and women's reproductive tract infections. *Chinese Medical Journal* 112(11): 1044-1048.

Guo SF, Wang LH et al. (2002) Health service needs of women with reproductive tract infections in selected areas of China. *Chinese Medical Journal* 115(8): 1253-1256.

Handsfield HH (1997) Clinical presentation and natural course of anogenital warts. *American Journal of Medicine* 102(5A): 16-20.

Havercamp S, Scandlin D, Roth M (2004) Health disparities among adults with developmental disabilities, adults with other disabilities, and adults not reporting disability in North Carolina. *Public Health Report*, 119(4): 418-426.

Hawkes S, Morison L et al. (1999) Reproductive-tract infections in women in low-income, low-prevalence situations: assessment of syndromic management in Matlab, Bangladesh. *Lancet* 354(9192): 1776-1781.

Hernandez-Giron CA, Cruz-Valdez A et al. (1998) Prevalence and risk factors associated with syphilis in women. *Review Saude Publica* 32(6): 579-86.

Hilton P (2001) Vesico-vaginal fistula: new perspectives. *Current Opinion in Obstetrics and Gynecology*, 13: 513-520.

Hilton P, Ward A (1998) Epidemiological and surgical aspects of urogenital fistula: a review of 25 years experience in south-east Nigeria. *International Urogynecology Journal and Pelvic Floor Dysfunction*, 9: 189-194.

Hoekstra, CEL, Riedijk M et al. (2006) Prevalence of HIV and syphilis in pregnant women in Leon, Nicaragua. *American Journal of Tropical Medicine and Hygiene* 75(3): 522-525.

Holmes M (1999). Sexually transmitted infections in female rape victims. *AIDS, Patient Care and STDS* 13(12): 703-708.

Holtgrave DR, Crosby RA (2003) Social capital, poverty, and income inequality as predictors of gonorrhoea, syphilis, chlamydia and AIDS case rates in the United States. *Sexually Transmitted Infections* 79(1): 62-64.

Hunt J, Geia L (2002) Can we better meet the healthcare needs of Aboriginal and Torres Strait Islander women? *Medical Journal of Australia*, 177(18 November): 533-534.

Ibrahim T, Sadiq A, Daniel S (2000) Characteristics of vesico-vaginal fistula patients as seen at the specialist hospital Sokoto, Nigeria. *West African Medical Journal*, 19: 59-63.

Irving, G, Miller D et al. (1998) Psychological factors associated with recurrent vaginal candidiasis: a preliminary study. *Sexually Transmitted Infections* 74(5): 334-8.

Jaswal S (2001) Gynaecological morbidity and common mental disorders in low-income urban women in Mumbai. In: Davar B, ed., *Mental health from a gender perspective*, New Delhi, Sage Publications: 138-154.

Jewkes R (2000) Violence against women: an emerging health problem. *International Clinical Psychopharmacology* 15: S37-S45.

Johnston A, Fernando D et al. (2005) Sexually transmitted infections in New Zealand in 2003. *New Zealand Medical Journal* 118(1211): U1347.

Judlin PG (2002) Genital herpes and health-related quality of life. *Pathologie Biologie* 50(8): 493-495.

Kahn JA, Slap GB et al. (2005) Psychological, behavioral, and interpersonal impact of human papillomavirus and Pap test results. *Journal of Womens Health* 14(7): 650-9.

Karapetyan AF, Sokolovsky YV et al. (2002) Syphilis among intravenous drug-using population: epidemiological situation in St Petersburg, Russia. *International Journal of STD and AIDS* 13(9): 618-23.

Kawsar M, Anfield A et al. (2004) Prevalence of sexually transmitted infections and mental health needs of female child and adolescent survivors of rape and sexual assault attending a specialist clinic. *Sexually Transmitted Infections* 80(2): 138-141.

Kerani RP, Handsfield HH et al. (2006) Rising Rates of Syphilis in the Era of Syphilis Elimination. *Sexually Transmitted Diseases.*

Kildea S, Bowden FJ (2000) Reproductive health, infertility and sexually transmitted infections in Indigenous women in a remote community in the Northern Territory. *Australian and New Zealand Journal of Public Health* 24 (4): 382-386.

Koenig M et al. (1998) Investigating women's gynaecological morbidity in India: not just another KAP survey. *Reproductive Health Matters*, 6(11): 84-96.

Kumari S, Walia I, Singh A (2000) Self-reported uterine prolapse in a resettlement colony of North India. *Journal of Midwifery and Women's Health*, 45(4): 343-350.

Leggatt GR, Frazer IH (2007) HPV vaccines: the beginning of the end for cervical cancer. *Current Opinions in Immunology.*

Lewis LM, Rosenthal SL et al. (1999) College students' knowledge and perceptions of genital herpes. *International Journal of STD & AIDS* 10(11): 703-708.

Li LK, Dai M et al. (2006) Human papillomavirus infection in Shenyang City, People's Republic of China: A population-based study. *British Journal of Cancer* 95(11): 1593-7.

Linnehan M, Groce NE (2000) Counseling and educational interventions for women with genital human papillomavirus infection. *AIDS Patient Care and STDS* 14(8): 439-445.

Longo D, Koehn K (1993) Psychosocial Factors and Recurrent Genital Herpes - a Review of Prediction and Psychiatric-Treatment Studies. *International Journal of Psychiatry in Medicine* 23(2): 99-117.

Luber K, Boero M, Choe J (2001) The demographics of pelvic floor disorders: current observations and future projections. *American Journal of Obstetrics and Gynaecology*, 184(7): 1496-1503.

Mak DB, Johnson GH et al. (2004) A syphilis outbreak in remote Australia: epidemiology and strategies for control. *Epidemiology of Infections* 132(5): 805-12.

Manhart LE, Dialmy A et al. (2000) Sexually transmitted diseases in Morocco: gender influences on prevention and health care seeking behavior. *Social Science & Medicine* 50 (10): 1369-1383.

Markovic M, Manderson L et al. (2006) Treatment decisions: A qualitative study with women with gynaecological cancer. *Australian & New Zealand Journal of Obstetrics & Gynaecology* 46(1): 46-48.

Martin SL, Matza LS et al. (1999) Domestic violence and sexually transmitted diseases: The experience of prenatal care patients. *Public Health Reports* 114(3): 262-268.

Mason L (2001) Evidence-based midwifery in action. Guidelines on the teaching of pelvic floor exercises. *British Journal of Midwifery*, 9(10): 608-611.

McCaffery K, Waller J et al. (2006) Social and psychological impact of HPV testing in cervical screening: a qualitative study. *Sexually Transmitted Infections* 82(2): 169-74.

Melville J, Sniffen S et al. (2003) Psychosocial impact of serological diagnosis of herpes simplex virus type 2: a qualitative assessment. *Sexually Transmitted Infections* 79(4): 280-285.

Messer E (1997) Intra-household allocation of food and health care: current findings and understandings-introduction. *Social Science and Medicine*, 44(11): 1675-1684.

Miller SM, Mischel W et al. (1996) From human papillomavirus (HPV) to cervical cancer: Psychosocial processes in infection, detection, and control. *Annals of Behavioral Medicine* 18(4): 219-228.

Miller K, Rosenfield A (1996) Population and women's reproductive health: an international perspective. *Annual Review of Public Health*, 17: 359-382.

Mindel A (1996) Psychological and psychosexual implications of herpes simplex virus infections. *Scandinavian Journal of Infectious Diseases* 100: 27-32.

Moerman M (1982) Growth of the birth canal in adolescent girls. *American Journal of Obstetrics and Gynecology*, 143(5): 528-532.

Muleta M (2004) Socio-demographic profile and obstetric experience of fistula patients managed at the Addis Ababa Fistula Hospital. *Ethiopian Medical Journal*, 42(1): 9-16.

Nigro L, Larocca L et al. (2006) Prevalence of HIV and other sexually transmitted diseases among Colombian and Dominican female sex workers living in Catania, Eastern Sicily. *Journal of Immigrant and Minority Health* 8(4): 319-23.

Norton P et al. (1995) Genitourinary prolapse and joint hypermobility in women. *Obstetrics and Gynecology*, 85: 225-228.

Nuwaha F, Faxelid E et al. (2000) Psychosocial determinants for sexual partner referral in Uganda: qualitative results. *International Journal of STD & AIDS* 11(3): 156-161.

O'Keefe EJ, Gardner A et al. (2006) Prevalence of genital human papillomavirus DNA in a sample of senior school-aged women in the Australian Capital Territory. *Sex Health* 3(2): 91-4.

Oliveira LH, Rosa ML et al. (2006) Human papillomavirus status and cervical abnormalities in women from public and private health care in Rio de Janeiro State, Brazil. *Review Institute of Medicine Tropica* Sao Paulo 48(5): 279-85.

Olsen A et al. (1997) Epidemiology of surgically managed pelvic organ prolapse and urinary incontinence. *Obstetrics and Gynecology*, 89: 501-506.

Pagliusi S. Vaccine Research and Development ([2001] 2003) *Vaccines against human papillomavirus*. Geneva, World Health Organization. 2007.

Pajaro MC, Barberis IL et al. (2001) Epidemiology of sexually transmitted diseases in Rio Cuarto, Argentina. *Review Latinoam Microbiology* 43(4): 157-60.

Papreen N, Sharma A et al. (2000) Living with infertility: Experiences among urban slum populations in Bangladesh. *Reproductive Health Matters* 8(15): 33-44.

Paris M, Gotuzzo E et al. (1999) Prevalence of gonococcal and chlamydial infections in commercial sex workers in a Peruvian Amazon city. *Sexually Transmitted Diseases* 26(2): 103-107.

Parkin DM (1994) Cancer in developing countries. *Cancer Survey* 19-20: 519-61.

Parkin DM, Bray F et al. (2005) Global Cancer Statistics, 2002. *Cancer Journal Clinics* 55(2): 74-108.

Parkin DM, Pisani P et al. (1999) Global cancer statistics. *Cancer Journal Clinics* 49(1): 33-64.

Patel V, Oomman N (1999) Mental health matters too: gynaecological symptoms and depression in South Asia. *Reproductive Health Matters*, 7(14): 30-38.

Patel V et al. (1999) Women, poverty and common mental disorders in four restructuring societies. *Social Science and Medicine*, 49: 1461-1471.

Paz-Bailey G, Ramaswamy M et al. (2007) Herpes simplex virus type 2: epidemiology and management options in developing countries. *Sexually Transmitted Infections* 83(1): 16-22.

Pereira DB, Antoni MH et al. (2003) Stress as a predictor of symptomatic genital herpes virus recurrence in women with human immunodeficiency virus. *Journal of Psychosomatic Research* 54(3): 237-244.

Petchesky R (1998) Cross-country comparisons and political visions. In: Petchesky R, Judd K, eds., *Negotiating reproductive rights. Women's perspectives across countries and cultures,* London, Zed Books: 295-323.

Philips Z, Avis M et al. (2005) Knowledge of cervical cancer and screening among women in east-central England. *International Journal of Gynecological Cancer* 15(4): 639-45.

Piot P, Islam MQ (1994) Sexually transmitted diseases in the 1990s. Global epidemiology and challenges for control. *Sexually Transmitted Diseases* 21(2 Suppl): S7-13.

Pitts M, Bowman M et al. (1995) Reactions to Repeated STD Infections - Psychosocial-Aspects and Gender Issues in Zimbabwe. *Social Science & Medicine* 40(9): 1299-1304.

Plazaola-Castano J, Perez IR (2004) Intimate partner violence and physical and mental health consequences. *Medicina Clinica* 122(12): 461-467.

Posner TN, Boyle FM et al. (2006) Prevalence and risk factors for lifetime exposure to Pap smear abnormalities in the Australian community. *Sex Health* 3(4): 275-9.

Potterat JJ, Zimmerman-Rogers H et al. (1999) Chlamydia transmission: Concurrency, reproduction number, and the epidemic trajectory. *American Journal of Epidemiology* 150(12): 1331-1339.

Prasad J, Abraham S et al. (2003) Symptoms related to the reproductive tract and mental health among women in rural southern India. *National Medical Journal of India* 16(6): 303-308.

Purevdawa E, Moon TD et al. (1997) Rise in sexually transmitted diseases during democratization and economic crisis in Mongolia. *International Journal of STD & AIDS* 8(6): 398-401.

Ramasubban R, Rishyasringa B (2001) Weakness ('ashaktapana') and reproductive health among women in a slum population in Mumbai. *Cultural Perspectives on Reproductive Health.* C. M. Obermeyer. Oxford, Oxford University Press.

Rein M (2000) Stress and genital herpes recurrences in women. *Journal of the American Medical Association* 283(11): 1394.

Resl V, Kumpova M (2005) Interaction of legislation and prevalence of sexually transmitted diseases with focus on syphilis and gonorrhoea in the Czech Republic - review to year 2003. *Journal of European Academy of Dermatology and Venereology* 19(6): 692-5.

Reynolds SJ, Risbud AR et al. (2006) High rates of syphilis among STI patients are contributing to the spread of HIV-1 in India. *Sexually Transmitted Infections* 82(2): 121-6.

Roche P et al (2001) Australia's notifiable disease status, 1999: annual report of the National Notifiable Diseases Surveillance System. *Communicable Diseases Intelligence* 25 (4): 7pp.

Rosenthal SL, Biro FM (1991) A Preliminary Investigation of the Psychological Impact of Sexually-Transmitted Diseases in Adolescent Females. *Adolescent and Pediatric Gynecology* 4(4): 198-201.

Ross JL, Laston SL et al. (2002) Exploring explanatory models of women's reproductive health in rural Bangladesh. *Culture Health & Sexuality* 4(2): 173-190.

Shrier LA, Harris SK et al. (2001) Associations of depression, self-esteem, and substance use with sexual risk among adolescents. *Preventive Medicine* 33(3): 179-189.

Singh V, Sehgal A et al. (1995) Clinical presentation of gynecologic infections among Indian women. *Obstetrics and Gynecology* 85(2): 215-9.

Smacchia C, Parolin A et al. (1998) Syphilis in prostitutes from Eastern Europe. *Lancet* 351(9102): 572.

Spencer B, Leplege A et al. (1999) Recurrent genital herpes and quality of life in France. *Quality of Life Research* 8(4): 365-371.

Stewart DE et al. (1990) Psychosocial aspects of chronic, clinically unconfirmed vulvovaginitis. *Obstetrics and Gynecology,* 75: 852-856.

Stoler MH (1996) A brief synopsis of the role of human papillomaviruses in cervical carcinogenesis. *American Journal of Obstetrics and Gynecology* 175(4 Pt 2): 1091-8.

Sundari Ravindran T, Savitri R, Bhavani A (1999) Women's experiences of utero-vaginal prolapse: a qualitative study from Tamil Nadu, India. In: Berer M, Sundari Ravindran T, eds., *Safe motherhood: critical issues,* London, Blackwell Science: 166-172.

Suris JC, Resnick MD et al. (1996) Sexual behavior of adolescents with chronic disease and disability. *Journal of Adolescent Health* 19(2): 124-131.

Taboulet F, Halioua B et al. (1999) Quality of life and use of health care among people with genital herpes in France. *Acta Dermato-Venereologica* 79(5): 380-384.

Thirumoorthy T (1990) The epidemiology of sexually transmitted diseases in Southeast Asia and the western Pacific. *Seminars Dermatology* 9(2): 102-4.

Tichonova L, Borisenko K et al. (1997) Epidemics of syphilis in the Russian Federation: trends, origins, and priorities for control. *Lancet* 350(9072): 210-3.

Tinkle MB (1990) Genital human papillomavirus infection. A growing health risk. *Journal of Obstetric Gynecological and Neonatal Nursing* 19(6): 501-7.

Trollope-Kumar K (2001) Cultural and biomedical meanings of the complaint of leukorrhea in South Asian women. *Tropical Medicine & International Health* 6(4): 260-266.

Upchurch DM, Kusunoki Y (2004) Associations between forced sex, sexual and protective practices, and sexually transmitted diseases among a national sample of adolescent girls. *Women's Health Issues* 14(3): 75-84.

UNFPA. (2001) *Report on the meeting for the prevention and treatment of obstetric fistula. London.* New York, United Nations Population Fund.

UNFPA. (2002) *Mending torn lives: initiatives against obstetric fistula.* New York, United Nations Population Fund (http://www.unfpa.org/mothers/ fistula/index.htm).

Uribe-Salas F, Conde-Glez CJ et al. (2003) Sociodemographic dynamics and sexually transmitted infections in female sex workers at the Mexican-Guatemalan border. *Sexually Transmitted Diseases* 30(3): 266-71.

Uuskula A, Silm H et al. (1997) Sexually transmitted diseases in Estonia: past and present. *International Journal of STD and AIDS* 8(7): 446-50.

Vangeenderhuysen C, Prual A, Ould el Joud D (2001) Obstetric fistulae: incidence estimates for sub-Saharan Africa. *International Journal of Gynecology and Obstetrics*, 73: 65-66.

Voeten H, O'Hara HB et al. (2004) Gender differences in health care-seeking behavior for sexually transmitted diseases - A population-based study in Nairobi, Kenya. *Sexually Transmitted Diseases* 31(5): 265-272.

Wade AS, Kane CT et al. (2005) HIV infection and sexually transmitted infections among men who have sex with men in Senegal. *Aids* 19(18): 2133-40.

Wall L (1999) Birth trauma and the pelvic floor: lessons from the developing world. *Journal of Women's Health,* 8(2): 149-155.

Wall L et al. (2004) The obstetric vesicovaginal fistula: characteristics of 899 patients from Jos, Nigeria. *American Journal of Obstetrics and Gynecology,* 190(4):1011-1019.

Waller J, McCaffery K et al. (2004) Beliefs about the risk factors for cervical cancer in a British population sample. *Preventive Medicine* 38(6): 745-53.

Walraven G et al. (2001) The burden of reproductive-organ disease in rural women in The Gambia, West Africa. *Lancet,* 357(9263): 1161-1167.

Walraven G, Scherf C et al. (2001) The burden of reproductive-organ disease in rural women in The Gambia, West Africa. *Lancet* 357(9263): 1161-1167.

Walters MD (2004) Pelvic floor disorders in women: an overview. *Revista de Medicina de la Universidad de Navarra,* 48(4): 9-12.

Wathne B et al. (1994) Vaginal discharge: comparison of clinical, laboratory and microbiological findings. *Acta Obstetrica et Gynecologica Scandinavica,* 73(10): 802–808.

Whittaker M (2002) Negotiating care: Reproductive tract infections in Vietnam. *Women & Health* 35(4): 43-57.

Whitten KL, Rein MF et al. (2003) The emotional experience of intercourse and sexually transmitted diseases - A decision-tree analysis. *Sexually Transmitted Diseases* 30(4): 348-356.

World Health Organization (WHO) (2001) *Progress in Reproductive Health Research*, No. 57. Geneva, World Health Organization.

WHO, (2001) *Global Prevalence and Incidence of Selected Curable Sexually Transmitted Infections: Overview and Estimates*. Geneva, Department of Communicable Disease Surveillance and Response, WHO.

WHO, (2006) *Prevention and control of sexually transmitted infections: draft global strategy*. Secretariat. Geneva, World Health Organization: 67.

Wild D, Patrick D et al. (1995) Measuring health-related quality of life in persons with genital herpes. *Quality of Life Research* 4(6): 532-539.

Wiley D, Masongsong E (2006) Human papillomavirus: the burden of infection. *Obstetric and Gynecological Survey* 61(6 Suppl 1): S3-14.

Williams KM, Wingood GM et al. (2002) Prevalence and correlates of Chlamydia trachomatis among sexually active African-American adolescent females. *Preventive Medicine* 35(6): 593-600.

Winter AJ, Sriskandabalan P et al. (2000) Sociodemography of genital Chlamydia trachomatis in Coventry, UK, 1992-6. *Sexually Transmitted Infections* 76(2): 103-109.

Yakubovsky A, Sokolovsky E et al. (2006) Syphilis management in St. Petersburg, Russia: 1995-2001. *Sexually Transmitted Diseases* 33(4): 244-9.

Zakoucka H, Polanecky V et al. (2004) Syphilis and gonorrhoea in the Czech Republic. *European Surveillance* 9(12): 18-20.

Zurayk H et al. (1995) Comparing women's reports with medical diagnoses of reproductive morbidity conditions in rural Egypt. *Studies in Family Planning,* 26(1): 14-21.

Chapter 7

Women's mental health in the context of HIV/AIDS

Mridula Bandyopadhyay

The epidemic of human immunodeficiency virus (HIV) infection and acquired immunodeficiency syndrome (AIDS) is a major international public health problem, especially in contexts where access to health services is difficult and social inequalities are marked. The patterns of transmission of HIV and development of AIDS reflect the socioeconomic context of infection and disease: disproportionately, the populations affected are poor, marginalized, ethnic minorities, and people living in resource-poor settings and countries (Dodds et al., 2000; Tiamson, 2002). Worldwide, the number of women living with HIV is the highest it has been in the history of the epidemic (UNAIDS, 2006b). Poverty is a major factor in risk of infection, and in the impact of infection on a person's general health. At the same time, the increase in the extent and severity of poverty that occurs with AIDS is felt most acutely by women. Rights violations, economic dependence, lack of decision-making power, conflicting gender roles, disproportionate domestic responsibilities, and gender-based violence are also closely linked to, and contribute to, reproductive and mental health problems for women (Gulcur, 2000). There is, however, a marked lack of evidence on women's mental health and how it interacts with vulnerability, risk of HIV infection, response to diagnosis, and subsequent health care (Patel & Oomman, 1999). Most research on HIV/AIDS and its effects on mental health has been conducted in the United States; there is some from other rich countries, but very little from developing countries.

Gender and the risk of contracting HIV/AIDS

Since the HIV epidemic began, more than 60 million people have been infected with the virus, and globally 39.5 million people are currently living with HIV/AIDS. In 2006, there were 4.3 million new infections, and 2.9 million deaths from HIV/AIDS, making it the fourth leading cause of death in the world (UNAIDS, 2006b). The AIDS epidemic is highly concentrated in Africa, with especially high prevalence in the sub-Saharan region. In 2006, 63% of people living with HIV and 72% of all deaths from AIDS occurred in sub-Saharan Africa.

Worldwide, at the end of December 2006, 17.7 million adult women (aged 15 years and over) were living with HIV, an increase from 16.5 million in 2004 and 17.3 million in 2005 (UNAIDS, 2006a, 2006b). In 2006, worldwide, 48% of all HIV-infected adults were women; this rate reaches almost 60% in sub-Saharan Africa. Three-quarters of all HIV-positive women live in sub-Saharan Africa. One-third of pregnant women visiting clinics for antenatal checkups are HIV-positive (UNAIDS, 2006a).

HIV/AIDS has spread particularly rapidly among women because of entrenched and pervasive gender inequality. Clinical research has shown that women who contract HIV/AIDS have shorter survival times than men do because they tend to seek treatment later, if at all (Bury, Morrison & McLachlan, 1992). Studies of women's particular vulnerability to various infections, including HIV, have until recently concentrated on clinical and physiological aspects, while the psychological and mental health ramifications have received less research attention. There have been few investigations of the social epidemiology of HIV infection and its interaction with mental health in women, particularly in resource-poor settings. However, there appears to be an intricate relationship between mental health and disease progression, quality of life and disease outcome. Clark (1998), in a review of the literature on the emotional impact of HIV/AIDS, described qualitative differences between women and men in terms of grief, shame, and depression. In addition, women experienced gender-specific social stigma, a greater sense of isolation, and oppression related to gender, stigma, ethnicity, poverty, and route of infection.

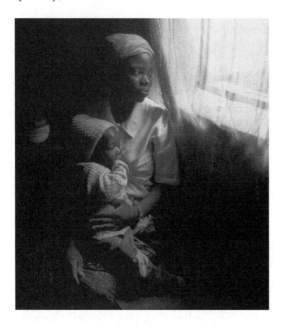

Worldwide in 2006, 2.3 million children under 12 years of age were infected with HIV, two million of them in sub-Saharan Africa (UNAIDS, 2006a). In 2005, half of all new adult HIV infections were in young people between the ages of 15 and 24 years (UNAIDS, 2006b). In particular, the incidcence of HIV among female adolescents is increasing steadily, affecting their life circumstances and potential by predisposing them to poor physical and mental health (Brady et al., 2002). Young women are particularly vulnerable to HIV infection, because their vaginal wall is thinner than that of older women, and they have a higher risk of epithelial lesions through which infection can occur. Girls and women are often dependent on men for financial security, and the combination of dependence and subordination makes it difficult for them to insist on safe sex

(even from their partner or husband), or to end relationships that increase their risk of infection (UNAIDS, 2002a, 2002b; UNIFEM, 2001). Young women are also more at risk of HIV infection for social and economic reasons, including poor access to education, information, employment, and health care. For example, in northern Thailand, commercial sex work is the "choice" of many young women in the face of family debt, landlessness and poverty, or as a way of escaping from unhappy or abusive relationships. These young women may risk assault if they insist on condom use, and may be dependent on drugs and alcohol to deal with the circumstances of their work (Bond, Celentano & Yaddhanaphuti, 1996).

In cultures where early marriage is common, young married women often have a higher risk of HIV infection, because of its association with early sexual debut, high frequency of intercourse, low condom use, and women's limited right to refuse sex. Recent research in urban settings in Kenya and Zambia, which sought to explain the higher rates of HIV infection in young married women than in single women, found that their husbands were three times more likely to be HIV-positive than the boyfriends of the single women (Clarke, 2004). Ulin, Cayemittes & Gringle (1996) reported that between 80% and 90% of HIV-infected Haitian women attending antenatal clinics had "no possible source of infection other than their own husbands" (WHO, 2001). While women have the right, in theory, to refuse sex, in reality their partners might not recognize this right; alternatively, they may turn to sex workers, where they risk contracting the virus and bringing it back to infect their wife. "Women tend to agree that refusing sex amounts to little less than a death warrant for themselves." "People say that when you like the skin, you should like the seed. In these times – with AIDS on the streets – you have to accept when your husband says, 'Let's make love'" (Ulin, Cayemittes & Gringle, 1996).

Women may also be subject to reprisals if they refuse sex, such as the withdrawal of financial support or domestic violence: (Ulin, Cayemittes & Gringle, 1996). A history of trauma has also been found to be a general risk factor for HIV in women (Jones et al., 2001; Wyatt et al., 2002).

Sociocultural, economic and educational barriers impede effective communication between partners (Gupta, Weiss & Mane, 1996). Lack of information about reproductive anatomy may also contribute to fears and pressures experienced by women: one review revealed that women from several countries, including Brazil, India, Jamaica and South Africa, did not like using condoms because they feared the condom might fall off inside the vagina and harm them (Gupta, Weiss & Mane, 1996).

Gender-based violence and HIV/AIDS

Gender-based violence can be both a contributor to, and a consequence of, HIV infection. Sexual violence and abuse are now recognized as a significant public health concern, placing women at high risk of sexually transmitted infections (STIs), including HIV, and a range of post-traumatic stress disorders, with adverse effects on physical and mental health (Carballo, Grocutt & Hadzihasanovic, 1996; McMahon, Goodwin & Stringer, 2000; Fikree & Bhatti, 1999). Reproductive tract infections, including STIs and HIV, contribute to a significant level of ill-health in women of reproductive age, and continue to pose a threat beyond the menopause (Sadik, 1997). The best predictors of HIV risk for women are limited material resources, previous exposure to violence, and high-risk sexual behaviour (Wyatt et al., 2002).

In December 1998, a young South African woman, Gugu Dlamini, was beaten to death by members of her community after disclosing her HIV status, because she was seen to be a disgrace to the community (Vetten & Bhana, 2001). Recently, an Indian women's rights group investigated the death of a woman with HIV/AIDS in Andhra Pradesh, India, and concluded that she had been stoned after being turned out of her family home. The National Commission for Women said they had not been able to determine the exact cause of death, but there were suggestions that she had been burned alive. However, the National AIDS Control Authority said that she had died of natural causes (BBC, 2003).

Sexual violence by men against women and girls of all ages is found in all societies. Violence and sexual exploitation increase women's and girls' exposure to, and risk of, multiple infections, including HIV, and have serious implications for women's ability to protect themselves from HIV infection (Institute of Development Studies, 2002). Women and girls are extremely vulnerable in coercive situations, where they have little power to insist on condom use or otherwise control the terms on which sex takes place. Several studies from South Africa, for example, have found that more than one in four women report that their first sexual encounter was forced (Astbury, 2002). .Furthermore, in a study involving 48 countries, WHO found that 10–69% of women had been abused by an intimate partner (WHO, 2002).

The HIV pandemic has reinforced gender-based violence, stigmatization and discrimination against women. Women who are HIV-positive, or who are perceived to be HIV-positive, may be subject to discriminatory treatment, abandoned and shunned by their families and communities, dismissed from employment, assaulted, and even killed if their husband or partner dies. Women are more likely than men to be blamed for spreading the disease and stigmatized as promiscuous (UNIFEM, 2001).

HIV-positive women experience high rates of sexual and physical violence (Gielen et al., 2000; Vlahov et al., 1998; Zierler, Witbeck & Mayer, 1996), often have inadequate social support (Catalan et al., 1996; Linn et al., 1996), and express concerns about stigma, discrimination and hopelessness (Gielen et al., 1997; Pizzi, 1992; Quinn, 1993; Sowell et al., 1997). A study by Kimerling, Armistead & Forehand (1999) found that HIV-positive women were more likely to report a violent victimization experience, and had higher levels of psychological distress, depressive symptoms, and distress regarding physical symptoms (see also Linn et al., 1996).

Various studies have reported that women and girls living with HIV/AIDS are significantly more likely to have experienced traumatic life events, such as incest, sexual assault, significant physical abuse, and substance abuse (Brady et al., 2002; Emlet & Gusz, 1998; Moser, Sowell & Phillips, 2001). Wyatt et al. (2002), in their investigation of HIV-related risk factors in a community sample in the United States, found that HIV-positive women had had more sexual partners and more sexually transmitted infections, and had suffered more severe abuse than HIV-negative women. Sexual abuse, incidents of rape and attempted rape since the age of 18, and physical abuse in childhood and adulthood increase the risk of HIV infection. Several other factors are also linked to HIV risk, including racial or ethnic group affiliation, socioeconomic status, overall health, sexual risk-taking, and prevalence of sexually transmitted infections (Newcomb et al., 1998; Wyatt, Forge & Guthrie, 1998; Wyatt et al., 1999). Women who report early and chronic sexual abuse have a sevenfold higher prevalence of HIV-related risk behaviour and markers of risk than women with no history of abuse (Allers et al., 1993; Arnow et al., 1999; Bensley, Van Eenwyk & Simmons, 2000; Parillo et al., 2001; Thompson et al., 1997; Zierler et al., 1991). The associations between child sexual abuse and HIV-related risks in adulthood have been well documented (Allers et al., 1993; Heise, Moore & Toubia, 1995; Zierler et al., 1991).

In war and conflict situations, the risk and incidence of violence against women escalate, because of breakdown of law and order, large-scale population movements, particularly of women and children, rape of young girls and women by opposing forces, and increased "survival sex", as women try to survive the loss of income, home and family (Institute of Development Studies, 2002). These factors all have an immense impact on women's psychological well-being and coping mechanisms.

Women who have sex in exchange for goods, services, security or money are at an especially increased risk of infection. Some employers may also try to exact sexual services in exchange for job security (Gordon & Crehan, 1999; Institute of Development Studies, 2002; UNAIDS, 2002a, 2002b; UNIFEM, 2001). In resource-poor settings, the context of most sex work and sexual transactions is poverty-driven, and the priority for many women is to make money to keep themselves and their families alive, rather than avoiding becoming infected.

In addition, in many countries, women have little access to treatment, and post-exposure prophylaxis (PEP) is not available. PEP is the administration of antiretroviral medication after a high-risk exposure in order to reduce the likelihood of HIV infection. Theoretically, PEP may prevent establishment of infection (Anderson, 2000). Currently, in most countries, PEP is available only to health care professionals, and is not available to women, children and men who have been sexually assaulted or raped. Recommendations have recently been developed for PEP after non-occupational exposure to HIV. So far, limited data are available regarding the type of exposures for which PEP is prescribed, and little is known about the population most likely to seek PEP (Kwong et al., 1999). Even when PEP is available (e.g. in the industrialized countries), many women have no knowledge or information about it and no means of accessing it.

Domestic violence is also associated with increased HIV-related risks (Kimerling, Armistead & Forehand, 1999; Wingood & DiClemente, 1997a, 1997b). Women in violent relationships tend to have more partners, are less able to negotiate sexual decisions, and are more at risk of HIV infection (Amaro, 1995; Wyatt et al., 2002). Kalichman et al. (2002), in a study in the USA, found that 68% of women and 35% of men living with HIV/AIDS reported having been sexually assaulted since the age of 15. They reported greater anxiety, depression, and symptoms of borderline personality disorder, and were more likely to have unprotected intercourse and to have traded sex than HIV-negative subjects. Women with HIV/AIDS who had been sexually assaulted reported more symptoms of trauma, depression, emotional distress, HIV symptoms, opportunistic infections and AIDS-defining conditions than HIV-infected women who had not been sexually assaulted (Kimerling, Armistead & Forehand, 1999; Simoni & Ng, 2000). Similar conclusions were drawn by Gielen et al. (2001), although they also found that a supportive social network was associated with better mental health and overall quality of life.

Research by Wyatt et al. (2002) showed that being HIV-positive is associated with significantly lower income for women of all ethnic groups. Regardless of ethnicity, women who are seropositive are more likely to report being victims of adult sexual abuse and to report a more severe history of trauma than other women. Women who had had more sexual partners, were unemployed, had had more STIs, had a history of more severe trauma, or were less educated were also more likely to be HIV-positive.

Low socioeconomic resources, exposure to violence, and risky sexual behaviour increase vulnerability to infection (Wyatt et al., 2002). In most societies, racial and ethnic minorities are marginalized and underprivileged, have less access to education, information and knowledge, have fewer economic resources, live in poorer sections of the society, engage in high-risk behaviour or engage in transactional sex for survival, and have unaddressed psychosocial problems. Indirectly, therefore, HIV/AIDS risk is a function of race and ethnicity.

Inability to access socioeconomic resources, especially employment and education, may be more important than income in increasing risk of HIV infection (Schifrin, 2001). A growing number of women are being diagnosed as having both HIV infection and substance abuse problems, particularly in industrialized countries (Moser, Sowell & Phillips, 2001); substance abuse is classified as a psychiatric disorder.

Sexual and physical abuse are frequently associated with physical and psychological co-morbidities. For example, Wingood, DiClemente & Raj (2000) found that women experiencing both sexual and physical abuse were more likely to have a history of multiple STIs, be worried about being infected with HIV, use marijuana and alcohol to cope, attempt suicide, feel as though they had no control in their relationships, and experience more episodes of physical abuse. Such traumatic life experiences are often associated with high rates of psychiatric co-morbidity, clinical depression or anxiety, substance abuse, and possible non-compliance with recommended health care and treatment (Brady et al., 2002; Weingourt et al., 2001).

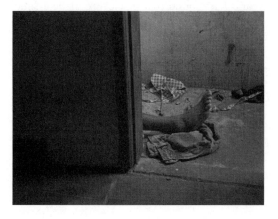

Other studies on violence and its relationship to mental health have come to similar conclusions, particularly that women exposed to physical and sexual abuse are more likely to have a high level of depressive symptoms and psychiatric disorders (Hall et al., 1993; Mullen et al., 1988). Roberts et al. (1998a, 1998b) found that women in Australia who experienced abuse as adults had elevated rates of mental disorders compared with non-abused women; women who had experienced abuse both in childhood and as adults had still higher rates. Women who reported sexual abuse in adulthood had increased rates of anxiety, dysthymia, depression, phobias, harmful alcohol consumption and psychoactive drug dependence. Doubly abused women (as a child and as an adult) also had a significantly higher risk of harmful alcohol consumption and drug dependence.

A recent study investigating violence among HIV-infected women in Zambia found three major problems; domestic violence, symptoms of depression, and alcohol abuse (Murray et al., 2006). The authors highlighted the important overlap between violence and HIV infection, and identified the potential for a cyclical pattern to materialize, in which exposure to violence in childhood leads to risky sexual behaviour, which leads to increased risk of HIV infection, which leads back to the initial risk of violence related to HIV status (Murray et al., 2006).

Migration and HIV/AIDS

Globally, each year, nearly 95 million women migrate, comprising almost 50% of all international migrants (UNFPA, 2006). Social and economic factors play a major role in migration (Institute of Development Studies, 2002). In many cases, women dominate migration flows, because female migration has increased as a survival strategy for families (Wolffers & Fernandez, 1999). The governments of a number of developing countries, e.g. Bangladesh, Indonesia, the Philippines, and Sri Lanka, help their people to migrate (Fernandez, 1998).

Most migrant workers travel without their sexual partners. They often have to deal with the disruption of social support, poor living conditions and poor provision of care for their health needs (Bandyopadhyay & Thomas, 2002; Fernandez, 1998; UNAIDS, 1998). Migrant women face double problems, as women and as migrants (Long & Ankrah, 1996; Lukalo, 1998). Being a migrant is not in itself a risk factor for infections, but circumstances can lead to increased personal risk. Two quite different sources of risk may be present in a migrant's life: stress, and sexual abuse and exploitation. In these situations, stress is associated with low wages, poor working and housing conditions and lack of autonomy. Unwelcome sexual attention and sexual abuse by employers are often reported (Bandyopadhyay & Thomas, 2002; Institute of Development Studies, 2002; Singhanetra-Renard, 1997).

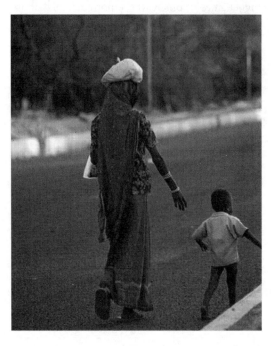

Sexual abuse and exploitation are under-acknowledged features of the working environment, particularly for women working in the entertainment industry, as domestic servants, or in the sex industry. Women are particularly vulnerable in work situations involving isolation and low levels of social support. Their low status, low pay, and isolation from family and social support networks make them vulnerable to abuse and infection, and increase their dependence on others for survival. Migrant women are regularly confronted with sexual harassment, discrimination and exploitation. They are often trapped in situations where they cannot refuse to provide sexual services (Fernandez, 1998). They may have few negotiation skills and little or no bargaining power. During the initial period of adaptation, migrants are particularly vulnerable to STIs and HIV infection. Migrant workers are generally concerned first with their livelihood and survival, rather than HIV risk (Bandyopadhyay & Thomas, 2002). Stress often

contributes to the greater vulnerability of migrants to STIs and HIV/AIDS, as well as to emotional and mental health problems.

Mental health and HIV/AIDS

The mental health problems experienced by women who have HIV infection are considerable and have multiple causes (Tostes, 2004; Murray, 2004). A study in Bangkok, Thailand, documented the profound negative impact of HIV infection on women who had given birth and their families (Manopaiboon et al., 1998). The women experienced depressive symptoms and anxiety, primarily related to being HIV-infected, but also to their children's and partner's health. Other adverse family impacts that women faced were reduced income, separation from or death of partner, shifting child care responsibilities, and family migration.

An estimated one in four women newly infected with HIV is between 35 and 44 years of age, (Kalichman, Heckman & Kochman, 2000). Little is known about the impact of HIV/AIDS on these women and their partners and families. However, VanDevanter et al. (1999), in a study on the impact of a diagnosis of HIV on serodiscordant heterosexual couples, identified four major sets of issues: (1) the emotional and sexual impact on the relationship; (2) reproductive decisions; (3) the future of children and the non-infected partner; and (4) disclosure of the infection to friends and family. Specific links have been found between stigma, disclosure and the mental health status of women. Comer et al. (2000) studied the relationship between disclosure of infection and mental health among an ethnically diverse group of 176 women with mean age 36.5 years. They found that disclosure made a small but independent contribution to mental health status. In stigmatized groups, disclosure was predictive of poorer mental health status. The researchers also explored an alternative model, that poor mental health might predict lower levels of disclosure. They looked at one particular study of Hispanic women in the United States, where greater disclosure was related to higher levels of depression, psychological distress, and reported pain (although this finding did not hold up for African-American or European women) (Comer et al., 2000).

Throughout their lives, women may face a variety of challenges: fear of unwanted pregnancy, partner infidelity, HIV infection, family rejection, loss of economic support and domestic violence. Married women often face considerable difficulty in attempting to assert their reproductive rights. If they request their partner to use a condom as a preventive measure, they may be seen as promiscuous or unfaithful (Long & Ankrah, 1996). On the other hand, if they contract HIV, they face being accused of causing it. "My wife at home cannot ask me to use condoms, but sometimes you sleep with a young girl. This young girl can ask you, because she doesn't want to get pregnant and have problems with her parents" (Ulin, Cayemittes & Gringle, 1996).

Women's disclosure of their HIV infection often triggers a downward spiral to destitution. In addition to the physical effects of the infection, women often lose their jobs and the support of their husbands, and are forced to turn to prostitution to feed, clothe, and educate their children. The multiple difficulties, including loss of physical and financial independence, discrimination, and other HIV-related problems, can often lead to significant distress and a risk of suicide (Heckman et al., 1999). Suicide is one of the ten leading causes of death for women aged 35–44 years, and the risk of suicide is significantly higher among those with HIV infection (Kalichman, Heckman & Kochman, 2000).

A emerging trend has been the increase in HIV infection among people aged over 50 years, reaching approximately 2.8 million cases in 2005 (UNAIDS, 2006a). The dominant risk factor for older women is heterosexual sex. Older women are particularly vulnerable, both because of the sexual behaviour of their husband or partner, and because of physiological changes that occur during menopause, such as thinning of the vaginal wall and reduced lubrication. A study of HIV-positive women over 45 years of age identified five risk factors for contracting HIV: poor mental health, substance abuse, ignorance of the earlier HIV risk behaviour of sexual partners, risk-taking in order to preserve the relationship, and lack of information on HIV prevention (Neundorfer, 2005). Mental health issues, often related to childhood or domestic abuse, were found to contribute to an increased risk of HIV. In many societies, multiple partner relationships are condoned for men, further increasing women's vulnerability to STIs, including HIV (Institute of Development Studies, 2002; Kalichman, Heckman & Kochman, 2000).

Globally, HIV/AIDS still carries a stigma, and discrimination and religious and other forms of social condemnation and sanctions persist. Depression is common among those who are infected, and is associated with a variety of other problems, including lowered immune response, disease progression to AIDS, shorter survival time, increased disability, and a lower quality of life (Chesney et al., 1996; Leserman et al., 2000; Sambamoorthi et al., 2000). Generally, patients are more likely to develop depression at two specific times: when they are diagnosed and when the first symptoms appear. HIV patients with untreated depression have higher medical costs than those treated with antidepressants.

HIV-infected patients also experience varying levels of anxiety, ranging from mild unease to full-blown panic. Inability to cope, altered body image, isolation and grief may trigger feelings of anger, despair and frustration. As a result, the patient may develop chronic generalized anxiety disorder, acute anxiety attacks, insomnia, hypochondria, major depression or brief psychosis. Dementia may be prominent, with manifestations ranging from mild forgetfulness to severe disorientation. Delirium too can be caused by a variety of organic disorders, as well as by mental distress (Abrams, Parket-Martin & Unger, 1989; Nichols, 1985; Perry, Jacobsberg & Fishman., 1990; WHO, 1987). A study in the United States found that half of HIV-positive adults had symptoms of mental disorder, including major depression, dysthymia, generalized anxiety disorder and panic attacks. A large number of these patients visited mental health specialists, participated in group treatment, used psychotherapeutic medication and discussed their emotional problems with their medical practitioners. However, few of those with low income, with little education, or from an ethnic minority attended mental health outpatient services (Bing, 2001).

Symptoms of depression are common, not only in those with HIV infection (Kalichman, Heckman & Kochman, 2000; Kalichman, Rompa & Cage, 2000), but also in people close to them (Sikkema et al., 2000). Biggar & Firehand (1998), for example, found more symptoms of depression in HIV-infected mothers and their children than in non-infected mothers and their children. People with HIV infection, particularly in small towns and rural areas, may face barriers that prevent them from receiving important care services, resulting in anxiety and depression (Heckman et al., 1998). A study on access to and use of antenatal care by HIV-infected women reported that barriers included the unexpected and unplanned nature of the pregnancy, and mental health issues related to HIV infection, poverty, periodic homelessness, substance dependence, and lack of social support. Seropositive women perceived the health care system as threatening, and feared discrimination and breach of confidentiality. Women were mostly concerned with their mental health and well-being (Napravnik et al., 2000).

In a study of the physical and mental health of African-American mothers with a seropositive infant, the women reported infections, difficulty thinking and remembering, low energy, and gynaecological problems (Miles, Gillespie & Holditch-Davis, 2001). Women reported moderate levels of perceived stigma and high levels of depressive symptoms. Significant correlations between depressive symptoms and physical health status were found, suggesting a clear link between mental and physical health. Bennetts et al. (1999) found evidence of depressive symptoms and HIV-related worry among HIV-infected mothers in Bangkok, Thailand, at 18–24 months postpartum. Women who were no longer with their partner were at greater risk of depression; women whose babies were HIV-infected had greater worries, as did those who had not disclosed their HIV status to others and who reported that their family would be ashamed about their HIV infection. Similar observations were made by Comer et al. (2000), who found that one of the main concerns of seropositive men and women was disclosure; this led to greater stress because of the stigma surrounding HIV infection (Armistead & Forehand, 1995; Demas et al., 1995; Semple et al., 1993).

HIV symptoms are likely to have a negative impact on functioning and well-being, thereby increasing psychological distress and anxiety. Moreover, the presence of multiple HIV-related symptoms is predictive of psychiatric disorder (Bing, 2001; Bing et al., 2001). A study of 2864 HIV-positive adults found that the probability of screening positive for anxiety and depression was related to the number of HIV symptoms present (Tsao, 2004). As the disease progresses, there may be further psychiatric problems. AIDS dementia complex (ADC), a neurological dysfunction, has been found in 25–90% of AIDS patients and in 30–40% of HIV-infected patients; in some cases, it is the only manifestation of AIDS (Adams, 1997). Depression has a serious impact on the course of disease. For example, a study in the USA found that depression was associated with reduced quality of life and poor adherence to HIV treatment regimens (Tate et al., 2003). Despite this, women in one study (Ciambrone, 2001) did not consider HIV to be the most devastating event in their lives. Despite initial disruption, many women infected with HIV regarded family violence, drug use, or separation from their children as more significantly disruptive elements in their lives. Demi et al. (1998) studied a number of variables in women with HIV infection, such as health status, depressive mood, family cohesion and perceived stigma. They found that suicidal thoughts and suicide attempts were quite common among women with HIV infection, and those who reported suicidal thoughts had more HIV-related symptoms. Chibnall (2002) found "death distress" (death-related depression and anxiety) among younger patients with specific, diagnosable life-threatening conditions; the experience of death distress was associated with the psychosocial and spiritual dimensions of the patient's life. These psychosocial ramifications are especially relevant to patients living with AIDS.

HIV/AIDS and depression

Recent studies have tended to concentrate on the overall health and well-being of people with HIV (Brady et al., 2002; Dodds et al., 2000; Moser, Sowell & Phillips, 2001; Napravnik et al., 2000; Wingood, DiClemente & Raj, 2000). Women's health is frequently linked to inequality and generalized oppression (Travis & Compton, 2001). Women's sexual health is a direct reflection of their low status and lack of sexual autonomy, which increase the risk of sexual health problems and make it difficult for them to obtain appropriate treatment and support. This is evident in the HIV/AIDS epidemic, in which women's vulnerability is increased by male-controlled sexual decision-making, partner violence, and sexual assault (Amaro, Raj & Reed, 2001; Farmer, Connors & Simmons, 1996; WHO, 1993). Additonally, psychosocial stress may be greater in patients with AIDS than in those with other chronic diseases (WHO, 1987). Most research on psychosocial stress in HIV infection has focused on homosexual white males (Chesney, Folkman & Chambers, 1996; Chuang et al., 1989; Folkman et al., 1996; Leserman et al., 2000; Rabkin et al., 1997; Sambamoorthi et al., 2000; Williams et al., 1991). In particular, there has been little research on the psychosocial problems faced by women with HIV infection and the related issues of childbearing and parenting (Perry, Jacobsberg & Fishman, 1990).

A 2004 study of 1716 HIV positive women found that AIDS-related deaths were more common among those with depression, and that use of mental health services was associated with lower mortality rates (Cook et al., 2004). A study among female injecting drug users found similar results: those with chronic depression were 1.7 times more likely to die from AIDS-related causes than those without (James, 2004). Again, those who used mental health services were less likely to die than those who did not use such services.

A number of studies have investigated the impact of depressive symptoms on adherence to HIV treatment. Some studies have found depression to be one of the primary reasons for poor adherence to antiretroviral treatment (Bogart, 2000; Starace 2002). A study in 2006 examined the relationship between treated or untreated depression and adherence to antiretroviral therapy in HIV-positive women (Cook et al., 2006). Those given antidepressants in addition to psychotherapy were more likely to adhere to antiretroviral therapy than those not receiving any treatment for depression. Similar findings have been found in various HIV-positive groups, including injecting drug users. In a study of 5073 HIV-positive injecting drug users, women were less adherent to antiretroviral therapy than men, and were more likely to be diagnosed with depression (Turner et al., 2003). However, a study published in 2006 found that mental health disorders, such as substance abuse and affective disorders (including depression), were not associated with decreased adherence to antiretroviral therapy or with reduced survival. In fact, mental illness was positively associated with increased use of health care services and adherence to antiretroviral therapy (Mijch et al., 2006).

Conclusion

Factors associated with psychosocial stress among patients with HIV infection and AIDS include lack of family support, fear of discrimination, loss of friends, uncertainty about the course of the illness, and concerns about sexual activity and transmitting the disease (Sadvosky, 1991). Depression is the most common mental health problem in women, and is closely linked to the stressful life events associated with being female (Patel et al., 1999). For example, women are more likely to be victims of violence, both within and outside their home; they are more likely to be denied educational and employment opportunities; and they are more likely to have difficulties accessing health care, receiving quality care, accessing information, and satisfying their nutritional needs (Das Gupta, 1987, 1989; Patel et al., 1999). The prevalence of depression in HIV-infected clinic populations in the United States has been found to range from 22% to 32%, 2–3 times that in the general community (Brown et al., 1992; Evans et al., 1998; Ferrando et al., 1998; Rabkin et al., 1997; Williams et al., 1991). Neuropsychiatric syndromes, including dementia, delirium and depression, occur in 40–70% of AIDS patients during the later stages of the disease (Abrams, Parket-Martin & Unger, 1989; Sadvosky, 1991).

Summary

Future research

1. There have been few reports on the psychological problems of new mothers with HIV infection, in either developed or developing countries. Further research is required to complement the strong biomedical efforts to reduce mother-to-child transmission of HIV. This needs to consider the psychosocial aspects of being HIV positive and breastfeeding and of decisions about HIV treatment during the antenatal and postnatal periods.

2. Studies of distress and anxiety in HIV-positive women regarding the fate of their children are extremely rare. An estimated 14 million children have lost one or both parents to AIDS, and it is predicted that by 2010 one-third of all children in southern Africa will be orphans.

3. The impact on the mental health of girls orphaned as a result of AIDS has barely been studied; the predicted increase in their number indicates an urgent need for such research.

4. There are significant gaps in the literature on the mental health of migrant and refugee women, and its interaction with reproductive functioning. These women continue to be vulnerable to STIs, including HIV. The mental health problems of these highly vulnerable groups are either sidelined or disre-

garded at present. Next to nothing is known about how the vulnerability of these women affects their overall reproductive health, mental health and emotional well-being.

5. Another under-researched aspect of the mental health impact of the HIV epidemic on women relates to the fact that the burden of care falls primarily on them. Women may adopt or care for orphaned children of friends or relatives who have died of AIDS. In addition, women often care for partners with AIDS, regardless of their own health status. How they fulfil this responsibility, care for others, and maintain their own health is an important area for future research.

Implications for policy

1. Policies and strategies to identify psychosocial problems in HIV-infected girls and women, and mechanisms to provide support to them through integrated reproductive health services, need to be put in place.

2. Policies and strategies to help halt the widespread sexual exploitation of children, including orphaned children, are critical.

3. Protection of vulnerable girls and women, including widows, migrants and refugees, needs to be built into legal frameworks.

4. Laws to reduce prejudice, stigma and violence against girls and women are neede.d

Services

1. The need for mental health care and support of girls, women and orphans in communities affected by AIDS must be ascertained and addressed at all levels of routine care.

2. Victims of domestic and sexual violence and coercion should have access to confidential care and quality psychosocial support at all levels.

3. The special needs of vulnerable children and orphans for psychosocial support and protection must be sensitively addressed through all service points.

4. Health care workers at all levels, including in the community, should receive training in counselling and psychosocial support techniques.

References

Adams MA, Ferraro FR (1997) Acquired immunodeficiency syndrome dementia complex. *Journal of Clinical Psychology*, 53(7): 767-778.

Abrams DI, Parket-Martin J, Unger KW (1989) Psychosocial aspects of terminal AIDS. *Patient Care*, 23(19): 41-60.

Allers CT et al. (1993) HIV vulnerability and the adult survivor of childhood sexual abuse. *Child Abuse and Neglect*, 17(2): 291-298.

Amaro H (1995) Love, sex, and power: considering women's realities in HIV prevention. *American Psychologist*, 5(6): 437-447.

Amaro H, Raj A, Reed E (2001) Women's sexual health: the need for feminist analyses in public health in the decade of behaviour. *Psychology of Women Quarterly*, 25(4): 324-334.

Anderson J, ed. (2000) *A guide to the clinical care of HIV+ women*. Rockville, MD, Womencare.

Armistead L, Forehand R (1995) For whom the bell tolls: parenting decisions and challenges faced by mothers who are HIV seropositive. *Clinical Psychology: Science and Practice*, 2: 239-249.

Arnow BA et al. (1999) Childhood sexual abuse, psychological distress, and medical use among women. *Psychosomatic Medicine*, 61(6): 762-770.

Astbury J (2002) Intimate partner violence finally a "legitimate" public health issue. *Australian and New Zealand Journal of Public Health*, 26(5): 409-411.

Bandyopadhyay M, Thomas J (2002) Women migrant workers' vulnerability to HIV infection in Hong Kong. *AIDS care*, 14(4): 509-521.

Bogart LM et al. (2000) Impact of medical and non medical factors on physician decision making for HIV/AIDS antiretroviral treatment. *Journal of Acquired Immune Deficiency Syndrome*, 23: 396-404.

BBC (2003) *Mystery death of Indian AIDS woman*. London, British Broadcasting Corporation.

Bennetts A et al. (1999) Determinants of depression and HIV related worry among HIV positive women who have recently given birth, Bangkok, Thailand. *Social Science and Medicine*, 49(6): 737-749.

Bensley LS, Van Eenwyk J, Simmons KW (2000) Self-reported childhood sexual and physical abuse and adult HIV-risk behaviors and heavy drinking. *American Journal of Preventive Medicine*, 18(2): 151-158.

Biggar H, Firehand R (1998) The relationship between maternal HIV status and child depressive symptoms: Do maternal depressive syndromes play a role? *Behavior Therapy*, 29(3): 409-421.

Bing EG (2001) Psychiatric disorders and drug use among human immunodeficiency virus infected adults in the US. *Journal of the American Medical Association*, 286(20): 2524.

Bing EG et al. (2001) Psychiatric disorders and drug use among human immunodeficiency virus infected adults in the United States. *Archives of General Psychiatry*, 58(8): 721.

Bond KC, Celentano DD, Yaddhanaphuti C (1996) "I'm not afraid of life or death": Women in brothels in Northern Thailand. In: Long LD, Ankrah EM, eds, *Women's experiences with HIV/AIDS: an international perspective*, New York, Columbia University Press: 123-149.

Brady S et al. (2002) Physical and sexual abuse in the lives of HIV-positive women enrolled in a primary medicine health maintenance organization. *AIDS Patient Care and Standards*, 16(3): 121-125.

Brown GR et al. (1992) Prevalence of psychiatric disorders in early stages of HIV infection. *Psychosomatic Medicine*, 54(5): 588-601.

Bury J, Morrison V, McLachlan S (1992) *Working with women and AIDS: medical, social, and counseling issues*. London, Routledge.

Carballo M, Grocutt M, Hadzihasanovic A (1996) Women and migration: a public health issue. *World Health Statistics Quarterly*, 49(2): 158-164.

Catalan J et al. (1996) Women and HIV infection: investigation of its psychosocial consequences. *Journal of Psychosomatic Research*, 41(1): 39-47.

Chesney M, Folkman S, Chambers D (1996) Coping effectiveness training for men living with HIV: preliminary findings. *International Journal of STD and AIDS*, 7 (Suppl 2): 75-82.

Ciambrone D (2001) Illness and other assaults on self: the relative impact of HIV/AIDS on women's lives. *Sociology of Health and Illness*, 23(4): 517-540.

Chibnall JT et al. (2002) Psychosocial-spiritual correlates of death distress in patients with life-threatening medical conditions. *Palliative Medicine*, 16(4): 331-338.

Chuang HT et al. (1989) Psychosocial distress and well-being among gay and bisexual men with human immunodeficiency virus infection. *American Journal of Psychiatry*, 146(7): 876-880.

Clark AS (1998) HIV/AIDS: The emotional effects and psychotherapeutic implications for women. *Dissertation Abstracts International: Section B: The Sciences & Engineering*, 59(5-B): 2414.

Clark S (2004) Early marriage and HIV rates in sub-Saharan Africa. *Studies in Family Planning*, 35(3): 149-160.

Comer LK et al. (2000) Illness disclosure and mental health among women with HIV/AIDS. *Journal of Community and Applied Social Psychology*, 10(6): 449-464.

Cook J, Nygren-Krug H (2001) *Health and the Fifty-Seventh Session of the United Nations Commission on Human Rights, Geneva, Palais des Nations*. Geneva, United Nations.

Cook J et al (2004) Depressive symptoms and AIDS related mortality among a multisite cohort of HIV positive women. *American Journal of Public Health*, 94(7): 1133-1140.

Cook J et al (2006) Effects of treated and untreated depressive symptoms on highly active antiretroviral therapy use in a US multi-site cohort of HIV positive women. *AIDS Care*, 18(2): 93-100.

Das Gupta M (1987) Selective discrimination against female children in rural Punjab, India. *Population and Development Review*, 13(1): 257-270.

Das Gupta M (1989) *The effects of discrimination on health and mortality*. New Delhi, International Union for the Scientific Study of Population.

Demas P et al. (1995) Stress, coping, and attitudes toward HIV treatment in injecting drug users: a qualitative study. *AIDS Education and Prevention*, 7(5): 429-442.

Demi A et al. (1998) Suicidal thoughts of women with HIV infection: Effect of stressors and moderating effects of family cohesion. *Journal of Family Psychology*, 12(3): 344.

Dodds S et al. (2000) Integrating mental health services into primary care for HIV-infected pregnant and non-pregnant women: whole life. A theoretically derived model for clinical care and outcomes assessment. *General Hospital Psychiatry*, 22: 251-260.

Emlet CA, Gusz SS (1998) Service use patterns in HIV/AIDS case management: a five-year study. *Journal of Case Management*, 7(1): 3-9.

Evans S et al. (1998) Pain and depression in HIV illness. *Psychosomatics*, 39(6): 528-535.

Farmer P, Connors M, Simmons J, eds. (1996) *Women, poverty and AIDS: sex, drugs and structural violence.* Health and Social Justice, Monroe, Maine, Common Courage Press.

Fernandez I (1998) Migration and HIV/AIDS vulnerability in South East Asia. *Paper presented at the12th World AIDS Conference, June 28-July 3 Geneva.*

Ferrando S et al. (1998) Fatigue in HIV illness: relationship to depression, physical limitations and disability. *Psychosomatic Medicine,* 60(6): 759-764.

Fikree FF, Bhatti LI (1999) Domestic violence and health of Pakistani women. *International Journal of Gynaecology and Obstetrics,* 65(2): 195-201.

Folkman S et al. (1996) Post-bereavement depressive mood and its prebereavement predictors in HIV+ and HIV- gay men. *Journal of Personality and Social Psychology,* 70(2): 336-348.

Gielen AC et al. (2000) Women living with HIV: disclosure, violence, and social support. *Journal of Urban Health,* 77(3): 480-491.

Gielen AC et al. (1997) Women's disclosure of HIV status: experiences of mistreatment and violence in an urban setting. *Women and Health,* 25(3): 19-31.

Gielen AC et al. (2001) Quality of life among women living with HIV: the importance of violence, social support, and self care behaviours. *Social Science and Medicine,* 52(2): 315-322.

Gordon P, Crehan K (1999) Dying of sadness: gender, sexual violence and the HIV epidemic. Geneva, United Nations Development Programme.

Gulcur L (2000) Evaluating the role of gender inequalities and rights violations in women's mental health. *Health and Human Rights,* 5(1): 46-66.

Gupta GR, Weiss E, Mane P (1996) Talking about sex: a prerequisite for AIDS prevention. In: Long LD, Ankrah EM, eds, *Women's experiences with HIV/AIDS: an international perspective.* New York, Columbia University Press: 333-350.

Hall LA et al. (1993) Childhood physical and sexual abuse: their relationship with depressive symptoms in adulthood. *Image – The Journal of Nursing Scholarship,* 25(4): 317-323.

Heckman TG et al. (1999) Depressive symptomatology, daily stressors, and ways of coping among middle-age and older adults living with HIV disease. *Journal of Mental Health Aging,* 5: 311-322.

Heckman TG et al. (1998) Barriers to care among persons living with HIV/AIDS in urban and rural areas. *AIDS Care,* 10(3): 365-375.

Heise L, Moore K, Toubia N (1995) *Sexual coercion and reproductive health: a focus on research.* New York, The Population Council.

Institute of Development Studies (2002) Gender and HIV/AIDS: Raising awareness among policy makers and practitioners. Brighton (Bridge Brief No 11).

James J (2004) Chronically depressed women with HIV twice as likely as others to die from AIDS related causes; those with mental health services had half the death rate of those without. *AIDS Treatment News,* 403: 2-3.

Jones DJ et al. (2001) Disease status in African American single mothers with HIV: The role of depressive symptoms. *Health Psychology,* 20(6): 417-423.

Kalichman SC, Heckman TG, Kochman A (2000) Depression and thoughts of suicide among middle-aged and older persons living with HIV-AIDS. *Psychiatric Services,* 51(7): 903-907.

Kalichman SC, Rompa D, Cage M (2000) Distinguishing between overlapping somatic symptoms of depression and HIV disease in people living with HIV/AIDS. *Journal of Nervous and Mental Disease,* 188(10): 662-670.

Kalichman SC et al. (2002) Emotional adjustment in survivors of sexual assault living with HIV/AIDS. *Journal of Traumatic Stress,* 15(4): 289-296.

Kimerling R, Armistead L, Forehand R (1999) Victimization experiences and HIV infection in women: associations with serostatus, psychological symptoms, and health status. *Journal of Traumatic Stress,* 12(1): 41-58.

Kwong J et al. (1999) Non-occupational HIV post-exposure prophylaxis at a Boston community health centre. *Paper presented at the 1999 National HIV Prevention Conference, Atlanta, GA.*

Leserman J et al. (2000) Impact of stressful life events, depression, social support, coping and cortisol on progression to AIDS. *American Journal of Psychiatry,* 157(8): 1221-1228.

Linn JG et al. (1996) Perceived health, HIV illness, and mental distress in African American clients of AIDS counseling centers. *Journal of the Association of Nurses in AIDS Care,* 7: 43-51.

Long LD, Ankrah EM, ed. (1996) *Women's experiences with HIV/AIDS: an international perspective.* New York, Columbia University Press.

Lukalo R (1998) *People on the move fuel HIV/AIDS*. Geneva, PANOS.

Manopaiboon C et al. (1998) Impact of HIV on families of recently delivered HIV-infected women, Bangkok, Thailand. *Journal of Acquired Immune Deficiency Syndromes and Human Retrovirology*, 18: 54-63.

McMahon PM, Goodwin MM, Stringer G (2000) Sexual violence and reproductive health. *Maternal and Child Health Journal*, 4(2): 121-124.

Miles MS, Gillespie JV, Holditch-Davis D (2001) Physical and mental health in African American mothers with HIV. *Journal of the Association of Nurses in AIDS Care*, 12(4): 42-50.

Mijch A et al (2006) Increased health care utilization and increased antiretroviral use in HIV-infected individuals with mental health disorders. *HIV Medicine,* 7: 205-212.

Moser KM, Sowell RL, Phillips KD (2001) Issues of women dually diagnosed with HIV infection and substance use problems in the Carolinas. *Issues in Mental Health Nursing,* 22(1): 23-49.

Mukoyogo MC, Williams G (1991) *AIDS orphans: a community perspective in Tanzania*. Actionaid.

Mullen PE et al. (1988) Impact of sexual and physical abuse on women's mental health. *Lancet*, 1(8590): 841-845.

Murray LK et al. (2006) Violence and abuse among HIV-infected women and their children in Zambia: a qualitative study. *Journal of Nervous and Mental Disease*, 194(8): 610-615.

Napravnik S et al. (2000) HIV-1 infected women and prenatal care utilization: barriers and facilitators. *AIDS Patient Care and Standards*, 14(8): 411-420.

Neundorfer M et al. (2005) HIV-risk factors for midlife and older women. *The Gerontologist*, 45(5): 617-625.

Newcomb MD et al. (1998) Acculturation, sexual risk taking and HIV health promotion among Latinas. *Journal of Counselling Psychology*, 45(4): 454-467.

Nichols SE (1985) Psychosocial reactions of persons with the acquired immunodeficiency syndrome. *Annals of Internal Medicine*, 103(5): 765-767.

Parillo KM et al. (2001) Association between early sexual abuse and adult HIV-risky sexual behaviors among community-recruited women. *Child Abuse and Neglect*, 25(3): 335-346.

Patel V, Oomman N (1999) Mental health matters too: gynaecological symptoms and depression in South Asia. *Reproductive Health Matters*, 7(14): 30-38.

Patel V et al. (1999) Women, poverty and common mental disorders in four restructuring societies. *Social Science and Medicine*, 49: 1461-1471.

Perry S, Jacobsberg I, Fishman B (1990) Relationships between CD4 lymphocytes and psychosocial variables among HIV seropositive adults. *Paper presented at Sixth International Conference on AIDS, San Francisco*.

Pizzi M (1992) Women, HIV infection, and AIDS: tapestries of life, death, and empowerment. *American Journal of Occupational Therapy*, 46(11): 1021-1027.

Quinn SC (1993) AIDS and the African American woman: the triple burden of race, class, and gender. *Health Education Quarterly*, 20: 305-320.

Rabkin JG et al. (1997) Stability of mood despite HIV illness progression in a group of homosexual men. *American Journal of Psychiatry*, 154(2): 231-238.

Reid JB (1998) HIV/AIDS: the emotional impact on two young women whose mothers are HIV-infected. *Dissertation Abstracts International Section A: Humanities and Social Sciences*, 59(3-A): 0971.

Roberts GL et al. (1998a) The impact of domestic violence on women's mental health. *Australian and New Zealand Journal of Public Health*, 22(7): 796-801.

Roberts GL et al. (1998b) How does domestic violence affect women's mental health? *Women and Health*, 28(1): 117-129.

Sadik N (1997) Reproductive health/family planning and the health of infants, girls and women. *Indian Journal of Pediatrics*, 64(6): 739-744.

Sambamoorthi U et al. (2000) Antidepressant treatment and health services utilisation among HIV-infected Medicaid patients diagnosed with depression. *Journal of General Internal Medicine*, 15(5): 311-320.

Schifrin E (2001) An overview of women's health issues in the United States and United Kingdom. *Womens Health Issues*, 11(4): 261-281.

Semple S et al. (1993) Identification of psychobiological stressors among HIV-poitive women. *Women and Health*, 20(4): 15-36.

Sikkema KJ et al. (2000) Coping strategies and emotional wellbeing among HIV infected men and women experiencing AIDS related bereavement. *AIDS Care*, 12(15): 613-624.

Simoni JM, Ng MT (2000) Trauma, coping, and depression among women with HIV/AIDS in New York City. *AIDS Care*, 12(5): 567-580.

Singhanetra-Renard A (1997) Population movement and the AIDS epidemic in Thailand. In: Herdt G, ed., *Sexual cultures and migration in the era of AIDS*. Oxford, Clarendon Press.

Sowell RL et al. (1997) Quality of life in HIV-infected women in the Southeastern United States. *AIDS Care*, 95(5): 501-512.

Starace F et al (2002) Depression is a risk factor for suboptimal adherence to highly active antiretroviral therapy. *Journal of Acquired Immune Deficiency Syndrome*, 31:S136-S139.

Tate D et al. (2003) The impact of apathy and depression on quality of life in patients infected with HIV. *AIDS Patient Care and STDs*, 17(3): 115-120.

Human Rights Watch (2002) *Suffering in silence: human rights abuse and HIV transmission to girls in Zambia*. New York.

Thompson NJ et al. (1997) The relationship of sexual abuse and HIV risk behaviors among heterosexual adult female STD patients. *Child Abuse and Neglect*, 21(2): 149-156.

Tiamson ML (2002) Challenges in the management of the HIV patient in the third decade of AIDS. *Psychiatric Quarterly*, 73(1): 51-58.

Travis CB, Compton JD (2001) Feminism and health in the decade of behaviour. *Psychology of Women Quarterly*, 25(4): 312-323.

Tsao JCI et al. (2004) Stability of anxiety and depression in a national sample of adults with human immunodeficiency virus. *Journal of Nervous and Mental Disease*, 192(2): 111-118.

Turner BJ et al. (2003) Relationships of gender, depression, and health care delivery with antiretroviral adherence in HIV-infected drug users. *Journal of General Internal Medicine*, 18:248-257.

Ulin PR, Cayemittes M, Gringle R (1996) Bargaining for life: women and the AIDS epidemic in Haiti. In: Long LD, Ankrah EM, eds, *Women's experiences with HIV/AIDS: an international perspective*. New York, Columbia University Press: 91-111.

UNAIDS (1998) *Migration and HIV/AIDS*. New Delhi, Joint United Nations Programme on HIV/AIDS.

UNAIDS (2002a) *AIDS epidemic update*. Geneva, Joint United Nations Programme on HIV/AIDS.

UNAIDS (2002b) *Report on the global HIV/AIDS epidemic*. Geneva, Joint United Nations Programme on HIV/AIDS.

UNAIDS (2006a) *Report on the global AIDS epidemic*. Geneva, Joint United Nations Programme on HIV/AIDS.

UNAIDS (2006b) *AIDS epidemic update 2006*. Geneva, Joint United Nations Programme on HIV/AIDS, World Health Organization.

UNICEF (2002) *The state of the world's children*. New York, United Nations Children's Fund.

UNIFEM (2001) *Turning the tide: CEDAW and the gender dimension of the HIV/AIDS pandemic*. New York, United Nations Development Fund for Women.

UNFPA (2006) *The State of World Population 2006. A passage to hope: women and international migration*. New York, United Nations Population Fund.

VanDevanter N et al. (1999) Heterosexual couples confronting the challenges of HIV infection. *AIDS Care*, 11(2): 181-193.

Vetten L, Bhana K (2001) *Violence, vengeance and gender: a preliminary investigation into the links between violence against women and HIV/AIDS in South Africa*. Johannesburg and Cape Town, Centre for the Study of Violence and Reconciliation.

Vlahov D et al. (1998) Violence among women with or at risk for HIV infection. *AIDS and Behaviour*, 2(1): 53-60.

Weingourt R et al. (2001) Domestic violence and women's mental health in Japan. *International Nursing Review*, 48: 102-108.

WHO (1987) *Report from consultation on psychosocial research needs in HIV infection and AIDS*. Geneva, World Health Organization.

WHO (1993) *Psychosocial and mental health aspects of women's health*. Geneva, World Health Organization.

WHO (2001) *Integration of the human rights of women and the gender perspective*. Geneva, World Health Organization.

WHO (2002) *World report on violence and health*. Geneva, World Health Organization.

Williams JB et al. (1991) Multidisciplinary baseline assessment of homosexual men with and without human immunodeficiency virus infection, II: Standardized clinical assessment of current and lifetime psychopathology. *Archives of General Psychiatry*, 48(2): 124-130.

Wingood GM, DiClemente RJ (1997a) Child sexual abuse, HIV sexual risk, and gender relations of African-American women. *American Journal of Preventive Medicine*, 13(5): 380-384.

Wingood GM, DiClemente RJ (1997b) The effects of an abusive primary partner on the condom use and sexual negotiation practices of African-American women. *American Journal of Public Health*, 87(6): 1016-1018.

Wingood GM, DiClemente RJ, Raj A (2000) Adverse consequences of intimate partner abuse among women in non-urban domestic violence shelters. *American Journal of Preventive Medicine*, 19(4): 270-275.

Wolffers I, Fernandez J (1999) *Female migrants from Bangladesh: two studies, one from Bangladesh and one from Malaysia.* Kuala Lumpur: Coordination of Action Research on AIDS and Mobility (CARAM)

Wyatt GE, Forge NG, Guthrie D (1998) Family constellation and ethnicity: current and lifetime HIV-related risk taking. *Journal of Family Psychology.* 12(1): 93-101.

Wyatt GE et al. (1999) The prevalence and circumstances of child sexual abuse: changes across a decade. *Child Abuse and Neglect*, 23(1): 45-60.

Wyatt GE et al. (2002) Does a history of trauma contribute to HIV risk for women of color? Implications for prevention and policy. *The American Journal of Public Health*, 92(4): 660-665.

Zierler S et al. (1991) Adult survivors of childhood sexual abuse and subsequent risk of HIV infection. *American Journal of Public Health*, 81(5): 572-575.

Zierler S, Witbeck B, Mayer K (1996) Sexual violence against women living with or at risk for HIV infection. *American Journal of Preventive Medicine*, 12(5): 304-310.

Chapter

8

Infertility and assisted reproduction

Jane Fisher

Estimating the prevalence of fertility difficulties, infertility or involuntary childlessness is hampered by variations in the definitions of these conditions (Schmidt & Munster, 1995; Kols & Nguyen, 1997). The central difficulty is in defining both the population with compromised fertility and the appropriate comparison population. The former may be conceptualized as either individuals or couples who are unable to conceive after a specified period of regular unprotected sexual intercourse or those seeking medical assistance in order to conceive. The specified time of trying to conceive has varied from 12 months to more than 24 months. Some studies have included people with primary infertility (the inability to conceive at all), secondary infertility (those who have at least one living child but are unable to conceive again), and sub-fecundity (the capacity to conceive but not to sustain a pregnancy to term). The comparison populations have sometimes included those who have never tried to conceive and large groups of young women who may not yet have tried to conceive.

The definition of infertility has a significant impact on clinical outcomes, including those reported in research studies. Definitions vary in terms of whether the condition is identified by self-report, or based on a life calendar of reproductive events, a physician consultation or a physician diagnosis. Infertility can be regarded as a heterogeneous group of health problems, influenced by a range of risk factors (Marchbanks et al., 1989).

It has been estimated, on the basis of investigations in several clinical services, that 8–12% of women in North America are unable to conceive spontaneously (Beral et al., 1994). Postal surveys of a national sample in Australia suggest that the equivalent figure there is 15% (Australian Bureau of Statistics, 2004). Kols & Nguyen (1997) summarized the available estimates of infertility in developing countries, and found wide variations, e.g. 11–20% in sub-Saharan Africa and 14–32% in Namibia. There have been relatively few population-based investigations of the prevalence of fertility difficulties in developing countries. While this reflects local research capacity, it is also argued that it reflects predominant concerns about overpopulation and the costs of unrestrained fertility in these areas (Inhorn & Buss, 1994). Most women with infertility live in the developing world, and have limited access to diagnostic tests or treatment and, often, no access to assisted reproductive technologies (Fathalla, 1992; Vayena, Rowe & Griffin, 2002). A population survey in Gambia, using randomly selected census areas, found that primary infertility was relatively uncommon (3%), but secondary infertility following the birth of at least one child was more common (6%) (Sundby, Mboge & Sonko, 1998). Half of those affected had not sought treatment and both investigative testing and treatment were limited. Larsen (2000) used linked population census data, which included childbirth history, to examine infertility in 28 African countries. Primary infertility was assumed in those who had been married for at least seven years without having a child, and secondary infertility in those aged 20–44 years whose most recent birth was more than five years ago. Primary infertility was low (less than 3% in the countries surveyed), but there was a wide range in secondary infertility (5–23%). In a survey using random sampling in a rural community in Nigeria, the prevalence of primary infertility was 9.2% and of secondary infertility 21.1% (Adetoro & Ebomoyi, 1991). In a single survey of one urban region in Viet Nam, 5.7% of couples were reported to be infertile (Thwaites, 2002). In countries where treatment for reproductive tract infections is not widely available, more than 30% of women develop secondary infertility caused by tubal occlusion resulting from infection (Vayena, Rowe & Peterson, 2002).

In reviewing prevalence surveys, Schmidt & Munster (1995) found that current and lifetime prevalence of infertility ranged from 3.6% to 32.6%. They concluded that, overall, about 24% of the global population experiences either primary or secondary infertility, and that about 15% of the population of reproductive age will seek medical assistance to conceive.

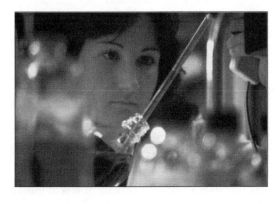

Causes of infertility

Male and female factors are each believed to account for 40% of cases of infertility; the remaining 20% are either unexplained – so-called idiopathic infertility – or of shared etiology. In women, the most common causes of fertility difficulties are obstructed fallopian tubes and ovulation dysfunction, while in men low sperm viability and dysfunction of sperm motility are most common (Johnson & Everitt, 2000). It has been suggested that 5% of infertility is caused by constitutional problems, including genetic conditions, anatomical defects, and endocrinological or immunological dysfunction (Kols & Nguyen, 1997). The balance is attributable to infection, unhygienic health care practices, particularly in obstetrics, and exposure to environmental toxins. Reproductive tract infections, especially sexually transmitted infections, are the predominant cause of infertility, leading to the

formation of scar tissue which obstructs the fallopian tubes (Kols & Nguyen, 1997). In a case-control study of 60 women with infertility and 53 matched controls in Ile-Ife, Nigeria (Okonofua et al., 1997), the infertile group had higher rates of *Neisseria gonorrhoeae* antibodies and of a history of other sexually transmitted infections than the controls. Infections secondary to abortion or childbirth are also implicated (Kols & Nguyen, 1997; Sundby, Mboge & Sonko, 1998). In a comparison of consecutive women presenting with fertility problems and female hospital workers in Nigeria, Aghanwa et al. (1999) found that the patients were significantly more likely to be married to polygamous men and to have had an abortion. It has also been suggested that inappropriate treatment of undiagnosed conditions, including curettage in Gambia (Sundby, Mboge & Sonko, 1998) and cervical electrocauterization in Egypt (Inhorn & Buss, 1994) may contribute to infertility. Female fertility may be reduced following genital mutilation, as a result of chronic pelvic infections leading to obstruction of the fallopian tubes, or because narrowing of the introitus may lead to the anus or urethra being used for intercourse (Ng, 2000). Normal vaginal intercourse may be impossible if the introitus is narrowed through infibulation (Okonofua et al., 2002). Female genital schistosomiasis, which is common in sub-Saharan Africa, leads to granulomatous inflammation of the cervix and increases the likelihood of other reproductive tract infections (Poggensee et al., 2001; Poggensee & Feldmeier, 2001). Infectious causes appear to be less common in male factor infertility, but parasitic infections (including schistosomiasis, which damages the male genital tract) have been implicated in some countries (Kols & Nguyen, 1997). In developing countries, occupational exposure, for example to heavy metals, biological metabolites, pesticides and heat, may also contribute to infertility (Inhorn & Buss, 1994; Kols & Nguyen, 1997). The assessment of male factors is limited because many men refuse to participate in studies, which may mean that cause is misattributed (Aghanwa et al., 1999).

In groups with limited education, poor access to services or little general knowledge of physiological functioning, superstitious attribution is common. Anthropological investigations of women in Botswana (Upton, 2001), southern Nigeria (Koster-Oyekan, 1999) and Mozambique (Mariano, 2004), using in-depth interviews and field observations, concluded that women are usually regarded as responsible for infertility. In these investigations, infertility was attributed to: transgression of sexual taboos or rituals relating to burial of a dead child; supernatural factors, including witchcraft or a curse by ancestors or deities; and prior abortions or use of orthodox contraceptives (Koster-Oyekan, 1999; Upton, 2001). Egyptian women of low socioeconomic status living in rural areas, who cannot conceive, are regarded as having been subjected to *kabsa,* or the constraint of reproductive capacity by exposure to contaminated individuals (Inhorn, 1994). Upton (2001) and Mariano (2004) identified a contemporary paradox in some African countries, where men in poor rural communities migrate to urban areas to work and are absent for prolonged periods, but their wives are still expected to have children and are responsible when this does not occur.

People who cannot have children may be stigmatized and socially marginalized in strongly pro-natal settings. Infertility exerts a significant adverse effect on the mental health of couples who want to have children.

Psychological causation of infertility?

There has been a long-standing belief that female infertility, particularly of unknown etiology, is attributable to psychological factors – so-called "psychogenic infertility". This has commonly been defined as fertility difficulties for which no organic cause can be identified and in which psychological mechanisms are assumed to be operating. Studies have attempted to find personality or psychiatric factors that would explain infertility. Almost all have focused on women, and most have made retrospective attribution of the observed differences between fertile and infertile women (usually those seeking treatment) to pre-existing factors. The issues proposed as etiologically involved have included uncertain gender identity, external locus of control, infertility as a defence against inner conflicts, ambivalence about having children, psychiatric symptoms, in particular, depression and anxiety, marital problems "masquerading as infertility" and sexual dysfunction (Callan & Hennessey, 1988b; Moller & Fallstrom, 1991; Greil, 1997).

There have been no population-based prospective studies that have followed women from adolescence and investigated pre-existing psychological differences between fertile and infertile groups. However, a number of cohort compari-son studies have used more adequate methodology, including systematic sampling, adequate sample size and standardized measures. These studies have found no significant difference in rates of psychiatric illness, other psychopathology or personality factors between presumed fertile groups and those seeking infertility treatment, or between infertile groups and population norms, or between groups with infertility of different origin and duration (Edelmann et al., 1991; Downey & McKinney, 1992; Visser et al., 1994). It has been argued that women who seek treatment may be psychologically robust and not representative of the population with fertility difficulties, but this assertion has not been tested (Eugster & Vingerhoest, 1999). The observed differences in mood and self-regard between fertile and infertile groups are more accurately regarded as secondary to the infertility, rather than etiologically involved (Edelmann et al., 1991; Downey & McKinney, 1992; Eugster & Vingerhoest, 1999). As understanding of the complex physiology and biology of reproduction has grown over the past three decades, the proportion of infertility attributed to unexplained origins has decreased from about 50% of cases to between 5% and 15% (Moller & Fallstrom, 1991).

One of the criticisms of efforts to ascribe infertility to psychological factors is that they have led to misattribution of responsibility and "blaming" of victims, especially women; little research has investigated this hypothesis in recent years. While agreeing with this view, some authors have argued that certain psychiatric illnesses and behaviours make individuals more vulnerable to infertility and that these should continue to be investigated (Rosenthal & Goldfarb, 1997). In particular, the severe weight loss associated with the eating disorder, anorexia nervosa, can lead to suppression of ovulation; cigarette smoking, and alcohol and drug use, can also lead to decreased fertility. Sexual difficulties, especially erectile dysfunction and vaginismus, can impair the completion of intercourse (Rosenthal & Goldfarb, 1997). The links between behavioural factors and fertility pathology were examined in a substantial epidemiological study, which found that, while there were few differences between fertile and infertile women, tubal obstruction was associated with a higher incidence of previous sexually transmitted disease. Women with this condition had a lower age of sexual debut and more sexual partners, were more likely to have used an intrauterine contraceptive device, and were less likely to have used condoms than those with other fertility difficulties (Beral et al., 1994). The study also found that obesity was associated with polycystic ovarian disease (Beral et al., 1994). The contribution to fertility difficulties of a delay in the age of marriage and reproduction has been identified as a concern in many industrialized countries, but the complex social and economic factors involved are not well understood (Rosenthal & Goldfarb, 1997).

Psychological impact of infertility

By definition, infertility can be identified only when it has lasted at least a year. The experience and eventual diagnostic confirmation of infertility can have a profound psychological impact (Menning, 1982), which has been conceptualized and assessed in different ways.

Psychiatric illness or normal psychological reaction to an abnormal circumstance?

There is debate about whether the psychological disturbance observable in people with infertility is more accurately conceptualized as a psychiatric illness or as an intense psychological reaction to abnormal personal circumstances. High rates of clinically significant symptoms of depression and anxiety have been reported in surveys of cohorts of women and, to a lesser extent, men seeking fertility treatment (Beaurepaire et al., 1994). More than 20% of women attending an infertility support group reported that they had experienced episodic suicidal ideation (Kerr, Brown & Balen, 1999). However, the labelling of these conditions as psychiatric illness has been criticized, because psychiatric symptom checklists include somatic symptoms (e.g. "Something is wrong with my body...") that are normal among those with infertility. As psychological state is dynamic following diagnosis and during treatment for infertility, it has been argued that a syndrome approach to conceptualization is inaccurate and that a psychological profile, along which individuals are ranged, would be more accurate (Berg & Wilson, 1990). Unlike other adverse life events, which may have a clear resolution, infertility is regarded as uniquely stressful because it can last for many years and for many will not be resolved (Berg & Wilson, 1990). Berg & Wilson (1990) have identified an infertility strain profile, characterized by increased anxiety, irritability, profound sadness, self-blame, lowered energy levels, social isolation and heightened interpersonal sensitivity.

Almost all women presenting for treatment have been found to demonstrate some of these features (Berg & Wilson, 1990).

Two approaches have been taken to describing the psychological sequelae of infertility (Greil, 1997). The first is qualitative investigation and clinical description of the experiential responses to infertility. In this approach, infertility is described as a profound life crisis or existential blow and a number of common themes are identified (Menning, 1982; Mahlstedt, 1985). Guilt is prominent among women, together with fears that earlier sexual experiences, the use of contraceptives, or delaying procreation while pursuing professional goals has compromised fertility (Mahlstedt, 1985). Other less rational beliefs – of being punished for past misdeeds or of intrinsic unworthiness – have also been reported, particularly if infertility is of unexplained origin. The frustration associated with being unable to control conception and physiological functioning commonly leads to feelings of anger (Becker, 1994). This may be directed towards a number of people, including the infertile partner, friends and associates who have been able to conceive easily, and people who offer unsolicited advice (Mahlstedt, 1985).

Reaction to infertility is also conceptualized as grief, including for many intangible or disenfranchised losses (Menning, 1982). The losses include: the experiences of pregnancy, childbirth and breastfeeding; the children and grandchildren who will not exist; a generation and genetic continuity; the state of parenthood and the activities and relationships it entails; and an element of adult and gender identity which will never be realized and is substituted with a flawed infertile identity (Menning, 1982; Olshansky, 1987; Dunnington & Glazer, 1991; Nachtigall, Becker & Wizny, 1992). In addition, individuals may fear losing significant relationships, in particular with the partner, physical attractiveness, or a positive sexual relationship (Mahlstedt, 1985; Nachtigall, Becker & Wizny, 1992). Some may offer to allow their spouse to partner someone else in order to have a child. Fertility difficulties can exert a pervasive negative effect on quality of life, compromising planning and commitment to other life activities. The effect is observable in both men and women, but more so in women (Abbey, Andrews & Halman, 1992).

Quantitative investigations have used psychometric measures, standardized in general populations, to examine whether the incidence of particular symptoms or syndromes is different in infertile and presumed fertile populations (Greil, 1997). This approach has two potential limitations. First, standardized measures of psychological dysfunction may not be sufficiently sensitive to capture the complexities of the infertility experience (Greil, 1997). Second, the group of women who experience infertility is heterogeneous, in both gynaecological and socioeconomic terms, and it is unlikely that any control or comparison group can be matched in these terms and in length of time to conceive (Hearn et al., 1987). Despite these limitations, there has been substantial research comparing infertile women and couples with presumed fertile controls or already pregnant women. Perhaps because of the limitations, the findings are inconsistent.

Significantly higher levels of depressive symptoms have been found among women seeking treatment for infertility than in presumed fertile controls (Bernstein, Potts & Mattox, 1985; Berg & Wilson, 1990; Domar et al., 1992; Beaurepaire et al., 1994). However, other investigators have reported no significant differences in levels of depression between infertile and comparison groups (Connolly et al., 1992; Downey & McKinney, 1992; Hynes et al., 1992). It has been suggested that there are, nevertheless, differences in distress between the two groups, but that the severity of this distress is not clinically significant (Greil, 1997). This is supported by the findings of significantly more nonspecific emotional distress (Moller & Fallstrom, 1991) and less life satisfaction and happiness (Callan & Hennessey, 1988b) in infertile populations. More severe depression is associated with increasing age and being childless (Morrow, Thoreson & Penney, 1995). The findings regarding anxiety are similar, with some studies finding significantly higher levels among infertile groups (Beaurepaire et al., 1994; Visser et al., 1994), and others finding no differences from controls (Connolly et al., 1992). However, Connolly et al. (1992) acknowledge that individuals have differing degrees of dispositional anxiety and that these may lead to varying anxious responses to infertility. Lower levels of self-esteem and self-regard have been reported, although the differences remain within a normal range (Callan & Hennessey, 1988b; Edelmann et al., 1991; Hynes et al., 1992; Nachtigall, Becker & Wizny, 1992; Beaurepaire et al., 1994). Similarly, heightened guilt and self-blame are common, but not pathological (Bernstein, Potts & Mattox, 1985; Morrow, Thoreson & Penney, 1995).

There have been few systematic studies of the psychological impact of infertility in developing countries, and relatively little is known about the psychological functioning of women with fertility difficulties in these settings. This situation has been described as reflecting the eurocentric focus of most research in this field (Inhorn & Buss, 1994). In a single study, Aghanwa, Dare & Ogunniyi, (1999) reported that 29.7% of infertile patients in Nigeria were depressed or had an anxiety disorder, compared with 2.7% of fertile non-matched hospital staff controls.

It has been suggested that in highly pro-natalist societies, where women may have few occupational choices and motherhood is the only identifier of adult status, infertility is highly stigmatizing (Inhorn, 2003; Koster-Oyekan, 1999; Mariano, 2004; Upton, 2001). The inability to have children damages both cultural and adult identity, and the attribution of responsibility leads to social rejection and marginalization. Infertile women may have their gender identity questioned, experience social exclusion, be suspected of having evil potential and be subject to harassment, especially from their in-laws (Koster-Oyekan, 1999; Upton, 2001). In settings where women are subordinated, they are highly likely to be blamed for infertility (Mariano, 2004). They may be divorced because of their failure to bear children, which itself is highly stigmatizing, or their husband may marry a second wife (Koster-Oyekan, 1999; Mariano, 2004; Upton, 2001). Divorced and childless women are highly vulnerable when old, because adult children are the usual primary supporters of older people. Given the very limited access to assisted reproductive treatments in these settings, infertility has been described as leading to profound human suffering (Inhorn, 2003). Upton (2001) has argued that the presumption that infertility is rare in countries with high fertility rates, and the inaccurate understanding of its determinants, have led to the condition being "invisible" to policy-makers. As a result, there has been insufficient consideration of the psychological and social costs to women of infertility in these contexts.

Gender differences in the psychological sequelae of infertility

Although infertility exerts adverse psychological effects on both men and women, there is evidence that they react differently (Abbey, Andrews

& Halman, 1991; Nachtigall, Becker & Wizny, 1992; Cook, 1993). Women have been found to experience more emotional distress and depressive symptoms associated with infertility than men, except in cases of male factor infertility where the degree of distress is similar (Nachtigall, Becker & Wizny, 1992; Beaurepaire, et al., 1994; Morrow, Thoreson & Penney, 1995). Similarly, there are adverse effects on the gender identity of all women with infertility regardless of the etiological factor; but male gender identity is adversely affected only by male factors (Nachtigall, Becker & Wizny, 1992). Even when male factors are implicated, women experience more guilt and self-blame than their male partners (Abbey, Andrews & Halman, 1991). This may be because, even when male factors are involved, most of the investigation and treatments focus on the female partner. Women's lives are more disrupted by infertility than men's (Abbey, Andrews & Halman, 1991). It also appears that the loss of sex role identity and the experiences of childbirth and parenthood is more profound for women than for men (Abbey, Andrews & Halman, 1991; Nachtigall, Becker & Wizny, 1992; Cook, 1993). Both men and women are more likely to believe that the woman is responsible if unexplained or combined factors are etiologically involved (Abbey, Andrews & Halman, 1991). Men are more likely than women to experience infertility as a sign of compromised potency and sexual adequacy (Nachtigall, Becker & Wizny, 1992).

Individuals respond to disturbing life events in different ways. Women who are able to take an active part in seeking information and making decisions about treatment have lower levels of depression and attract more social support than those who passively submit to medical recommendations (Woods, Olshansky & Draye, 1991). Individuals with high self-esteem and dispositional optimism are better protected against severe depression (Litt et al., 1992). Denial and avoidance are elements of a normal response to adverse experiences, including infertility (Menning, 1982). Some individuals may appear to be more persistently unaffected emotionally by the diagnosis of infertility, but denial is not an effective defence against severe emotional distress. Individuals who use avoidant coping and deny the emotional impact of infertility may seek multiple medical opinions, in order to find an optimistic assessment. They are at higher risk of becoming depressed and may also be vulnerable to exploitation by extravagant claims for treatments, including those for which there is

scant scientific evidence (Woods, Olshansky & Draye, 1991; Litt et al., 1992; Morrow, Thoreson & Penney, 1995).

Impact of infertility and infertility treatment on the marital relationship

Infertility can exert adverse effects on the emotional and sexual relationship between partners (Andrews, Abbey & Halman, 1992; Greil, 1997; Eugster & Vingerhoest, 1999; Hart, 2002). Guilt and inexpressible blame can have insidious effects on intimacy. The infertile partner may fear rejection or may feel obliged to offer the other a divorce so that he or she can achieve genetic parenthood with someone else (Hart, 2002). The expression of anger and frustration about the predicament may be constrained in order to protect the infertile partner (Hart, 2002). Sexual spontaneity can be impaired by the need for sexual intercourse to be carefully timed and by the clinical scrutiny to which the relationship is subjected. Both partners may experience emotional pain seeing other couples with children (Hart, 2002). However, systematic psychometric investigations have revealed few differences in quality of marital relationship between infertile and comparison groups. Rather they suggest that marital intimacy and cohesion can be strengthened and enhanced through confronting the experience of infertility together (Dennerstein & Morse, 1988; Berg & Wilson, 1991; Greil, 1997).

Psychological aspects of treatment of infertility using assisted reproductive technology

Psychological sequelae of diagnosis and treatment

In the past 25 years, technologies to treat both male and female infertility have developed rapidly. In industrialized countries with well developed infertility treatment services, it is estimated that more than 60% of couples with fertility difficulties will seek treatment (Dawson, 1994). Although the need for assisted reproductive technologies in poor countries is high, the public provision of these highly sophisticated services has to be weighed against the competing demands of major infectious and chronic disease burdens, and limited obstetric and perinatal health services (Vayena, Rowe & Griffin, 2002; WHO, 2003). Private infertility treatment services are being established in many poor countries, but are likely to be accessible and available only to socioeconomically advantaged groups (Vayena, Rowe & Peterson, 2002; WHO, 2003). Teaching hospitals in some developing countries are starting to offer public infertility treatment services (Vayena, Rowe & Griffin, 2002). Overall, the situation in developing countries varies considerably, in terms of availability of appropriately trained health professionals and essential laboratory services, and it is not possible to generalize (Vayena, Rowe & Griffin, 2002).

Rates of pregnancy and live births following assisted conception depend on the experience of the treating centre (Eugster & Vingerhoest, 1999). While rates continue to improve, on average only 20% of couples conceive at each embryo transfer cycle (Kovacs, MacLachlan & Brehny, 2001). Using life-table calculations to review 4225 couples who had undergone 8207 cycles over six years, Kovacs, MacLachlan & Brehny (2001) reported that half the women became pregnant within three cycles and two-thirds became pregnant over six cycles. There is a theoretical debate about whether infertility should be considered a disease that requires medical treatment or an unfortunate life circumstance on which public resources should not be spent. Bewley (1995) argues that the physical and mental health risks of treating an individual, in whom the expected successful outcome of a living child is low, may outweigh the benefits. Others have suggested that the availability of assisted reproductive technologies means that both patients and clinicians try to seek a cure for the condition, rather than exploring other means of establishing a fulfilling life (Becker & Nachtigall, 1994). Critics assert that women are coerced into participating in and persisting with treatment, rather than making a free choice (Shattuck & Schwarz, 1991).

There is now substantial evidence that the nature and intensity of emotional distress vary over the course of infertility treatment. At diagnosis, symptoms of acute distress may increase; there then appears to be a decrease in symptoms once treatment starts (Beaurepaire et al., 1994). Severity of depression at this stage has been linked to having a confirmed diagnosis and a history of surgery for investigation or treatment of infertility (Domar et al., 1992). The initiation of treatment arouses optimism that the condition may be alleviated. However, there is evidence that women hold unrealistically high expectations at this stage of the likely success of treatment (Callan & Hennessey, 1988a; Beaurepaire et al., 1994; Hammarberg, Astbury & Baker, 2001). Injections, scans, blood tests and waiting to know whether eggs have been fertilized are all regarded as more psychologically than physically demanding (Callan & Hennessey, 1988a; Hammarberg, Astbury & Baker, 2001). There is consistent evidence that the moment of embryo transfer arouses optimism, but that the interval between transfer and pregnancy testing to confirm whether implantation and conception have occurred is highly anxiety arousing (Callan & Hennessey, 1988a; Yong, Martin & Thong, 2000; Franco et al., 2002). The onset of menstruation or a negative pregnancy test leads to intense sadness, despair and a sense of lost control (Litt et al., 1992; Franco et al., 2002). Dispositional optimism and active coping are protective against depression following implantation failure; women who use avoidant coping are generally more distressed (Litt et al., 1992).

Repeated unsuccessful treatment cycles can erode the increase in confidence and hope that comes at the start of treatment. It has been shown that, after two years of unsuccessful treatment, distress returns to a higher level than before treatment and can develop into chronic and severe depression (Berg & Wilson, 1990; Domar et al., 1992). Optimism gradually diminishes over repeated cycles and few couples persist for more than six (Callan & Hennessey, 1988a; Kovacs, MacLachlan & Brehny, 2001). Making the decision to stop fertility treatment is not straightforward, as there is no clear terminal point if conception has not yet occurred (Covington, 1995). Among other factors, the decision not to attempt another treatment cycle is strongly influenced by social forces, including the opinions of family members and friends (Callan et al., 1988). One qualitative study suggested that a state of dissociation between the physical treatment and its psychological consequences is necessary in order for couples to persist with repeat cycles (Benjamin & Ha'elyon, 2002). The authors argued that this is a response to the violation of privacy and time that diagnosis and treatment involve, and that once this detachment cannot be sustained, individuals cease treatment.

In many settings, the costs of infertility treatment are not subsidized by the state and fall on the individual. This can add substantially to the burden of emotional distress, and have a marked effect on decision-making about persistence with treatment; couples have to weigh the financial costs of diagnostic tests and treatment cycles against their yearning for a child (Abbey, Halman & Andrews, 1992; Franco et al., 2002). It has been asserted that couples cannot make a fully informed choice about participation in infertility treatment, because the risks of procedures (including ovarian hyperstimulation and multiple gestations), the economic costs, the limited success rates, and the possible adverse health effects on women and their offspring are generally understated (Pfeffer, 1991; Collins, 1994). Some support for this view has been provided by evidence that, after prolonged infertility, multiple gestations can be idealized and the associated hazards underestimated (Franco et al., 2002). Couples may actively seek a multiple birth in order to create an instant family (Leiblum, Kemmann & Taska, 1990; Gleicher et al., 1995; Goldfarb et al., 1996). Although couples may have significant fears about fetal well-being and doubts about their own capacity to care for more than one infant, they can feel prohibited from expressing this ambivalence because they consented to the transfer of multiple embryos (Leiblum, Kemmann & Taska, 1990; Gleicher et al., 1995; Goldfarb et al., 1996).

Psychological components of treatment

It has been cogently argued that, given the intensity and severity of distress that can be apparent during treatment, infertility clinicians need to have both medical and psychological skills (Covington, 1995). The promotion of optimism and personal control during treatment reduces psychological distress (Abbey, Halman & Andrews, 1992). As irritability, anxiety and depressive symptoms are most intense during the period between embryo transfer and pregnancy-testing, it has been argued that supportive counselling should be available at this time (Yong, Martin & Thong, 2000).

General social support has been found to have a more positive effect on women's distress than on men's (Abbey, Halman & Andrews, 1992). There have been a number of attempts to relieve the psychological distress of infertility and to examine whether this can increase conception rates. Individual, couple and group therapy approaches have been tried (Hart, 2002). A behavioural group treatment approach, including

relaxation training, cognitive therapy, exercise and nutritional counselling, reduced psychological symptoms in women, 34% of whom conceived; however, there was no untreated comparison group (Domar, Seibel & Benson, 1990; Domar, 1994). This psychological improvement was replicated in a subsequent study, (Domar et al., 1992b) but the group did not include women with severe psychological dysfunction. Having a peer counsellor who had experienced infertility, as well as a group leader, was found to be beneficial (Domar, Seibel & Benson, 1990). Fewer men than women want to participate in self-help support groups, although participation has been shown to provide emotional support and practical information and to reduce social isolation. Men who attended such groups to support their wives ultimately found them personally helpful (Lentner & Glazer, 1991).

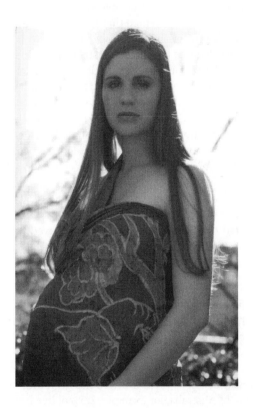

Termination of infertility treatment

Not all couples with fertility difficulties will conceive following infertility treatment; significant proportions have to adjust to life without a biological offspring. Long-term follow-up studies have examined women's views about, and recollections of, the experience of infertility treatment. Combining a survey of past patients at a hospital in Oslo, Norway with a medical record audit, Sundby, Olsen & Schei (1994) showed that most women had experienced discontinuity of treatment in the public sector, seeing different doctors at each consultation. One-third had stopped treatment without its being formally documented. Those who had a child were satisfied with their treatment, but less than half who did not conceive were satisfied. Independent of whether a child had been born, 70% were dissatisfied with the emotional support that had been provided by health staff (Sundby, Olsen & Schei, 1994). A follow-up study six years after cessation of treatment found that it was recalled as a traumatic life event. Overall, long-term psychological functioning was in the normal range, with greater well-being among those with a child compared with those without a child. Those with a hostile marital relationship, pre-existing psychiatric illness, or low level of education were more vulnerable in the long term. The authors commented that people undergoing infertility treatment should be encouraged, and counselled that psychological stability will eventually be restored and that adoption is often a satisfactory outcome (Sundby, 1992). Similarly, fewer than half the women in a study in Finalnd were satisfied with their infertility treatment. Dissatisfaction was higher among older women who had not conceived, and the doctor's capacity for empathy and kindness was central to satisfaction (Malin et al., 2001). In an Australian study of 116 women, 2–3 years after ceasing infertility treatment, Hammarberg et al. (2001) found that women who had not conceived were less satisfied with the treatment and clinical care and with their life than those who had a baby.

Psychological aspects of pregnancy, childbirth and the postpartum period after assisted conception

In recent years, the number of children born as a result of assisted reproduction has been increasing. In Australia, for example, 2.5% of live births now follow assisted conception (Waters, Dean & Sullivan, 2006). Pregnancies that have been assisted in this way carry higher risks for both mother and infant. These include increased risk of antepartum haemorrhage, multiple gestation, pregnancy hypertension, caesarean delivery, premature birth, low or very low birth weight, and the infant requiring oxygen at birth (Tallo et al., 1995; Wang et al., 1994; Waters et al., 2006). However, these risks are predominantly those associated with pregnancy at an advanced ma-

ternal age and multiple gestations (Olivennes et al., 1993). Many pregnancies following assisted conception are regarded as high risk (Dulude et al., 2002).

Pregnancy

Multiple gestations are more likely following induction of ovulation, or after the transfer of multiple embryos (McKinney & Leary, 1999). Multiple gestations are usually diagnosed very early after assisted conception, and parents may not think about the possibility of losing one fetus. Grief in those who have a single baby after having lost another fetus during the pregnancy is intense, but can be unrecognized by both health professionals and friends (Kollantai & Fleischer, 2001; Swanson, Pearsall-Jones & Hay, 2002; Fisher & Stocky, 2003). The coincidence of bereavement and pregnancy presents a psychological paradox, which is not easily resolved and may lead to delayed or disturbed grief reactions or disrupt the mother–infant attachment (Bryan & Denton, 2001; Pector & Smith-Levitin, 2002).

Very little is known about the long-term psychological consequences of what is termed planned fetal reduction or selective abortion of one or more fetuses in multiple pregnancy. In a study comparing 42 women who had undergone fetal reduction with women who had conceived a singleton pregnancy after in vitro fertilization (IVF), the rates of depression were equal in those who ultimately had a baby, but was high in those from either group who miscarried the pregnancy. However, many described fetal reduction as extremely stressful, 98% experienced anxiety, 69% sadness and 57% guilt as a result of the procedure. Grief, mourning and underlying feelings of shame were apparent in most (McKinney & Leary, 1999). Perhaps reflecting this, fetal reduction is rarely widely disclosed and may be kept secret. However, it is known that keeping secrets harms family relationships through fear of discovery and mistrust (Covington & Burns, 1999; Bryan, 2002). Qualitative investigations have reported complicated grief reactions in which multiple disenfranchised losses are experienced (Collopy, 2002). The potential impact on the living infant remains unknown, but the possibility of a "survivor syndrome", characterized by guilt, perplexity and grief for a lost sibling, has been suggested (Bryan & Denton, 2001; Fisher & Stocky, 2003).

Pregnancies in which a heightened risk to maternal or fetal health is identified are more psychologically distressing (Dulude et al., 2002). Women who become pregnant following assisted conception have been described as: having heightened anxiety about pregnancy loss and infant health, less self-confidence, and greater difficulty in acknowledging ambivalence, anxiety or sadness; using avoidant coping; becoming hypervigilant; feeling unable to complain or seek support and denying the pregnant state as self-protection against loss (Dunnington & Glazer, 1991; Bernstein, Lewis & Seibel, 1994; van Balen, Naaktgeboren & Trimbos-Kemper, 1996; Covington & Burns, 1999; Eugster & Vingerhoest, 1999; McMahon, 1999; Hjelmstedt et al., 2003). Concern about fetal development is high even in women whose pregnancies are known to be low-risk (Reading, Chang & Kerin, 1989; Gibson et al., 2000b) and preparation of a home environment for the baby is delayed (Dunnington & Glazer, 1991; Bernstein, Lewis & Seibel, 1994). The universal psychological challenge of pregnancy is to form a maternal identity, and this process appears to be more problematic in women who have a history of infertility. The relinquishing of an infertile identity and the adoption of a fertile and maternal one have to happen rapidly, but may in reality be complicated and prolonged (Covington & Burns, 1999; McMahon, 1999). Motherhood following infertility has usually been idealized and the losses and adverse experiences it inevitably entails may be unexpected (Covington & Burns, 1999; McMahon, 1999). Although women report increased anxiety about intrapartum damage to the baby, they have often underestimated the potential risks of childbirth to themselves (Connolly et al., 1992; McMahon, 1999). In contrast, two studies reported no differences in anxiety or depressive symptoms measured with standardized instruments between women who had conceived spontaneously and those who had conceived after IVF (Stanton & Golombok, 1993; Klock & Greenfield, 2000). None of the studies controlled for the particular effects of multiple gestation, and most studies excluded multiple gestations and women who already had a child.

No differences in the intensity or quality of self-reported maternal–fetal emotional attachment have been reported, although women anticipated that their infants might have more difficulties than those conceived spontaneously. In a single longitudinal study, anxiety was reported to decrease more as pregnancy progressed in those who had had assisted conception than in those who had conceived spontaneously (Stanton & Golombok, 1993; McMahon, 1999; Klock & Greenfield, 2000). It has been suggested that women may need additional support and sensitized care in pregnancy after assisted conception (McMahon et al. 1995; McMahon, 1999; Hjelmstedt et al., 2003).

Childbirth

Although women are at greatly elevated risk of caesarean birth after assisted conception (Wang et al., 1994), there has been little investigation of the interactions between these two procedures. There is consistent evidence that both instrumental intervention in vaginal birth and caesarean surgery are associated with increased anxiety, disappointment, grief and dissatisfaction (Boyce & Todd, 1992; Fisher, Astbury & Smith, 1997). Although mode of delivery does not appear to make an independent contribution to postpartum depression when other risk factors are taken into account (Johnstone et al., 2001), caesarean surgery can induce post-traumatic stress reactions (Fisher, Astbury & Smith, 1997). After caesarean childbirth, the first encounter between mother and infant and the initiation of breastfeeding are disrupted, with adverse effects on maternal confidence that are still measurable eight months later (Rowe-Murray & Fisher, 2001, 2002). In one study, childbirth was reported as "more exceptional" after assisted conception, but this descriptor was not defined and is difficult to interpret (van Balen, Naaktgeboren & Trimbos-Kemper, 1996).

Operative delivery and premature birth are both more common among women with multiple gestation, which occurs in 20% of pregnancies after assisted conception (Barrett & Ritchie, 2002). Premature birth typically involves separation of the mother from her infants, sometimes for prolonged periods. Intense anxiety about the infants' health and development and about the separation is universal, and is more severe among those whose infants are seriously unwell; and the anxiety can persist for up to three years (Singer et al., 1999). When babies are kept in neonatal intensive care units, mothers report uncertainty about whether the health professional or the parent has authority over the baby (Bryan & Denton, 2001; Loo et al., 2003). A cooperative approach to decision-making, respecting parental rights, can be helpful (Carter & Leuthner, 2002). Fear about the infants' health and viability can persist and lead to hypervigilance in relation to infant care, and delayed formation of a secure affectionate emotional attachment (Klock, 2001; Loo et al., 2003). No studies have examined the interacting emotional effects of assisted conception, operative birth, prematurity, neonatal hospitalization and multiple birth. However, the established difficulties are further magnified if the infants are separated, for example by discharge of one infant ahead of another or by care in different hospitals (Bryan & Denton, 2001). Maintaining a supply of breastmilk and establishing breastfeeding are difficult and anxiety-arousing with premature and very low-birthweight infants.

Parenthood after infertility and assisted reproduction

Most of the investigations into the long-term impact of assisted conception have focused on women's capacity to mother, the quality of mother–infant attachment and the developmental outcomes of the children. Few have focused on maternal mental and physical health in itself.

Descriptive and exploratory studies claim that, after assisted conception, mothers are more likely to be overprotective and to recall infertility as an influential negative life event. Burns (1990) concluded that infertility is not transient, continues after conception and may be experienced as long-term adjustment difficulties in the family. Further, parents may be less conscious of the challenges of parenthood and, although the quality of parenting is high, have to make an extraordinary effort to feel effective. Burns (1990) suggested that parents may have formed unrealistic and "utopian fantasies", which make it difficult for them to adjust to the unique demands and unavoidable ambivalence of parenting. She also suggested that they are particularly likely to have difficulties separating from their infants and with the developmental process of individuation, and may be less able to foster the child's capacity for self-sufficiency (Burns, 1990, 1999). In Australia, there is an excess (6.3–9% compared with 1.2–1.7% of live births) of mothers who have experienced fertility difficulties or assisted conception among those admitted to residential early parenting services because of infant sleep or feeding disorders and mater-

nal exhaustion or mild to moderate depression (Barnett et al., 1993; Fisher et al., 2002; Fisher, Hammarberg & Baker, 2005). A group of mothers who were members of an infertility support group were found to confide less and have fewer acquaintances and friendships than a comparison group who had conceived spontaneously (Munro, Ironside & Smith, 1992). Mothers who had had assistance to conceive anticipated that their infants would have more problems and rated their infants as having more difficult temperaments than a group of controls (McMahon et al., 1997). In contrast, Golombok et al. (1995) found no adverse psychological consequences and "superior parenting" among children conceived with assisted reproductive technologies. Systematic investigations have used the Strange Situations Test, which assesses the quality of mother–child attachment through videotaped observations of the mother and child, while playing together and when separated from each other. These studies have found no differences in mother–child attachment between children conceived spontaneously or with assistance, and that most mothers were sensitive and responsive to their children (Gibson et al., 2000a). None of these studies included infants conceived by use of donor gametes or multiple births (Fisher & Stocky, 2003). In reviewing the early studies, McMahon et al. (1995) concluded that there was little evidence of differences in quality of parenting between families formed with assisted conception and others, but conceded that most of the available studies had methodological limitations.

There is consistent evidence that the emotional health of mothers of multiple infants is poorer than that of mothers of single infants, and that they are at higher risk of becoming depressed, anxious and clinically exhausted after childbirth. Hay et al. (1990) found that 29.7% of mothers of 3-month-old twins reported depression (a rate five times higher than among mothers of single 3-month-old infants); 42% had high anxiety (three times higher than among mothers of single infants). Even higher rates of depression have been reported among mothers of triplets. Robin et al. (1991) found that 40% were depressed 4 months postpartum, while Garel, Salobir & Blondel (1997) found that all reported significant distress and a quarter were being treated for depression one year postpartum. Two studies of the health and social circumstances of women admitted to Australian residential early parenting services for treatment of unsettled infant behaviour and maternal exhaustion, anxiety and depression found an excess of mothers with multiple infants (3.7–5%, compared with the general population rate of 1.4%) (Barnett et al., 1993; Fisher et al., 2002). In a longitudinal study of more than 13 000 women who gave birth in one month in 1970, Thorpe et al. (1991) found that, five years after the birth, independent of other explanatory factors, mothers of twins were three times more likely to be depressed than those with a single child. In a small comparative study, higher parenting stress was associated with having twins, regardless of mode of conception (Cook, Bradley & Golombok, 1998). This effect may lessen as the children grow older. In examining 158 sets of twins entering preschool, Munro, Ironside & Smith (1990) found less psychiatric disturbance among mothers of twins conceived by IVF than mothers of spontaneously conceived twins.

New technologies and their implications

Donated fresh sperm has been used to treat male factor infertility for 100 years. The use of cryopreservation to store sperm for later donation is a newer technological development. The donation of embryos and oocytes has become possible more recently, and involves the donor undergoing a stimulated cycle and the surgical removal of oocytes for either transfer, cryopreservation or fertilization with donated sperm (Barrero, 2002). The new technologies now available to treat fertility difficulties may themselves carry sequelae for mental health, but very little evidence is so far available (Kirby, 1994).

Issues arising with use of the new technologies include: the ethical, legal and psychological complexities of the use of donated genetic material; payments to donors for their genetic material; debates about the maintenance of secrecy and disclosure, and the impact of legislation regarding children's rights to know their biological heritage versus parents' rights to secrecy. Gestational surrogacy and the use of donor gametes lead to complex considerations of what constitutes a parent–infant relationship (Kirkman, 1996, 1999; Barrero, 2002; Vayena, Rowe & Griffin, 2002). Relatively little is known about the motives and psychological functioning of donors, including those who donate genetic material anonymously

(Rosenthal, 1998). However, it has been established that, over time, donors may change their minds about remaining anonymous or allowing their identity to be disclosed to offspring (Blyth, Crawshaw & Daniels, 2004). In general, people conceived from donated genetic material want to know their genetic heritage and the identity of the donor, and believe that secrecy is harmful to individuals and to families (Blyth, Crawshaw & Daniels, 2004).

A shortage of donated eggs places significant limitations on treatment in most settings. In order to donate ova, women have to undergo ovarian stimulation and surgical aspiration, and the number willing to do so is limited (Cleland, 1994; Murray et al., 1994). Depending on local legislation, eggs may be donated by someone known to the recipient or by an anonymous donor, voluntarily or in exchange for payment. In some European countries, a strategy termed egg sharing is available, in which women undergoing fertility treatment requiring ovarian stimulation and oocyte retrieval can donate half the resulting ova anonymously to another couple in exchange for reduced fees and rapid access to treatment (Ahuja et al., 2003). Investigation of the psychological implications of donating ova to other women has only recently begun. However, in-depth interviews with small samples in the United Kingdom have found that the decision to participate as a donor in egg sharing schemes is influenced by the waiting time for treatment, costs of treatment, individual perceptions of the donated gametes as "tissue" or as a "potential baby", and a complex existential notion of altruism combined with a desire to achieve a personal life goal (Rapport, 2003; Blyth, 2004). There is ongoing debate about the ethics of this option, in particular since the evidence in its favour has been generated to a large extent by providers. The short- and long-term psychological and emotional sequelae have not been examined systematically by independent investigators (Ahuja et al, 2003; Blyth, Crawshaw & Daniels, 2004).

There is debate about whether tissues with reproductive potential should be treated differently from those donated post mortem. Consideration is being given to whether cadavers, aborted fetuses or live donors may be the best source of eggs (Murray et al., 1994). In order to investigate attitudes to this theoretical possibility, women attending for pregnancy termination, contraception or infertility treatment were surveyed. In general, there was strong support for methods to increase the supply of donated ova, from all sources, but women having abortions did not in general support post-mortem donation of ova. Neither potential donors nor potential recipients disapproved of the use of fetal ovarian tissue for research (Murray et al., 1994).

There is wide variation internationally regarding record-keeping and access to records following the use of donated genetic material (Kirby, 1994). There is a need for considered public and expert debate regarding a number of issues, e.g. quality control to protect against consanguinity, legal acknowledgment of the social rather than the genetic parent, and the rights of the children and not just the adults exposed to these procedures. The disposal of, and experimentation on, surplus frozen embryos or other genetic material remain controversial (Kirby, 1994). In considering the allocation of health resources, there is debate about whether individuals should bear the cost or whether it is a social cost to be born publicly. The complex economics of the cost-effectiveness of treatment have to be considered (Kirby, 1994; Neumann, Gharib & Weinstein, 1994).

There is also debate about whether treatment should be offered to all who seek it, or whether there should be criteria for inclusion in treatment programmes The debate regarding the rights of the child is sometimes used to withhold treatment from post-menopausal women, because of the complex ethics relating to being born to parents who may die before the child reached maturity (Hope, Lockwood & Lockwood, 1995). Older women are generally less likely to conceive, and it has been suggested that health professionals who offer fertility treatment to older women are assisting them to act irresponsibly (Jackson, 1995). There is debate about whether these decisions, especially whether women over 50 years of age should be refused treatment, should be made by an ethics committee (who may not know the individual patient) or by a single clinician (Craft, 1995).

The psychological implications of the preservation of tissue to protect fertility in those undergoing chemotherapy are yet to be investigated.

For many women, being a mother is core to the formation of their adult identity, and the availability of technologies means that some will persevere in their efforts to have a child, even to the extent of putting their own health at risk (Kirkman, 1996). Health professionals face significant difficulties in interpreting social and ethical dilemmas in individual cases. Nurses rated the emotional distress associated with infertility treatment as worse than either patients or physicians did, and patients rated it as worse than physicians did. However, all agreed that infertility treatment was one of the most difficult professional fields in which to practise (Kopitzke et al., 1991). Patients' irritability and frustration may be directed at health professionals, who may be perceived as lacking sensitivity and ability to communicate, or blamed for the limitations of existing knowledge and techniques. Covington (1995) stated that, because of the multiple losses, prolonged treatment, complexities in defining the end of treatment, and high failure rate, all professionals in this field need to integrate psychological with medical care.

The psychosocial sequelae of infertility and the complex psychological responses to technologically assisted conception are central to the health of people facing these life experiences, and should be considered in research and clinical services.

Summary

Future research

1. Causes of infertility differ, and in each country an accurate understanding is needed of the fertility problems of the population.

2. In most countries, the prevalence, etiology and mental health effects of fertility problems have not been established.

3. Research is needed into the demand for, and nature of, infertility treatment services in developing countries.

4. The long-term psychological consequences of infertility, including after the birth of a child, should be investigated.

5. There is a need for data on the short- and long-term psychosocial and medical consequences for both donors and recipients of gametes, including women in egg-sharing programmes.

6. There is a need for long-term comprehensive follow-up of the physical and mental health of offspring of assisted conception, with disaggregation by method of conception.

7. Multiple pregnancies, which are more common after assisted conception, carry greater psychological hazards. The interaction between infertility and multiple gestations in influencing perinatal mental health should be clarified.

8. The short- and long-term psychological effects of fetal reduction in multiple-gestation pregnancy need to be systematically investigated.

9. The potential of psychological treatments to relieve the distress associated with infertility and assisted reproduction should be investigated in randomized controlled trials.

Policy

1. Attention to population control in countries with high fertility rates should not preclude identification and treatment of infertility.

2. The causes of infertility should be accurately ascertained.

3. Specialized diagnostic and treatment services are needed for people with fertility problems.

4. Infertility services need to have clear policies about disclosure of mode of conception, maintenance of donor registries, and protection of the needs of children conceived by assisted reproduction. These policies should be informed by public and professional debate.

Services

1. Infertility treatment services in all settings need to be based on evidence about local causes and best practice in treatment.

2. Infertility treatment services should include mental health care as a component of routine care.

3. Mental health care should be focused on: assisting the person to make a realistic appraisal of the chance of treatment success; providing emotional support in the interval between embryo transfer and pregnancy-testing; and assisting the person to make a clear choice about when to stop treatment.

References

Abbey A, Andrews F, Halman L (1991) Gender's role in responses to infertility. *Psychology of Women Quarterly*, 15: 295-316.

Abbey A, Andrews F, Halman L (1992) Infertility and subjective well-being: the mediating roles of self-esteem, internal control, and interpersonal conflict. *Journal of Marriage and the Family*, 54(May): 408-416.

Abbey A, Halman L, Andrews F (1992) Psychosocial, treatment, and demographic predictors of the stress associated with infertility. *Fertility and Sterility,* 57(1): 122-128.

Adetoro OO, Ebomoyi EW (1991) The prevalence of infertility in a rural Nigerian community. *African Journal of Medicine and Medical Science* 20: 23-27.

Aghanwa HS, Dare FO, Ogunniyi SO (1999) Sociodemographic factors in mental disorders associated with infertility in Nigeria. *Journal of Psychosomatic Research*, 46(2): 117-123.

Ahuja KK et al. (2003) Minimizing risk in anonymous egg donation. *Reproductive Biomedicine Online*, 7: 504-505.

Andrews FM, Abbey A, Halman L (1992) Is fertility problem stress different? The dynamics of stress in fertile and infertile couples. *Fertility and Sterility*, 46: 1247-1253.

Australian Bureau of Statistics (2004) *Women in Australia.* Canberra, Commonwealth of Australia.

Barnett B et al. (1993) Mood disorders among mothers of infants admitted to a mothercraft hospital. *Journal of Paediatrics and Child Health*, 29:270-275.

Barrero C (2002) Gamete and embryo donation. In: Vayena E, Rowe PJ, Griffin PD, eds., *Current practices and controversies in assisted reproduction. Report of a meeting on medical, ethical and social aspects of assisted reproduction.* Geneva, World Health Organization.

Barrett JF, Ritchie WK (2002) Twin delivery. *Best Practice and Research in Clinical Obstetrics and Gynaecology*, 16(1): 43-56.

Beaurepaire J et al. (1994) Psychososocial adjustment to infertility and its treatment: male and female responses at different stages of IVF/ET treatment. *Journal of Psychosomatic Research*, 38(3): 229-240.

Becker G (1994) Metaphors in disrupted lives: infertility and cultural constructions of continuity. *Medical Anthropology Quarterly*, 8: 383-410.

Becker G, Nachtigall RD (1994) Born to be a mother: the cultural construction of risk in infertility treatment. *Social Science and Medicine*, 39(4): 507-518.

Benjamin O, Ha'elyon H (2002) Rewriting fertilization: trust, pain, and exit points. *Women's Studies International Forum*, 25(6): 667-678.

Beral V et al. (1994) Primary infertility: characteristics of women in North America according to pathological findings. *Journal of Epidemiology and Community Health*, 48: 576-579.

Berg B, Wilson J (1990) Psychiatric morbidity in the infertile population: a reconceptualization. *Infertility and sterility*, 53(4): 654-661.

Berg B, Wilson J (1991) Psychological functioning across stages of treatment for fertility. *Journal of Behavioural Medicine*, 14: 11-26.

Bernstein J, Lewis J, Seibel M (1994) Effect of previous infertility on maternal-fetal attachment, coping styles, and self-concept during pregnancy. *Journal of Women's Health*, 3(2): 125-133.

Bernstein J, Potts N, Mattox JH (1985) Assessment of psychological dysfunction associated with infertility. *Journal of Obstetric, Gynecologic and Neonatal Nursing*, 14: 63-66.

Bewley S (1995) In vitro fertilisation is rarely successful in older women. *British Medical Journal*, 310: 1457.

Blyth E (2004) Patient experiences of an "egg sharing" programme. *Human Fertility*, 7: 157-162.

Blyth E, Crawshaw M, Daniels K (2004) Policy formation in gamete donation and egg sharing in the UK: a critical appraisal. *Social Science and Medicine*, 59: 2617-2626.

Boyce PM, Todd AL (1992) Increased risk of postnatal depression after emergency caesarean section. *Medical Journal of Australia*, 157(3 August): 172-174.

Bryan E (2002) Loss in higher multiple pregnancy and multifetal pregnancy reduction. *Twin Research*, 5(3): 169-174.

Bryan E, Denton J (2001) Education for parents. In: Blickstein I, Keith LG, eds., *Iatrogenic multiple pregnancy: clinical implications*. New York, Parthenon Publishing: 211-222.

Burns LH (1990) An exploratory study of perceptions of parenting after infertility. *Family Systems Medicine*, 8(2): 177-189.

Burns LH (1999) Parenting after infertility. In: Burns LH, Covington SN, eds., *Infertility counselling: a comprehensive handbook for clinicians*. London, Parthenon Publishing.

Callan VJ, Hennessey JF (1988a) Emotional aspects and support in in vitro fertilization and embryo transfer programs. *Journal of In Vitro Fertilization and Embryo Transfer*, 5(5): 290-295.

Callan VJ, Hennessey JF (1988b) The psychological adjustment of women experiencing infertility. *British Journal of Medical Psychology*, 61: 137-140.

Callan VJ et al. (1988) Towards understanding women's decisions to continue or stop in vitro fertilization: the role of social, psychological and background factors. *Journal of In Vitro Fertilization and Embryo Transfer*, 5(6): 363-369.

Carter BS, Leuthner SR (2002) Decision making in the NICU – strategies, statistics, and "satisficing". *Bioethics Forum*, 18(3-4): 7-15.

Cleland JGF (1994) Ovum donation: move slowly. *Lancet*, 344: 142, 204.

Collins JA (1994) Reproductive technology: the price of progress. *New England Journal of Medicine*, 331(4): 270-271.

Collopy KS (2002) We didn't deserve this: bereavement associated with multifetal reduction. *Twin Research*, 5(3): 231-235.

Connolly K et al. (1992) The impact of infertility on psychological functioning. *Journal of Psychosomatic Research*, 36(5): 459-468.

Cook R (1993) The relationship between sex role and emotional functioning in patients undergoing assisted conception. *Journal of Psychosomatic Obstetrics and Gynaecology*, 14: 31-40.

Cook R, Bradley S, Golombok S (1998) A preliminary study of parental stress and child behaviour in families with twins conceived by in-vitro fertilization. *Human Reproduction*, 13(11): 3244-3246.

Covington SN (1995) The role of the mental health professional in reproductive medicine. *Fertility and Sterility*, 64(5): 895-897.

Covington SN, Burns LH (1999) Pregnancy after infertility. In: Burns LH, Covington SN, eds., *Infertility counselling: a comprehensive handbook for clinicians*. London, Parthenon Publishing.

Craft I (1995) The role of ethics committees. *British Medical Journal*, 310: 1457-1458.

Dawson K (1994) *Reproductive technology, the science, the ethics, the law, and the social issues*. Melbourne, VCTA Publishing.

Dennerstein L, Morse C (1988) A review of psychological and social aspects of *in vitro* fertilization. *Journal of Psychosomatic Obstetrics and Gynaecology*, 9: 159-170.

Domar AD (1994) A behavioral approach to infertility treatment. *Clinical Consultations in Obstetrics and Gynecology*, 6(2): 116-121.

Domar AD, Seibel MM, Benson H (1990) The mind/body program for infertility: a new behavioral treatment approach for women with infertility. *Fertility and Sterility*, 53(2): 246-249.

Domar A et al. (1992a) The prevalence and predictability of depression in infertile women. *Fertility and Sterility*, 58(6): 1158-1163.

Domar AD et al. (1992b) Psychological improvement in infertile women after behavioral treatment: a replication. *Fertility and Sterility*, 58(1): 144-147.

Downey J, McKinney M (1992) The psychiatric status of women presenting for infertility evaluation. *American Journal of Orthopsychiatry*, 62(2): 196-205.

Dulude D et al. (2002) High-risk pregnancies, psychological distress, and dyadic adjustment. *Journal of Reproductive and Infant Psychology*, 20(2): 101-123.

Dunnington RM, Glazer G (1991) Maternal identity and early mothering behaviour in previously infertile and never infertile women. *Journal of Obstetric, Gynecologic and Neonatal Nursing*, 20(4): 309-333.

Edelmann RJ et al. (1991) Psychogenic infertility: some findings. *Journal of Psychosomatic Obstetrics and Gynaecology*, 12: 163-168.

Eugster A, Vingerhoest AJJM (1999) Psychological aspects of in vitro fertilization: a review. *Social Science and Medicine*, 48: 575-589.

Fathalla MF (1992) Reproductive health – a global overview. *Early Human Development*, 29(1-3): 35-42.

Fisher JRW, Stocky AJ (2003) Maternal perinatal mental health and multiple birth: implications for practice. *Twin Research*, 6: 506-513.

Fisher J, Astbury J, Smith A (1997) Adverse psychological impact of operative obstetric interventions: a prospective study. *Australian and New Zealand Journal of Psychiatry*, 31: 728-738.

Fisher JRW, Hammarberg K, Baker HWG (2005) Assisted conception is a risk factor for perinatal mood disturbance and early parenting difficulties *Fertility and Sterility*, 84: 426-430.

Fisher JRW et al. (2002) Health and social circumstances of women admitted to a private mother baby unit. A descriptive cohort study. *Australian Family Physician*, 31(10): 966-969.

Franco JG et al. (2002) Psychological evaluation test after use of assisted reproduction technologies. *Journal of Assisted Reproduction and Genetics*, 19(6): 274-278.

Garel M, Salobir C, Blondel B (1997) Psychological consequences of having triplets: a 4-year follow-up study. *Fertility and Sterility*, 67(6): 1162-1165.

Gibson FL et al. (2000a) The mother-child relationship following in vitro fertilisation (IVF): infant attachment, responsivity, and maternal sensitivity. *Journal of Child Psychology and Psychiatry*, 41(8): 1015-1023.

Gibson FL et al. (2000b) Parental adjustment and attitudes to parenting after in vitro fertilization. *Fertility and Sterility*, 73(3): 565-574.

Gleicher N et al. (1995) The desire for multiple births in couples with infertility problems contradicts present practice patterns. *Human Reproduction*, 10(5): 1079-1084.

Goldfarb JD et al. (1996) Attitudes of in vitro fertilization and intrauterine insemination couples toward multiple gestation pregnancy and multifetal pregnancy reduction. *Fertility and Sterility*, 65(4): 815-820.

Golombok S et al. (1995) Families created by the new reproductive technologies: quality of parenting and social and emotional development of the children. *Child Development*, 66: 285-298.

Greil A (1997) Infertility and psychological distress: a critical review of the literature. *Social Science and Medicine*, 45(11): 1679-1704.

Hammarberg K, Astbury J, Baker HWG (2001) Women's experience of IVF: a follow-up study. *Human Reproduction*, 16(2): 374-383.

Hart VA (2002) Infertility and the role of psychotherapy. *Issues in Mental Health Nursing*, 23(1): 31-41.

Hay DA et al. (1990) What information should the multiple birth family receive before, during and after the birth? *Acta Geneticae Medicae et Gemellologiae*, 39: 259-269.

Hearn MT et al. (1987) Psychological characteristics of in vitro fertilization participants. *American Journal of Obstetrics and Gynecology*, 156(2): 269-274.

Hjelmstedt A et al. (2003) Personality factors and emotional responses to pregnancy among IVF couples in early pregnancy: a comparative study. *Acta Obstetrica et Gynecologica Scandinavica*, 82: 152-161.

Hope T, Lockwood G, Lockwood M (1995) Should older women be offered in vitro fertilization? The interests of the potential child. *British Medical Journal*, 310: 1455-1456.

Hurst T, Lancaster P (2001) *Assisted conception Australia and New Zealand 1999 and 2000*. Sydney, Australian Institute of Health and Welfare.

Hynes GJ et al. (1992) The psychological wellbeing of infertile women after a failed IVF attempt: the effects of coping. *British Journal of Medical Psychology*, 65: 269-278.

Inhorn MC (1994) *Kabsa* (a.k.a. *Mushara*) and threatened fertility in Egypt. *Social Science and Medicine*, 39(4): 487-505.

Inhorn MC (2003) Global infertility and the globalization of new reproductive technologies: illustrations from Egypt. *Social Science and Medicine*, 56(9): 1837-1851.

Inhorn M, Buss K (1994) Ethnography, epidemiology and infertility in Egypt. *Social Science and Medicine*, 39(5): 671-686.

Jackson J (1995) Can older women cope with motherhood? *British Medical Journal*, 310: 1456-1457.

Johnson MH, Everitt BJ (2000) *Essential reproduction*. Oxford, Blackwell Science.

Johnstone S et al. (2001) Obstetric risk factors for postnatal depression in urban and rural community samples. *Australian & New Zealand Journal of Psychiatry*, 35(1): 69-74.

Kerr J, Brown C, Balen AH (1999) The experience of couples who have had infertility treatment in the United Kingdom: results of a survey performed in 1997. *Human Reproduction*, 14: 934-938.

Kirby MD (1994) Reproductive technology and law reform. *Medical Journal of Australia*, 161: 580-581.

Kirkman L (1999) Still not maternal: giving birth to my niece (10 years on). In: *Fertility and Genetics Beyond 1999. The Plenary Proceedings of the 11th World Congress on In Vitro Fertilization and Human Reproductive Genetics*. Sydney, Parthenon Publishing.

Kirkman M (1996) "Life doesn't go according to plan." Narratives of infertility. *Sixth International Interdisciplinary Congress on Women*, Adelaide.

Klock SC (2001) The transition to parenthood. In: Blickstein I, Keith LG, eds., *Iatrogenic multiple pregnancy: clinical implications*. New York, Parthenon Publishing: 225-234.

Klock SC, Greenfield DA (2000) Psychological status of in vitro fertilization patients during pregnancy: a longitudinal study. *Fertility and Sterility*, 73(6): 1159-1164.

Kollantai J, Fleischer LM (2001) Insert 16.3. Realities: coping with the impact of death in a multiple pregnancy. In: Blickstein I, Keith LG, eds., *Iatrogenic multiple pregnancy: clinical implications*. New York, Parthenon Publishing: 216-217.

Kols A, Nguyen T (1997) Infertility in developing countries. *Reproductive Health Outlook*, 15(3): 1-14.

Kopitzke EJ et al. (1991) Physical and emotional stress associated with components of the infertility investigation: perspectives of professionals and patients. *Fertility and Sterility*, 55(6): 1137-1143.

Koster-Oyekan W (1999) Infertility among Yoruba women: perceptions, causes, treatments and consequences. *African Journal of Reproductive Health*, 3: 13-26.

Kovacs G, MacLachlan V, Brehny S (2001) What is the probability of conception for couples entering an IVF program? *Australian and New Zealand Journal of Obstetrics and Gynaecology*, 41: 208-209.

Larsen U (2000) Primary and secondary infertility in sub-Saharan Africa. *International Journal of Epidemiology*, 29: 285-291.

Leiblum SR, Kemmann E, Taska L (1990) Attitudes toward multiple births and pregnancy concerns in infertile and non-infertile women. *Journal of Psychosomatic Obstetrics and Gynaecology*, 11: 197-210.

Lentner E, Glazer G (1991) Infertile couples' perceptions of infertility support-group participation. *Health Care for Women International*, 12: 317-330.

Litt MD et al. (1992) Coping and cognitive factors in adaptation to *in vitro* fertilization failure. *Journal of Behavioural Medicine*, 15(2): 171-187.

Loo KK et al. (2003) Using knowledge to cope with stress in the NICU: how parents integrate learning to read the physiologic and behavioral cues of the infant. *Neonatal Networks*, 22(1): 31-37.

Mahlstedt PP (1985) The psychological component of infertility. *Fertility and Sterility*, 43(3): 335-346.

Malin M et al. (2001) What do women want? Women's experiences of infertility treatment. *Social Science and Medicine*, 53(1): 123-133.

Marchbanks PA et al. (1989) Research on infertility: definition makes a difference. *American Journal of Epidemiology*, 130(2): 259-267.

McKinney M, Leary K (1999) Integrating quantitative and qualitative methods to study multifetal pregnancy reduction. *Journal of Women's Health*, 8(2): 259-269.

McMahon CA (1999) Does assisted reproduction make an impact on the identity and self-esteem of infertile women during the transition to parenthood? *Journal of Assisted Reproduction and Genetics*, 16(2): 59-62.

McMahon CA et al. (1995) Psychosocial outcomes for parents and children after *in vitro* fertilization: a review. *Journal of Reproductive and Infant Psychology*, 13: 1-16.

McMahon CA et al. (1997) Anxiety during pregnancy and fetal attachment after in-vitro fertilization conception. *Human Reproduction*, 12(1): 176-182.

Menning BE (1982) The psychosocial impact of infertility. *Symposium in Women's Health Issues*, 17(1): 155-163.

Moller A, Fallstrom K (1991) Psychological factors in the etiology of infertility: a longitudinal study. *Journal Psychosomatic Obstetrics and Gynaecology*, 12: 13-26.

Morrow KA, Thoreson RW, Penney LL (1995) Predictors of psychological distress among infertility clinic patients. *Journal of Consulting and Clinical Psychology*, 63(1): 163-167.

Munro JM, Ironside W, Smith G (1990) Psychiatric morbidity in parents of twins born after in vitro fertilization (IVF) techniques. *Journal of In Vitro Fertilization and Embryo Transfer*, 7(6): 332-336.

Munro JM, Ironside W, Smith G (1992) Successful parents of an in vitro fertilization (IVF): the social repercussions. *Journal of Assisted Reproduction and Genetics*, 9(2): 170-176.

Murray E et al. (1994) Donated ovarian tissue: the public's view. *Lancet*, 344: 204.

Nachtigall HD, Becker G, Wizny D (1992) The effects of gender-specific diagnosis on men's and women's response to infertility. *Fertility and Sterility*, 57(1): 113-121.

Neumann PJ, Gharib S, Weinstein MC (1994) The cost of a successful delivery with in vitro fertilization. *New England Journal of Medicine*, 331(4): 239-243.

Ng F (2000) Female genital mutilation; its implications for reproductive health. An overview. *British Journal of Family Planning*, 26(1): 47-51.

Okonofua FE et al. (1997) Serological and clinical correlates of gonorrhea and syphilis in fertile and infertile Nigerian women. *Genitourinary Medicine*, 73: 194-197.

Okonofua FE et al. (2002) The association between female genital cutting and correlates of sexual and gynaecological morbidity in Edo State, Nigeria. *BJOG: an International Journal of Obstetrics and Gynaecology*, 109: 1089-1096.

Olivennes F et al. (1993) The increased risk of complications observed in singleton pregnancies resulting from IVF does not seem to be related to the IVF method itself. *Human Reproduction*, 8: 1297-1300.

Olshansky EF (1987) Identity of self as infertile: an example of theory generating research. *Advances in Nursing Science*, 9(2): 54-63.

Pector EA, Smith-Levitin M (2002) Mourning and psychological issues in multiple birth loss. *Seminars in Neonatology*, 7(3): 247-256.

Pfeffer N (1991) The uninformed conception. *New Scientist*, (July 20th): 32-33.

Poggensee G, Feldmeier H (2001) Female genital schistosomiasis: facts and hypotheses. *Acta Tropica*, 79(3): 193-210.

Poggensee G et al. (2001) Diagnosis of genital cervical schistosomiasis: comparison of cytological, histopathological and parasitological examinations. *American Journal of Tropical Medicine and Hygiene*, 65(3): 233-236.

Rapport F (2003) Exploring the beliefs and experiences of potential egg share donors. *Journal of Advanced Nursing*, 43: 28-42.

Reading AE, Chang LC, Kerin JF (1989) Attitudes and anxiety levels in women conceiving through in vitro fertilization and gamete intrafallopian transfer. *Fertility and Sterility*, 52(1): 95-98.

Robin M et al. (1991) Maternal reactions to the birth of triplets. *Acta Geneticae Medicae et Gemellologiae*. 40: 41-51.

Rosenthal M (1998) Further needs in clinical assessment: women and infertility. *Psychopharmacology Bulletin*, 34(3): 307-309.

Rosenthal MB, Goldfarb J (1997) Infertility and assisted reproductive technology: an update for mental health professionals. *Harvard Review of Psychiatry*, 5(3): 169-172.

Rowe-Murray HJ, Fisher J (2001) Operative intervention in delivery is associated with disruptions to early mother-infant contact. *BJOG: an international journal of obstetrics and gynaecology,* 108: 1068-1075.

Rowe-Murray H, Fisher J (2002) Baby friendly hospital practices: cesarean section is a persistent barrier to early initiation of breastfeeding. *Birth,* 29(2): 124-130.

Schmidt L, Munster K (1995) Infertility, involuntary infecundity, and the seeking of medical advice in industrialized countries 1970-1992: a review of concepts, measurements and results. *Human Reproduction,* 10(6): 1407-1418.

Shattuck J, Schwarz K (1991) Walking the line between feminism and infertility: implications for nursing, medicine, and patient care. *Health Care for Women International,* 12(3): 331-339.

Singer LT et al. (1999) Maternal psychological distress and parenting stress after the birth of a very low-birth-weight infant. *Journal of the American Medical Association,* 281(9): 799-805.

Stanton F, Golombok S (1993) Maternal-fetal attachment during pregnancy following *in vitro* fertilization. *Journal of Psychosomatic Obstetrics and Gynaecology,* 14: 153-158.

Sundby J (1992) Long-term psychological consequences of infertility: a follow-up study of former patients. *Journal of Women's Health,* 1(3): 209-217.

Sundby J, Mboge R, Sonko S (1998) Infertility in the Gambia: frequency and health care seeking. *Social Science and Medicine,* 46(7): 891-899.

Sundby J, Olsen A, Schei B (1994) Quality of care for infertility patients. An evaluation of a plan for a hospital investigation. *Scandinavian Journal of Social Medicine,* 22(2): 139-144.

Swanson PB, Pearsall-Jones JG, Hay DA (2002) How mothers cope with the death of a twin or higher multiple. *Twin Research,* 5(3): 156-164.

Tallo CP et al. (1995) Maternal and neonatal morbidity associated with in vitro fertilization. *Journal of Pediatrics,* 127(5): 794-800.

Thorpe K et al. (1991) Comparison of prevalence of depression in mothers of twins and mothers of singletons. *British Medical Journal,* 302: 875-878.

Thwaites T (2002) Infertility treatment in Vietnam. *Orgyn, Organon's Magazine on Women and Health,* (4): 2-6.

Upton RL (2001) "Infertility makes you invisible": gender, health and the negotiation of fertility in northern Botswana. *Journal of Southern African Studies,* 27: 349-362.

van Balen F, Naaktgeboren N, Trimbos-Kemper TCM (1996) In-vitro fertilization: the experience of treatment, pregnancy and delivery. *Human Reproduction,* 11(1): 95-98.

Vayena E, Rowe PJ, Peterson HB (2002) Assisted reproductive technology in developing countries: why should we care? *Fertility and Sterility,* 78: 13-15.

Vayena E, Rowe PJ, Griffin PD, eds (2002) *Current practices and controversies in assisted reproduction. Report of a meeting on medical, ethical and social aspects of assisted reproduction.* Geneva, World Health Organization.

Visser AP et al. (1994) Psychosocial aspects of in vitro fertilization. *Journal of Psychosomatic Obstetrics and Gynaecology,* 15: 35-43.

Wang J et al. (1994) The obstetric outcome of singleton pregnancies following fertilization/gameter intra-Fallopian transfer. *Human Reproduction,* 9(1): 141-146.

Waters A-M, Dean JH, Sullivan EA (2006) *Assisted reproduction technology in Australia and New Zealand 2003.* Sydney, AIHW National Perinatal Statistics Unit.

WHO (2003) Assisted reproduction in developing countries: facing up to the issues. *Progress in Reproductive Health Research,* 63.

Woods NF, Olshansky EF, Draye MA (1991) Infertility: women's experiences. *Health Care for Women International,* 12(1991): 179-190.

Yong P, Martin C, Thong J (2000) A comparison of psychological functioning in women at different stages of in vitro fertilization treatment using the Mean Affect Adjective Check List. *Journal of Assisted Reproduction and Genetics,* 17(10): 553-556.

Chapter 9

Female genital mutilation

Jane Fisher

Female genital mutilation (FGM) or female genital cutting – sometimes termed female circumcision – is a common practice in some parts of the world (Ladjali, Rattray & Walder, 1993; Okonofua et al., 2002; UNICEF, 2005). Approximately 130 million women alive today have experienced some form of this procedure, and at least three million girls are at risk or are subjected to it each year (WHO, 1998, 2000a; UNICEF, 2005) The practice is most common in the countries of sub-Saharan Africa, parts of the Eastern Mediterranean, including Egypt, Oman, Sudan and Yemen, and Indonesia and Malaysia. It is also seen in other countries, including industrialized countries, among immigrants and refugees (Black & Debelle, 1995; UNICEF, 2005). Estimates of prevalence in different population groups range from 5% to 99%; in Egypt, Eritrea, Ethiopia, Somalia and Sudan, 70–98% of women have undergone the procedure (Dorkenoo, 1994; Toubia, 1994; Leonard, 1996; Sayed, Abd El-Aty & Fadel, 1996; Chelala, 1998; Eke, 2000; WHO, 2000a; Al-Hussaini, 2003; UNICEF, 2005). The rate of female genital mutilation is higher in settings where there are low levels of adult literacy and high rates of poverty. In general, prevalence is lower among better-educated women (Sayed, Abd El-Aty & Fatel, 1996; UNICEF, 2005).

Female genital mutilation is defined as any procedure that involves irremediable partial or total removal of, or injury to, external female genital organs for non-therapeutic reasons. WHO classifies this mutilation into a number of types, according to the severity of structural damage. Type I, or Sunna, is excision of the prepuce and part or all of the clitoris. Type II is removal of the clitoris and part or complete removal of the labia minora; this is anatomically equivalent to amputation of the penis (Toubia, 1994). Type III, or Pharaonic, also known as infibulation, is the excision of all external female genital organs and the use of stitches or other techniques to close the wound, leaving a narrow opening for the flow of urine and menstrual blood. Forms that do not fit the criteria for these three typologies are classified as Type IV. These include: pricking, piercing, cutting or distending the clitoris or labia; burning the external genital organs; cutting or scraping the vagina or placing herbs or corrosive agents into the vagina to cause bleeding or tissue damage and lead to tightening of the vaginal opening (Ng, 2000; Weir, 2000; WHO, 2000a) The most extreme forms of genital cutting are the least prevalent (Slanger, Snow & Okonofua, 2002).

As a result of migration and humanitarian programmes of relocation for refugees, Australia, Canada, some European countries and some states in the USA have now developed legislation, policies and clinical practice guidelines related to female genital mutilation (Allotey, Manderson & Grover, 2001). Accurate estimates of prevalence among immigrants in such countries are not available (Webb, 1995), but large numbers of people have migrated from the sub-Saharan African communities in which FGM is practised.

The age at which FGM is carried out varies, according to region, type of procedure and the existence of prohibiting legislation. It may be done a few days after birth, at the age of 8–10 years, prior to marriage, or after the birth of a first child (Dorkenoo & Elworthy, 1992; Toubia,

1994; Young, 2002). It is usually performed by untrained people, often traditional birth attendants or village barbers. They are likely to use unsterilized instruments, including razor blades, knives, broken glass, scissors or sharpened stones, without anaesthetic in unhygienic settings (Little, 2003; Odoi, Brody & Elkins, 1997). Recently, there has been a trend for FGM to be undertaken by medical personnel in medical settings (Toubia, 1994; UNICEF, 2005). This development has been strongly condemned by the World Health Organization and various professional bodies, which recommend that female genital mutilation should stop, and that it should never be performed by doctors or nurses (Wright, 1996; American Academy of Pediatrics Committee on Bioethics, 1998; WHO, 2000a).

Female genital mutilation is widely regarded as an ancient practice, which preceded the founding of both Christianity and Islam. However, there is evidence that FGM is not always a deeply embedded practice and that, in some settings, it has been practised for less than a century (Leonard, 1996). It is not consistently more common in one religious group than another (Little, 2003; UNICEF, 2005). It is deemed a tradition that is culturally and ethnically determined and is not mandated by religious doctrine (al-Sabbagh, 1996; Dorkenoo, 1994; Leonard, 1996; Cook, Dickens & Fathalla, 2002; UNICEF, 2005). The custom is rationalized and maintained by cultural beliefs. These include culturally defined rituals of initiation into adulthood; replication of the experience of previous generations; promotion of hygiene; maintenance of chastity through the construction of a physical barrier to sexual intercourse and reduction of potential sexual pleasure; and as an identifier of chaste status and thereby a prerequisite to marriage (Al-Hussaini, 2003; Dorkenoo, 1994; Ng, 2000; Sayed, Abd El-Aty & Fatel, 1996; Wright, 1996; Cook, Dickens & Fathalla, 2002; UNICEF, 2005). Other rationales for FGM are that it is performed for aesthetic reasons because the female genitals are regarded as intrinsically unattractive or may grow to an excessive length if left in a natural state (Dorkenoo, 1994; Ng, 2000; UNICEF, 2005). In some African groups there is a belief that removal of the clitoris clearly demarcates femininity, because its presence may lead to sexual confusion (Dorkenoo, 1994).

Marriageability is essential for economic security and social inclusion in settings where wom-

en have few occupational choices. Families are unlikely to break with tradition if it places their daughters at risk of remaining unmarried (Cook, Dickens & Fathalla, 2002; Lightfoot-Klein & Shaw, 1990; Missailidis & Gebre-Mehdin, 2000; Toubia, 1994). Ogunlola, Orji & Owalabi (2003) found that the father of a female child in Nigeria has the greatest power in making the decision to circumcise her, and that the decision is made before birth.

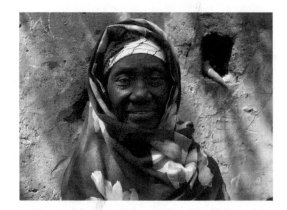

Health effects of female genital mutilation

The health effects of female genital mutilation, where the practice is widespread, are just starting to be documented. WHO (2000a) commissioned a systematic review of the health consequences of female genital mutilation, which retrieved 504 relevant articles published between 1925 and 1998. The review identified methodological limitations in many of the studies. Most of the publications were case reports or case series, while only a few studies compared women who had and had not had FGM. In some articles, the type of FGM was not defined, while in others type I and type II were combined. Often, results were given for all types of FGM combined. In addition, the age or developmental stage at which the procedure was performed was often not reported (WHO, 2000a). Many of the investigations did not include clinical examination of the perineum, and classification of FGM status may not be reliable under these circumstances (Odujinrin, Akitoye & Oyediran, 1989).

Most of the studies examining the complications of female genital mutilation have been done in Africa, but some evidence has been gathered in industrialized countries among immigrant populations. The adverse physical sequelae of female genital mutilation have been much more comprehensively investigated and described than the psychological effects.

Immediate and short-term health effects

The most common immediate adverse effects of the procedure are intense pain and haemorrhage, which can lead to hypovolaemic shock and death (Toubia, 1994; Johansen, 2002). Mortality rates are likely to be obscured by under-reporting, and qualitative investigations suggest that they are high (Lightfoot-Klein, 1991; Ng, 2000). Abscesses, wound contamination and local infections are common because of "gross disregard for asepsis" (Eke, 2000), the unhygienic circumstances in which the procedure is conducted, and the use of substances such as ash or crushed herbs to cover the wound (Toubia, 1994; Moller & Hansen, 2003; Rushwan, 2000). Adjacent anatomical structures, including the urethra, bladder, vagina and rectum, may be damaged because of poor technique or if the girl or woman struggles (Fox, de Ruiter & Bingham, 1997a; Ng, 2000). Systemic septicaemia, gangrene and tetanus infection can occur, and healing of the wound is often slow (Ng, 2000; Toubia, 1994).

In the short term, prolonged bleeding can cause anaemia, which has adverse effects on growth and development, especially in the presence of under-nutrition (Toubia, 1994). Slow-healing vulval abscesses may form (Rushwan, 2000) and dermoid cysts or keloids may grow on the clitoral stump or infibulation scar (Thabet & Thabet, 2003). Enlarged cysts and scar tissue can become grossly disfiguring (Toubia, 1994).

There are substantial long-term risks associated with female genital mutilation, especially following infibulation. The drainage of urine, vaginal secretions and menstrual blood is commonly obstructed, which can lead to chronic pelvic infections, menstrual dysfunction and menstrual pain (Fox, de Ruiter & Bingham, 1997b; Ng, 2000; Johansen, 2002). Urinary retention leads to chronic urinary tract infection and renal damage (Ng, 2000; Toubia, 1994). The procedure renders women vulnerable to chronic reproductive tract and pelvic infections, with associated abdominal pain and offensive vaginal discharge (Okonofua et al., 2002). Anecdotal reports describe young women developing abdominal swelling because menstrual blood is unable to flow out of the vagina. The lack of menstrual flow, coupled with abdominal distension, has

been misinterpreted as pregnancy, with anecdotal reports that it has led to unmarried women being killed in order to preserve the family's reputation (Dorkenoo, 1994). More recently, it has been suggested that genital cutting of women increases the risk of transmission of HIV, both through the use of unsterilized instruments and because cuts and tears are more likely to occur during intercourse (Rushwan, 2000).

The most obvious long-term adverse effects of FGM are on gynaecological health, especially sexual and obstetric functioning.

Effects on sexual and psychosexual functioning

Women who have been infibulated may have difficulty having sexual intercourse, as a result of a narrow introitus (Johansen, 2002; Okonofua et al., 2002). Absolute failure of penetration because of FGM, especially type III, has been reported (WHO, 2000a). Defibulation, by tearing or cutting, may be necessary before sexual penetration is possible (Lightfoot-Klein, 1991; Little, 2003; Wright, 1996). Studies of clinic populations have found that up to 25% of infibulated women require surgery before vaginal intercourse is possible (Fox, de Ruiter & Bingham, 1997b; Knight et al., 1999). However, it is difficult for women to seek health care for these problems. Mawad & Hassanein (1994) reviewed 934 patients attending Khartoum North Hospital between 1987 and 1989 with complications of genital mutilation. They found that women tended to seek health care only when they experienced severe pain, and that they were generally inhibited in discussing sexual matters. They concluded that fear of, and dissatisfaction with, sex were common, especially among those who had undergone type III FGM.

Sexual desire and frequency of intercourse may also be adversely affected. Although there have been few comprehensive studies, sexual problems, including persistent painful intercourse (13%), prolonged postcoital bleeding (5%) and anorgasmia (12%), were reported in a consecutive cohort study of women attending hospital clinics in northern Ghana (Odoi et al., 1997). The authors compared 76 women who had undergone FGM with 119 who had not. FGM was associated with a threefold increase in postcoital bleeding and a twelvefold increase in anorgasmia. In a systematic comparison of women who had experienced varying degrees of genital cutting with an unaffected comparison group in a Cairo University hospital, it was found that sexual desire and capacity for sexual arousal and orgasm were significantly adversely affected in those who had undergone type II mutilation, or who had developed clitoral cysts after any type of mutilation (Thabet & Thabet, 2003). El-Defrawi et al. (2001) selected 250 women at random among those attending maternal and child health centres in Ismailia, Egypt. Participants were given a gynaecological examination and interviewed; 80% had undergone FGM. These women were significantly more likely than those who had not undergone FGM to report one or more adverse psychosexual effects. These included painful menstruation (81%), low sexual desire (45%), sexual dissatisfaction (49%) and anorgasmia (61%). In contrast, Stewart, Morison & White (2002) undertook secondary analysis of data generated through a household survey in the Central African Republic, in which experience of female genital mutilation and frequency of sexual intercourse were ascertained through self-report. In total, data were available for 2188 married women. When other determinants, including length of marital relationship, level of education, being one of a number of wives, and desire to conceive, were taken into account, frequency of intercourse was not found to be associated with FGM. Similarly, Okonofua et al. (2002) compared 827 women who had experienced genital cutting and were attending family planning and antenatal clinics in Edo State, Nigeria, with 1009 women patients who had not been cut. Data were collected through gynaecological examination and self-report questionnaires. No differences were found between the two groups in terms of sexual arousal, frequency of intercourse and capacity for orgasm, although women who had experienced genital cutting were less likely to report high clitoral sensitivity than those who had not. However, women who had been cut were more likely to have had reproductive tract infections and premature births. These apparently conflicting findings may be related in part to the method of investigation, and be governed by women's capacity to report sexual impairment and to discuss sexual experiences freely (Morrison & Sherf, 2003). Lightfoot-Klein (1989) interviewed 300 Sudanese women who had experienced "extreme sexual mutilation", and found that most experienced sexual desire, arousal and orgasm. It has been suggested that the degree of cutting, consequent anatomic in-

jury, and women's capacity to derive sexual pleasure from non-genital stimulation or sexual fantasy interact to govern the degree of sexual impairment (Toubia, 1994).

Knight et al. (1999) found high rates of reported painful intercourse (76.5%) in a hospital cohort of women who had migrated to Australia after having experienced genital cutting, usually type III. Frequency of sexual intercourse and capacity for orgasm were reduced as a result of the pain. In a medical record audit of a small sample of 22 women who had experienced genital mutilation in their country of origin before migrating to the United Kingdom, 60% of those who had undergone infibulation had health problems, including perineal scarring, pain on intercourse and pelvic infections (Fox, de Ruiter & Bingham, 1997b).

Effects on fertility

Fertility may be diminished following genital mutilation, as a result of chronic pelvic infections leading to obstruction of the fallopian tubes. Narrowing of the introitus may lead to the anus or urethra being used for intercourse (Ng, 2000). Hormonal changes during pregnancy lead to increased vulnerability to genital and urinary tract infections, and risk is further increased in those who have undergone genital cutting (Rushwan, 2000). Vaginal examination is more difficult, which may mean that infections are difficult to diagnose (Rushwan, 2000). Cysts may develop or swell because of increased vulval vascularity (Rushwan, 2000). Almroth et al. (2005) conducted a meticulous case–control gynaecological, laparoscopic and laboratory test comparison of 99 women presenting for investigation of primary infertility in Khartoum, Sudan with 180 primigravid women. Women who had undergone extensive FGM, involving the labia majora, were more likely to be infertile than those who had not, probably as a result of recurrent tubal infections.

Obstetric effects

Significant obstetric difficulties are associated with genital cutting. In WHO's systematic review (WHO, 2000a), 67 of the 504 retrieved articles had primary data on obstetric sequelae. The authors concluded that the most significant adverse obstetric effects of FGM are usually scarring and vaginal obstruction. Jones et al. (1999) investigated self-reported obstetric complication rates in more than 3000 women attending for routine antenatal or gynaecological care in Burkina Faso (where 93% had experienced FGM) and Mali (where 94% had undergone FGM). Women who had experienced FGM were at significantly higher risk of obstetric complications. Larsen & Okonofua (2002) assessed 1851 women attending family planning and antenatal clinics in Nigerian hospitals, of whom 45% had undergone FGM. From interviews and physical examinations, they found that the prevalence of birth complications was higher among those who had had FGM. Slanger, Snow & Okonofua (2002) compared obstetric outcomes of first births among 1107 women in Nigeria, 56% of whom had experienced FGM. They found that adverse obstetric outcomes were no more common in the cut group, when socioeconomic status and place of birth were taken into account. Obstetric outcomes were worse in very poor women who gave birth without medical assistance regardless of whether they had had FGM. The authors concluded that the type of genital cutting has to be defined and coincidental social circumstances assessed in examining associations with obstetric outcome.

Antenatal and intrapartum vaginal examinations are more difficult in women who have had FGM, leading to difficulties in assessing pregnancy state and progress during labour (WHO, 2000a). De Silva (1989) compared obstetric outcomes in 167 Sudanese women who had undergone FGM (20 with type I, 76 with type II and 71 with type III) with those in 1990 Saudi women with no FGM. Duration of the second stage of labour was found to be significantly prolonged in the mutilated group. Rates of urinary retention during labour were also higher in women who had undergone FGM (WHO, 2000a).

Women who have been infibulated cannot give birth unassisted, since the scar has to be cut, in a procedure known as defibulation, in order to allow the fetus to pass (Rushwan, 2000). Episiotomy has been recommended as part of routine care for women whose genitals have been cut, but these women still have higher rates of perineal tears (WHO, 2000a; Al-Hussaini, 2003). Vaginal and perineal tears are common, and are associated with postpartum haemorrhage and high rates of postpartum perineal infection (WHO, 2000a; Rushwan, 2000). Together, these factors contribute to higher maternal mortal-

ity among women who have undergone FGM (WHO, 2000a). Obstructed or prolonged unassisted labour can lead to the formation of vesicovaginal or rectovaginal fistulae (Fox, de Ruiter & Bingham, 1997a; WHO, 2000a; Ng, 2000). These lead to urinary and faecal incontinence; it is common for incontinent women to be rejected by their partner and family (Rushwan, 2000). In countries with limited experience of managing childbirth in women who have been infibulated, caesarean sections are frequently performed (Fox, de Ruiter & Bingham, 1997a).

The newborn infants of women who have had FGM may also be adversely affected. WHO (2000a) reported higher rates of fetal distress during childbirth among women who had experienced FGM. Increased rates of stillbirth and neonatal death have been attributed to genital cutting, in particular infibulation, in some settings (Mella, 2003), but comparable, comprehensive international data are unavailable. Essen et al. (2002) reviewed perinatal deaths in Sweden between 1990 and 1996, including among women from Eritrea, Ethiopia and Somalia who had undergone genital cutting. They concluded that perinatal death was not associated with FGM per se, but with the women's refusal to accept caesarean delivery and difficulties in communicating with them, because of a lack of interpreters. Knight et al. (1999) also found that women who had experienced infibulation and who gave birth in a tertiary hospital in Melbourne, Australia, where caesarean section was readily available, had similar obstetric outcomes to the general population. Studies in industrialized countries with highly sophisticated medical care and where almost all women give birth in hospital cannot be generalized to settings with few trained medical personnel, in which many women give birth at home and maternal mortality rates are high.Following childbirth, many women who have been infibulated request re-infibulation, which can present ethical dilemmas for health professionals, especially in countries where it is illegal (Rushwan, 2000). Clinical practice guidelines usually discourage re-infibulation, but the physical and psychological health effects of not re-stitching the vulva are not known (Allotey, Manderson & Grover, 2001). It has been suggested that refusing to re-infibulate may cause women to avoid using the hospital for subsequent deliveries, to perceive institutional racism, or to resort to non-medical personnel to perform the procedure without anaesthetic in unhygienic settings (Gibeau, 1998; Rushwan, 2000, Allotey, Manderson & Grover, 2001). However, perhaps because of a desire for acculturation, neither infibulated women nor their partners requested re-infibulation after childbirth in one clinical practice in Canada (Lalonde, 1995). Almroth-Berggren et al. (2001) interviewed 60 women living in a rural setting in Sudan; many of the women reported that the decision to re-infibulate them after childbirth was made by senior female family members or by the birth attendant, because of a strong social belief that men preferred it. However, a small group of women had elected not to be re-infibulated, and were supported in this decision by their husbands.

Effects on mental health

There is an almost complete lack of systematic evidence about the psychological sequelae, including mental health effects, of female genital cutting. WHO's systematic review (WHO, 2000a) found that only 15% of the studies of the health effects of FGM considered mental health; most of these were case reports. It has been suggested that this situation has led to speculation about the psychological impact of FGM in the absence of scientific evidence. Toubia (1994) described the conflict faced by young women, who want to conform to parental and societal expectations by complying with FGM, but who are thereby exposed to fear, pain, complicated recovery and possible long-term health problems. She reported clinical observations of chronic depression and anxiety, associated with genital disfigurement and gynaecological dysfunction, as well as with specific fears that cysts or scars were cancer or that the genitals were re-growing (Toubia, 1994). Lightfoot-Klein & Shaw (1990) interviewed 300 women and health care providers, and found that anxiety was associated with obstructed menstrual flow and both anticipation of and actual experience of painful intercourse; some women reported intensely traumatic memories of their wedding night. Menage (1993, 1995) suggested that women might be traumatized by the procedure, on the basis of such responses having been observed in women who had undergone mutilating gynaecological procedures for clinical reasons. However, Black & Debelle (1996) have challenged the validity of this assertion for different cultural settings, considering that it cannot be inferred in the absence of supporting evidence.

Incontinence resulting from FGM may lead to ostracization and impede full social participation. Difficult vaginal penetration may be used as grounds for divorce (Rushwan, 2000). Women are reported to believe that their husband's sexual pleasure will be enhanced if they have been infibulated and re-infibulated. They fear being abandoned by their partner if they do not comply (Lightfoot-Klein, 1991). Depression following re-infibulation (in type III FGM) after childbirth has also been described (Lightfoot-Klein, 1983).

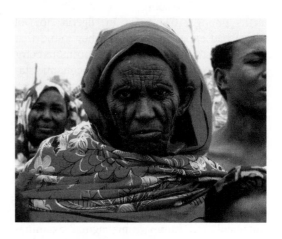

The most comprehensive study of the mental health effects of FGM reported the findings of structured interviews with 432 Somali women living in Canada, who had previously experienced genital cutting. The investigation focused on their experiences of childbirth, but also ascertained their recollections of the experience of genital cutting. Participants recalled intense fear, severe pain, and being seriously ill at the time of mutilation, but also recounted a sense of pride, happiness and enhanced purity and beauty (Chalmers & Hashi, 2000). It has been reported that, in countries where genital cutting is not commonly practised or is illegal, women who have had FGM fear that the quality of obstetric care provided by health professionals may be compromised by their lack of experience (Lightfoot-Klein & Shaw, 1990; Vangen et al., 2004). Pelvic examinations may be experienced as humiliating or offensive especially if conducted by male practitioners. These examinations need to be done with great sensitivity for women whose safety is predicated on modesty (Lightfoot-Klein & Shaw, 1990). Intense fear of caesarean surgery was universal in an interview study of 23 Somali women receiving antenatal care in Norway, who had been infibulated prior to migration (Vangen et al., 2004)

In 1959 the United Nations adopted the Convention on the Rights of the Child, which states that "all effective and appropriate measures to abolish traditional practices prejudicial to the health of children" should be taken (Black & Debelle, 1995). In 1979, the World Health Organization convened a round-table discussion on *Traditional practices affecting the health of women and children*, which concluded that female genital mutilation constituted a grave hazard to health and that the practice should end (Wright, 1996). Further, in 1997, WHO convened a technical consultation focusing on obstetric and postnatal health care "in the presence of FGM", which concluded that FGM carries grave consequences for the health and well-being of women and girl children, and reaffirming support for the United Nations Convention on the Rights of the Child. WHO, UNICEF and UNFPA issued a joint statement in 1997 outlining the need for cultures to adapt to knowledge about harmful practices, by relinquishing them.

There is debate about whether female genital mutilation constitutes a human rights violation or is an established cultural ritual that identifies social membership and should not be challenged (Aikman, 2001; Cook, Dickens & Fathalla, 2002).

Aikman (2001) and UNICEF (2005) concluded that the practice violates human rights to bodily integrity and freedom from torture, but that its elimination requires understanding of the cultural traditions that maintain it.

It has also been suggested that, by endangering the life and physical and mental health of children, genital cutting is a form of child abuse (Schroeder, 1994). An alternative view is that parents subject their daughters to this procedure to protect them and to ensure their social inclusion (Black & Debelle, 1995, 1996). In practice, it is difficult to prove child abuse under established legislation, because risk does not continue after

the mutilation has taken place (Webb, 1995). In Canada, specific sections of child protection acts identify FGM as assault causing actual bodily harm (Weir, 2000). It has been strongly argued that, in balancing these ethical dilemmas, health concerns should have absolute primacy (Wright, 1996).

The controversy about whether FGM constitutes a human rights violation or a tradition continues, and United Nations human rights procedures have had limited success in reducing the practice (Wright, 1996). Pilot programmes to reduce and ultimately eliminate female genital cutting have been implemented over the past 20 years, and have led to some reduction in incidence. The practice is now prohibited in some countries where it was previously common, but the initiative has had limited efficacy in reducing rates (Chelala, 1998; El Hadi, 1997). Walder (1995) argued that criminalizing the practice has driven it to become a clandestine activity in the United Kingdom. Health professionals in Egypt have objected to its prohibition, arguing that outlawing the procedure in health care settings increases the likelihood that it will be done without anaesthesia or hygiene precautions (American Academy of Pediatrics Committee on Bioethics, 1998; El Hadi, 1997). It has also been argued that, although women arrange the procedure for their daughters, it has little intrinsic value for them and is maintained because it is expected by men (El Hadi, 1997). It has been proposed that educational programmes for community members and health professionals are essential to promote change. Approaches that substitute alternative ceremonies or rituals combined with specific education to mark the transition to adulthood are beginning to have some success in replacing genital mutilation (Chelala, 1998; Shaaban & Harbison, 2005).

Gynaecological surgery, fertility difficulties, incontinence, operative interventions in childbirth, and chronic reproductive tract infections can each have adverse effects on women's mental health. It is likely, therefore, that the physical consequences of female genital mutilation will be psychologically problematic, although systematic investigations are needed to confirm this and to characterize the effects. The severe and lasting pain, coupled with the human rights transgression of performing a harmful procedure to which young girls cannot give voluntary and informed consent, is highly likely to have lasting adverse psychological sequelae (Johansen, 2002). Acceptance of social expectations and adherence to cultural norms may inhibit complaints or protests, and can lead to denial of associated difficulties (Toubia, 1994). Psychological reactions may be different in migrant or refugee populations, as they attempt to conform to different social norms (Toubia, 1994). Clinicians have recommended that sensitive health promotion and health education should be routinely done with women who have experienced genital cutting (Lalonde, 1995; Fox, de Ruiter & Bingham, 1997b; American Academy of Pediatrics Committee on Bioethics, 1998; Bayly, 1998; Knight et al., 1999). More specifically, Eke (2000) recommended psychological counselling for them. Overall, given the severity of physical damage and long-term adverse health effects, it is highly likely that genital cutting exerts an adverse effect on women's mental health. As long as the practice continues, systematic and comprehensive examination of these effects is urgently needed.

Summary

Future research

1. Research is urgently needed to determine:
   - the global extent and rates of the different forms of female genital mutilation;
   - the immediate, medium- and long-term consequences for mental health of female genital mutilation;
   - the complex interactions between the social position of women and the pressure to maintain tradition and to adhere to family expectations, and their effects on the psychological response to genital mutilation; and
   - the psychological effects of failing to comply with genital mutilation in settings where it as an established traditional practice.

2. There is a need to generate comprehensive international evidence regarding the psychological, psychosexual, psychosocial and cultural sequelae of female genital mutilation.

Implications for policy

1. Genital mutilation constitutes a risk to the health of women and girls, and a violation of their human rights.

2. Health professionals are in a unique position to advocate for the human rights of women in relation to female genital mutilation, and need to feel able to do so without fear of being criticised for challenging an established practice.

3. Female genital mutilation should not be undertaken by health personnel.

Services

1. Health professionals, in countries where female genital mutilation is practised or to which women who have experienced genital mutilation migrate, need to have specific knowledge and skills about the procedure in order to provide appropriate health care.

2. Obstetric health professionals should be trained to provide antenatal, intrapartum and postpartum health care for women who have undergone FGM, especially type III.

3. Health care for women who have experienced genital mutilation needs to be informed by cultural sensitivity, provision of choice, and an appreciation of human rights.

4. Women who have experienced genital mutilation should be counselled on its adverse health effects, encouraged to discuss the implications for their daughters, and helped to make intergenerational changes related to this practice.

References

Aikman P (2001) Female genital mutilation: human rights abuse or protected cultural practice. *Health Science Journal* (www.docs/vol1-1/fgm.html 1-6).

Al-Hussaini TK (2003) Female genital cutting: types, motives and perineal damage in labouring Egyptian women. *Medical Principles and Practice*, 12(2): 123-128.

Allotey P, Manderson L, Grover S (2001) The politics of female genital surgery in displaced communities. *Critical Public Health*, 11(3): 189-201.

Almroth L et al. (2005) Primary infertility after genital mutilation in girlhood in Sudan: a case-control study. *Lancet*, 366: 385-391.

Almroth-Berggren V et al. (2001) Reinfibulation among women in a rural area in central Sudan. *Health Care for Women International*, 22: 711-721.

al-Sabbagh ML (1996) Islamic ruling on female and male circumcision. Alexandria, WHO Regional Office for the Eastern Mediterranean.

American Academy of Pediatrics Committee on Bioethics (1998) Female genital mutilation. *Pediatrics*, 102(1): 153-156.

Bayly CM (1998) Female genital mutilation: responding to health needs. *Medical Journal of Australia*, 169: 455-456.

Black JA, Debelle GD (1995) Female genital mutilation in Britain. *British Medical Journal*, 310(6994): 1590-1592.

Black JA, Debelle GD (1996) Female genital mutilation. *British Medical Journal*, 312 (7027): 377-378.

Chalmers B, Hashi KO (2000) 432 Somali women's birth experiences after earlier female genital mutilation. *Birth*, 27: 227-234.

Chelala C (1998) An alternative way to stop female genital mutilation. *Lancet*, 352 (9122): 126.

Cook RJ, Dickens BM, Fathalla M (2002) Female genital cutting (mutilation / circumcision): ethical and legal dimensions. *International Journal of Gynaecology and Obstetrics*, 79: 281-287.

De Silva S (1989) Obstetric sequelae of female circumcision. *European Journal of Obstetrics, Gynaecology and Reproductive Biology*, 32: 233-240.

Dorkenoo E (1994) *Cutting the rose. Female genital mutilation: the practice and its prevention.* London, Minority Rights Publications.

Dorkenoo E, Elworthy S (1992) *Female genital mutilation: proposals for change.* London, Minority Rights Group.

Eke N (2000) Female genital mutilation: what can be done? *Lancet*, 356(suppl.): s57.

El-Defrawi MH et al. (2001) Female genital mutilation and its psychosexual impact. *Journal of Sex and Marital Therapy*, 27: 465-473.

El Hadi A (1997) A step forward for opponents of female genital mutilation in Egypt. *Lancet*, 349(9045): 129-130.

Essen B et al. (2002) Is there an association between female circumcision and perinatal death? *Bulletin of the World Health Organization*, 80(8): 629-632.

Fox E, de Ruiter A, Bingham J (1997a) Female genital mutilation. *International Journal of STD and AIDS*, 8(10): 599-601.

Fox E, de Ruiter A, Bingham J (1997b) Female genital mutilation in a genitourinary medicine clinic: a case note review. *International Journal of STD and AIDS*, 8(10): 659-660.

Gallard C (1995) Female genital mutilation in Britain: female genital mutilation in France. *British Medical Journal*, 310(6994): 1592-1593.

Gibeau AM (1998) Female genital mutilation: when a cultural practice generates clinical and ethical dilemmas. *Journal of Obstetric, Gynecologic and Neonatal Nursing*, 27(1): 85-91.

Johansen REB (2002) Pain as a counterpoint to culture: toward an analysis of pain associated with infibulations among Somali immigrants in Norway. *Medical Anthroplogy Quarterly*, 16(3): 312-340.

Jones H et al. (1999) Female genital cutting practices in Burkina Faso and Mali and their negative health outcomes. *Studies in Family Planning*, 30: 219-230.

Knight R et al. (1999) Female genital mutilation - experience of The Royal Women's Hospital, Melbourne. Australian and New Zealand *Journal of Obstetrics and Gynaecology*, 39(1): 50-54.

Ladjali M, Rattray TW, Walder RJW (1993) Female genital mutilation. *British Medical Journal*, 307(6902): 460.

Lalonde A (1995) Clinical management of female genital mutilation must be handled with understanding, compassion. *Canadian Medical Association Journal*, 152(6): 949-950.

Larsen U, Okonofua FE (2002) Female circumcision and obstetric complications. *International Journal of Gynaecology and Obstetrics*, 77: 255-265.

Leonard L (1996) Female circumcision in southern Chad: origins, meaning and cultural practice. *Social Science and Medicine*, 43(2): 255-263.

Lightfoot-Klein H (1983) Pharaonic circumcision of females in the Sudan. *Medicine and Law*, 2: 353-360.

Lightfoot-Klein H (1989) The sexual experience and marital adjustment of genitally circumcised and infibulated females in Sudan. *Journal of Sex Research*, 26(3): 375-392.

Lightfoot-Klein H (1991) *Prisoners of ritual:some contemporary developments in the history of female genital mutilation*. Second International Symposium on Circumcision, San Francisco.

Lightfoot-Klein H, Shaw E (1990) Special needs of ritually circumcised women patients. *Journal of Obstetric, Gynecologic and Neonatal Nursing*, 20(2): 102-107.

Little C (2003) Female genital circumcision: medical and cultural considerations. *Journal of Cultural Diversity*, 10(1): 30-34.

Mawad NM, Hassanein OM (1994) Female circumcision: three years expereince of common complaints in patients treated in Khartoum teaching hospitals. *Journal of Obstetrics and Gynaecology*, 14: 40-43.

Mella PP (2003) Major factors that impact on women's health in Tanzania: the way forward. *Health Care for Women International*, 24: 712-722.

Menage J (1993) Post-traumatic stress disorder in women who have undergone obstetric and/or gynaecologial procedures. *Journal of Reproductive and Infant Psychology*, 11: 221-228.

Menage J (1995) Female genital mutilation: professionals should not collude with abusive systems. *British Medical Journal*, 311 (7012): 1088-1089.

Missailidis K, Gebre-Mehdin M (2000) Female genital mutilation in eastern Ethiopia. *Lancet*, 356 (9224): 137-138.

Moller BR, Hansen UD (2003) Foreign bodies as a complication of female genital mutilation. *Journal of Obstetrics and Gynaecology* 23: 449-450

Morrison L, Scherf C (2003) The association between female genital cutting and correlates of sexual and gynaecological morbidity in Edo State, Nigeria. *BJOG: an International Journal of Obstetrics and Gynaecology*, 110: 1137-1140.

Ng F (2000) Female genital mutilation; its implications for reproductive health. An overview. *British Journal of Family Planning*, 26(1): 47-51.

Odoi A, Brody SP, Elkins TE (1997) Female genital mutilation in rural Ghana, West Africa. *International Journal of Gynecology and Obstetrics*, 56: 179-180.

Odujinrin OM, Akitoye CO, Oyediran MA (1989) A study on female circumcision in Nigeria. *West Afrian Journal of Medicine*, 8: 183-192.

Ogunlola O, Orji EO, Owolabi AT (2003) Female genital mutilation and the unborn female child in southwest Nigeria. *Journal of Obstetrics and Gynaecology*, 23: 143-145.

Okonofua FE et al. (2002) The association between female genital cutting and correlates of sexual and gynaecological mobidity in Edo State, Nigeria. *BJOG: an International Journal of Obsteterics and Gynaecology*, 109: 1089-1096.

Rushwan H (2000) Female genital mutilation (FGM) management during pregnancy, childbirth and the postpartum period. *International Journal of Gynecology and Obstetrics*, 70: 99-104.

Sayed GH, Abd El-Aty MA, Fadel KA (1996) The practice of female genital mutilation in Upper Egypt. *International Journal of Gynecology and Obstetrics*, 55: 285-291.

Schroeder P (1994) Female genital mutilation: a form of child abuse. *New England Journal of Medicine*, 33(11): 739-740.

Shaaban LM, Harbison S (2005) Reaching the tipping point against female genital mutilation. *Lancet*, 366: 347-349.

Slanger TE, Snow RC, Okonofua FE (2002) The impact of female genital cutting on first delivery in southwest Nigeria. *Studies in Family Planning*, 33(2): 173-180.

Stewart H, Morison L, White R (2002) Determinants of coital frequency among married women in Central African Republic: the role of female genital cutting. *Journal of Biosocial Science*, 34: 525-539.

Thabet SM, Thabet AS (2003) Defective sexuality and female circumcision: the cause and possible management. *Journal of Obstetric and Gynaecological Research*, 29(1): 12-19.

Toubia N (1994) Female circumcision as a public health issue. *New England Journal of Medicine*, 33(11): 712-716.

UNICEF (2005) *Female genital mutilation/cutting: a statistical exploration*. New York, United Nations Children's Fund.

Vangen S et al. (2004) Qualitative study of perinatal care experinces among Somali women and local health care professionals in Norway. *European Journal of Obstetrics and Gynaecology and Reproductive Biology*, 112: 29-35.

Walder RJW (1995) Female genital mutilation in Britain: why the problem continues in Britain. *British Medical Journal*, 310(6994): 1593-1594.

Webb E (1995) Female genital mutilation: cultural knowledge is the key to understanding. *British Medical Journal*, 311(7012): 1088.

Weir E (2000) Female genital mutilation. *Canadian Medical Association Journal*, 162(9): 1344.

WHO (1997) *Management of pregnancy, chidbirth and the postpartum period in the presence of female genital mutilation. Report of a WHO Technical Consultation.* Geneva, World Health Organization.

WHO (1998) *Female genital mutilation – an overview.* Geneva, World Health Organization.

WHO (2000a) *A systematic review of the health complications of female genital mutilation including sequelae in childbirth.* Geneva, World Health Organization.

WHO (2000b) *Female genital mutilation. Fact Sheet 241.* Geneva, World Health Organization.

WHO, UNICEF, UNFPA (1997) *Female genital mutilation: a joint WHO/UNICEF/UNFPA statement.* Geneva, World Health Organization.

Wright J (1996) Female genital mutilation: an overview. *Journal of Advanced Nursing*, 24(2): 251-259.

Young JS (2002) Editor's note: Female genital mutilation. *Journal of the American Medical Association*, 288(9): 1130.

Chapter

Conclusions

Meena Cabral de Mello & Shekhar Saxena

It is becoming increasingly clear that mental and physical health are closely linked, influencing each other in powerful and complex ways. This understanding is helping to break down some long-standing barriers to good health and is beginning to offer new hope of care and cure. This review has sought to increase understanding of the interaction of reproductive health with mental health, especially in relation to women's lives and well-being.

According to WHO (WHO, 2001), depression is the single largest contributor to years lived with disability in adults. Symptoms of depression and anxiety, as well as unspecified psychiatric disorder and psychological distress, are 2–3 times more prevalent among women than among men. There is considerable evidence that stressful life events and reproductive health problems are closely associated with depression and anxiety disorders. Such events and problems are more common in the lives of women; in particular, gender inequality leads to considerable stress for women. Nowhere is this more evident than in situations where girls and women are subject to violence, particularly from an intimate partner. The violence can include physical, sexual and emotional abuse, and is common throughout the world. Available data suggest that, in some countries, nearly one woman in four experiences sexual violence from an intimate partner. Large numbers of women experience violence during pregnancy, with adverse consequences both for them and for their baby, such as miscarriage, premature labour and low birth weight.

Reproductive and sexual ill-health is estimated to account for 20% of the global burden of ill-

health for women, and 14% for men. These figures, however, do not capture the full burden of ill-health. Reproductive problems may be linked to antenatal care, delivery, postpartum care, family planning; infertility, unsafe abortion, sexually transmitted infections, including HIV, reproductive tract infections, cervical cancer and other gynaecological problems. These can have major social, emotional and physical consequences, which are severely underestimated in global burden of disease estimates. WHO considers unsafe sex to be one of the most important risk factors for health in the world, particularly for girls and women, whose low social status in many parts of the world means they have little control over their sexual and reproductive lives.

Although mental health is widely recognized as closely linked to reproductive health, in many countries it remains, at best, a marginal concern. Nevertheless, the areas of interaction of reproductive and mental health are considerable, and include, for example, psychological issues related to sexuality, childbirth, sexual violence, adverse maternal outcomes (such as stillbirths and abortions), sexually transmitted infections, including HIV/AIDS, family planning, reproductive tract surgery, sterilization, premarital pregnancy, menopause and infertility. These issues relate to both men's and women's reproductive health, as well as their relationships.

It has not been possible to consider all these issues in this review, because the evidence base for many is simply non-existent at present. Nevertheless, the available evidence on a number of key issues has been consolidated and analysed to present as complete a picture as possible of the current situation. A considerable amount of research on reproductive and mental health has been reported in recent years, but most of this research has focused on a relatively small number of sexual and reproductive health conditions. More importantly, much of the research has been done in developed countries, with very little coming from developing countries. As an example, an electronic search revealed that, between 1992 and 2006, some 1500 research papers were published on postnatal depression, but none on depression following vaginal fistula. There is a complete lack of information on the mental health aspects of chronic health problems, such as vesicovaginal fistula, perineal tears and uterovaginal prolapse, which are much more common among women living in resource-poor and research-poor settings. This can lead to the erroneous conclusion that there are no mental health consequences of these conditions. Moreover, even in middle- and high-income countries, where many more data are available on the interaction between reproductive and mental health, the available evidence primarily concerns married women of childbearing age. The reproductive and mental health of men and of young, single women remains largely unexplored. Also seriously underinvestigated are the important inter-relationships between women's and men's reproductive health.

The developing countries have benefited from considerable research efforts on certain reproductive health issues, such as family planning, pregnancy, childbirth and lactation. Unfortunately, very few, if any, of these efforts have considered the mental health implications of these conditions to any significant extent. The gaps in the evidence have been highlighted throughout the present review.

From the available evidence, however, it is already clear that mental health needs to be an integral part of any programme that aims to address the major reproductive health priorities in developing countries. There is a high prevalence of depression and anxiety disorders in women attending gynaecological clinics in developing countries. Qualitative studies have demonstrated a strong relationship between psychological distress, depression and anxiety disorders, and aspects of reproductive health, such as sexually transmitted infections, HIV, childbirth and the postpartum period, pregnancy termination, spontaneous pregnancy loss, menopause, infer-

tility, and a number of gynaecological injuries and conditions. Mental health problems are also more frequent in women who are disproportionately exposed to risk factors and adverse life experiences that also affect their reproductive health.

The framework for analysis used in this review was informed by two interconnected concepts – namely, gender and human rights, especially reproductive rights – in identifying the risk factors and vulnerability of women to emotional distress associated with reproductive health conditions. The review draws attention to the critical importance of the dynamic interplay between women's reproductive and mental functioning. Even though the evidence presented is, of necessity, uneven, it is hoped that it will stimulate much-needed additional research, especially in developing countries, and that it will encourage policy-makers and reproductive health managers to expand the scope of existing services to embrace a holistic perspective. Policy-makers and service providers need to begin to address the mental health dimensions of many reproductive health conditions, and to look at how reproductive health services, and their treatment of women, can have profound effects on mental as well as physical health.

The burden of both reproductive and mental ill-health is greatest in the poorest countries, where health services tend to be dispersed or physically inaccessible, poorly staffed, resourced and equipped, and beyond the reach of many poor people. Increasing access to reproductive health services, and mainstreaming mental health concerns within them, are essential. The mental health of women is also closely linked to their capacity to give essential responsive care to their infants, children and other family members, and any initiative to improve family health must also seek to improve women's mental health. Mental health can no longer be considered an unaffordable "luxury" for women in resource-poor settings.

An obvious implication of these conclusions is that a two-pronged approach needs to be pursued: first, to give more attention to research on reproductive mental health in developing countries and to build the capacity of researchers in this neglected area; and second, to incorporate mental health considerations into reproductive health programmes and into the training of providers of reproductive health care at all levels.

Overview of key areas discussed

Some of the key findings from earlier chapters are presented below. The major gaps and needs for further research and action are highlighted.

Pregnancy, childbirth and the postpartum period

Research has shown that, although mental health is inextricably linked to maternal and child mortality and morbidity, it has so far been neglected in initiatives to improve maternal and child health. In high-income countries, 10–15% of women who have recently given birth suffer from depression. In addition to the distress caused to the woman herself, postnatal depression can interfere with interpersonal relationships and have a negative effect on the cognitive and emotional development of the child. In developing countries, attention has tended to focus on physical health problems, such as infectious diseases, which may appear to be more urgent, and postnatal depression has received little attention. Yet recent studies have shown that as many as 25–30% of new mothers in these countries suffer from postnatal depression – a prevalence double that in the developed world.

The underlying determinants of postnatal depression are complex, and include the low status of women relative to men in many countries, their lack of autonomy, the birth of a girl in regions where there is a strong preference for male children, poor housing, marital and family discord, including violence, poor health, lack of emotional and practical support, isolation and poverty. There is increasing evidence related to the predictors, prevalence and correlates of poor mental health postpartum in developing regions, but investigations are yet to be conducted in some of the poorest countries.

It is not just the woman who is at risk: postnatal depression in low-income countries also affects the infant's cognitive and emotional development, and appears to play a crucial – and previously unrecognized – role in physical growth and survival. As a consequence of the more difficult environmental conditions in developing countries, depression may have a greater effect on the mother and her capacity to give responsive care to her baby. Investigations of infant development following maternal depression should ascertain and control for the contribution of social adversity.

While effective treatments for postnatal depression, such as psychotherapy and antidepressant medications, are available in the developed world, interventions have so far focused almost exclusively on individual women. Evidence is emerging to suggest that strategies involving the partner may be more effective, but such strategies need to be designed and appropriately evaluated. It may not be possible to transfer existing approaches directly to developing countries, which have very different health care systems and cultural beliefs. Randomized controlled trials are needed to develop treatments for depression during pregnancy and after childbirth that are suitable for use in primary health care in resource-poor settings.

High rates of maternal depression constitute a major public health problem. It might appear anomalous to give attention to perinatal depression in developing countries, where other health problems seem so compelling, but it is likely that these are precisely the places where mental health is worst and contributes most significantly to the severity of other health problems. Programmes aimed at improving child health depend on the effective participation of mothers, but women who are depressed are less able to understand and respond to health-promoting interventions and education.

More generally, research attention has focused on mental health after childbirth rather than mental health during pregnancy, which warrants more comprehensive investigation.

Psychosocial aspects of family planning

Central to the discussion of the mental health implications of contraceptive use is the issue of women's agency, and how a gender-based lack of power and control affects women's ability to make contraceptive choices and undermines their mental health and emotional well-being. Women's ability to make decisions, including on participation in family planning programmes and use of contraception, is closely linked to their emotional well-being and their status in the family. Women who receive support from health professionals for autonomous decision-making have fewer psychosomatic complaints and depressive symptoms.

The relationship between broad situational and interpersonal determinants of contraceptive use, decision-making, and the development of emotional distress, depression and other psychological disorders that primarily affect women has not been adequately investigated. Extensive research on the characteristics of situations that trigger clinical depression has revealed many areas of overlap with situations of intimate partner violence. Family planning programmes need to extend their explanatory models for unmet need and non-use or inconsistent use of contraceptives to include the possibility that intimate partner violence and lack of autonomy may be major causes of low rates of contraceptive use and poor reproductive health outcomes. Programmes to increase contraceptive use need to be based on an accurate understanding of the multiple determinants of contraceptive use.

Much of the research on the psychological effects of different methods of contraception, including female sterilization and the intrauterine device, has found that negative effects on mood are usually attributable to a lack of confidence in the effectiveness of the method, coincidental adverse life events, relationship problems or a family history of psychiatric illness, rather than the method itself. Negative psychological effects have been found among women who were coerced into being sterilized, those who did not understand the consequences of sterilization or experienced complications after the procedure, those who disagreed with their partner about the sterilization, and those whose marriage was unstable before sterilization. Adverse psychological effects are more likely to be a consequence of violations of reproductive rights, including the rights to accurate health information and to give free and informed consent to medical intervention, than to the procedure itself.

More recent research has confirmed the importance to psychological well-being of women being given adequate information before sterilization, and feeling that they have been able to make their own decision without pressure from either the partner or health care providers. The timing of the sterilization procedure is also relevant; women who are sterilized immediately after delivery, abortion or Caesarean section have

an increased incidence of psychosomatic complaints and depressive symptoms.

Women who are mentally ill or who abuse alcohol or drugs may be unable to give meaningful consent to sexual activity, and are less likely to use contraception effectively; they are at high risk of sexual exploitation. Some hormonal contraceptives should not be prescribed to women who are currently depressed, because they might contribute to further worsening mood. However, health professionals are less likely to discuss contraception with women who have serious psychiatric illness, and provision of contraception is problematic for groups who do not attend routine medical or reproductive health services.

Further participatory research is required to establish accurately needs for contraception, and to examine the disparity between contraceptive intentions and contraceptive use, looking beyond women's "failure" to adhere to their intentions. Investigations are needed of the coercion and pressure women experience from family planning programmes regarding child-spacing and uptake of contraceptive methods, including sterilization.

The mental health aspects of elective abortion are linked to the particular context of reproductive health and rights, attitudes to sexuality, and specific attitudes and laws relating to abortion and to women. Specific issues include women's access to safe, timely and affordable abortion, and the degree to which they receive interpersonal and societal support. Psychiatric sequelae of elective, safe abortion are rare. Typically, women experience heightened distress before abortion, and show significantly improved mental health indices afterwards. Following abortion, approximately 10% of women report regret, guilt, or other symptoms of psychological intrusion or avoidance. Over a longer time span, up to 20% of women may report some abortion-related regret or distress. The mental health consequences of unsafe abortion are not known. Qualitative data suggest that unsafe abortion can be traumatic, and is likely to cause more psychological harm to considerably more women than safe abortion.

There is a need for systematic methodologically rigorous investigations into the psychological aspects of abortion, including decision-making, the procedure itself, post-abortion adjustment, and need for counselling and follow-up medical care. Comprehensive qualitative and quantitative investigations are needed in both developing and industrialized countries. The interactions between risk and protective factors in determining mental health in relation to abortion need to be clarified. Finally, the psychosocial aspects of sex-selective abortion are at present unknown and need to be systematically investigated.

Spontaneous pregnancy loss

There is an abundance of evidence documenting the wide range of psychological reactions to the experience of miscarriage. These reactions are mediated by differences in sociocultural as well as personal and health service factors. There is general agreement in the literature that many women experience miscarriage as highly distressing, and that subsequent rates of psychopathology, including depression and anxiety, are higher than in the general population. The particular factors that predispose some women to more intense psychological reactions have not yet been clearly identified, but vulnerability as a result of earlier adverse events appears salient and warrants additional investigation.

Although psychological reactions to miscarriage resolve spontaneously in most women, there appears to be a role for psychological intervention, immediately after treatment or in the long term. It is not clear whether some or all women would benefit from this type of intervention, or what form it should take, and there has been no evaluation of existing services. Medical services are routinely involved in preventing the potential complications of miscarriage, but are not generally perceived as providing psychological support at the time of treatment or at follow-up. In fact, the psychological component of medical care for miscarriage is largely neglected, and there is little agreement in the literature about the form that psychological intervention should take, or from which women would benefit most. It is, nevertheless, acknowledged that women who use health services after losing a pregnancy may benefit from a more psychologically informed model of care than currently exists in most settings. In practice, it is unlikely that a single approach to the psychological care of women after spontaneous pregnancy loss will be effective in all settings and for all cultural groups.

Menopause

It is necessary to look beyond menopausal status, hormone levels and menopausal symptoms to explain depression in women in midlife. A life course approach, rather than a cross-sectional one, is necessary to understand emotional distress in midlife. The "classical" social determinants of depression, as well as the presence of distressing somatic symptoms and reduced sexual functioning and pleasure, are likely to contribute to dysphoria and depression. A history of depression and high levels of psychosocial adversity may be more important than menopausal status in explaining emotional distress. It is important to evaluate the sources and impact of stress, and of social support, on women's emotional well-being. Family and friends may function as conduits of stress, as well as sources of support.

While there is considerable anthropological literature on the cultural construction of menopause in low- and middle-income countries, and on women's expectations and experiences of it, data on the links between mental health and menopause are more limited. Research on this relationship is needed to provide culturally specific data for decision-making at programme, policy and service-provision level. In particular, data are needed on whether the factors identified in high-income countries as critical to women's mental life in midlife are also relevant for women in low- and middle-income countries. Other relevant socioeconomic, cultural and interpersonal factors also need to be identified, and assessments made of the effectiveness of assistance given to women in low- and middle-income countries for health problems and physically or psychologically distressing symptoms related to menopause.

Gynaecological conditions

Gynaecological injuries and diseases are common, and yet women who develop these problems often feel isolated and distressed as a result of inadequate general understanding of their injury or disease, and inaccurate beliefs about the causes. If surgery is required, it may be deeply traumatic, adversely affecting the woman's body image, self-esteem, social confidence and sexual life, and having short- and long-term effects on mood and personal relationships. These potential effects have not yet been systematically investigated. Relatively little research has been conducted outside the United States on the mental health aspects of gynaecological injuries and diseases, and knowledge of the wider psychological and social factors associated with them is limited. Overall, many problems result in significant psychological stress and psychosexual morbidity, with a marked negative impact on quality of life. Distress is greater in those who are young and poor or socially disadvantaged, and who have a history of undergoing violence. The diagnosis of an STI or cancer is often associated with a range of psychological responses, including anguish, anger, lowered self-esteem, hostility, shame, depression, and anxiety.

There has been virtually no consideration of the mental health factors associated with the diagnosis or outcome of any of these conditions in developing countries, even though they have direct and significant effects on mental health and psychological functioning.

The psychosocial consequences of obstetric injury, reproductive tract morbidity and cancers in women should be included in all research into these conditions. The specific needs of women in culturally diverse settings for advice, support and counselling during treatment and rehabilitation for gynaecological conditions should be systematically ascertained.

Programmes for primary prevention of gynaecological morbidity need to be designed and evaluated. Where women's access to health services is constrained by social and cultural factors, strategies to reduce obstetric injury and gynaecological morbidity should be accompanied by efforts to improve women's social position. Obstetric injury and consequent gynaecological morbidity can also be reduced by: encouraging social changes that promote the value of girls and delay marriage and first birth; ensuring rapid access to trained personnel during labour and childbirth; and ensuring that women do not return to hard manual labour shortly after childbirth.

Gynaecological and obstetric health services need to be accessible, affordable and appropriate to women's needs. The staff of such services should be trained to manage sensitively gynaecological morbidity and obstetric injury; they should try to change cultural practices that reduce women's self-determination and to identify psychological distress and anxiety. Health serv-

ice staff should offer non-judgemental, empathic care, which encourages women to talk about their reproductive health concerns. They should also be capable of providing support to minimize the mental health impact associated with treatment and care. Gynaecological and cancer screening services should recognize that women may be embarrassed or ashamed of tests, treatment and possible disease, and should ensure that they understand the nature of screening.

Mental health in the context of HIV/AIDS

The psychological morbidity experienced by women who have HIV infection is considerable and has multiple causes. There is an intricate relationship between mental health, disease progression, quality of life and disease outcome. Qualitative differences have been found between women and men in the emotional impact of HIV infection, in terms of grief, shame, and depression.

Regardless of ethnicity, women who are seropositive are more likely to report being victims of sexual and physical violence. They often have inadequate social support and express concerns about stigma, discrimination and hopelessness. They are more likely to report psychological distress, symptoms of depression, and distress related to physical symptoms. In addition, women experience gender-specific social stigma, a greater sense of isolation, and oppression related to gender, stigma, ethnicity, poverty, and route of infection. In stigmatized groups, disclosure of HIV infection is predictive of poorer mental health status. Conversely, poorer mental health might also predict lower levels of disclosure. Women experiencing both sexual and physical abuse are more likely to have a history of multiple sexually transmitted infections, be worried about the fact that they are infected with HIV, use marijuana and alcohol to cope, attempt suicide, feel as though they have no control in their relationships, and experience more episodes of physical abuse. Such traumatic life experiences are often associated with high rates of psychiatric co-morbidity, clinical depression or anxiety, substance abuse, and possible non-compliance with recommended health care and treatment.

In addition to the physical effects of HIV infection, women often lose their jobs and the support of their husband, and may be forced to turn to prostitution to feed, clothe, and educate their children. The multiple problems, loss of physical and financial independence, discrimination, and other HIV-related difficulties can often lead to significant distress and a risk of suicide. Conversely, having a wide social network can be associated with better mental health and overall quality of life.

An emerging trend is the increase in HIV infection among people aged over 50 years, especially women, reaching approximately 2,8 million cases in 2005. Older people with HIV require special attention because they are likely to have a variety of other health, social, and emotional concerns. The mental health aspects of older women, in relation to sexual health, tend to be ignored except in terms of menopause. These women are often denied appropriate sexual health information, for instance regarding risk and vulnerability to reproductive tract and sexually transmitted infections, including HIV.

Depression is common among those who are HIV-infected, and is associated with a variety of other problems, including lowered immune response, shorter survival time, increased disability, and a lower quality of life. With the progression of the disease, there is the added risk of AIDS dementia complex.

Considerable attention, in terms of research, and policy and programme development, has been given to reducing mother-to-child transmission of HIV/AIDS. However, there have been few reports on the psychological well-being of new mothers with HIV, or on the mental health impact on young girls and boys of the death of their mother from AIDS in both developed and developing countries. This is an important area for research.

One of the most worrying and complex aspects of the spread of HIV/AIDS is its link to the widespread sexual exploitation of children, who are most vulnerable to contracting HIV/AIDS. Young girls whose parents have died of AIDS are often targeted by older men for sex. Another underresearched aspect is the mental health impact of the fact that the burden of care for people with HIV/AIDS falls primarily on women.

Rights violations, economic dependence, lack of decision-making power, conflicting gender roles, disproportionate domestic responsibilities, and gender-based violence contribute to reproductive and mental health problems for women. There is a marked lack of evidence on women's mental health and how it interacts with vulnerability, risk of HIV infection, response to diagnosis, and subsequent health care. Most research on AIDS and its effects on mental health has been conducted in the United States; there is some from other rich countries, but very little from developing countries. This should be corrected.

Infertility and assisted reproduction

Infertility is experienced by many women as a profound life crisis or existential blow, which is uniquely stressful because it can last for many years and for many will not be resolved. The experience and eventual diagnostic confirmation of infertility can have a profound psychological impact, which has been conceptualized and assessed in different ways.

Women have been found to experience more emotional distress and depressive symptoms associated with infertility than men, and their lives are more disrupted by infertility than men's. Almost all women presenting for treatment for infertility have been found to demonstrate some of the following characteristics: increased anxiety, irritability, anger, profound sadness, self-blame, lowered energy levels, social isolation and heightened interpersonal sensitivity. Many women fear that earlier sexual experiences, the use of contraceptives or delaying procreation while pursuing professional goals may have compromised their fertility. Other less rational beliefs – of being punished for past misdeeds or of intrinsic unworthiness – have also been reported, particularly when infertility is of unexplained origin. Reaction to infertility is also conceptualized as grief, including for many intangible or disenfranchised losses, such as: the experiences of pregnancy, childbirth and breastfeeding; the children and grandchildren who will not exist; a generation and genetic continuity; the state of parenthood and the activities and relationships it entails; and an element of adult and gender identity which will never be realized and is substituted with a flawed infertile identity In addition, individuals may fear losing significant relationships, in particular with the partner, physical attractiveness, or a positive sexual relationship. Fertility difficulties can exert a pervasive negative effect on quality of life, compromising planning and commitment to other life activities. The effect is observable in both men and women, but more so in women.

The inability to bear children is highly stigmatized in strongly pro-natalist settings, and people who cannot have children may be socially marginalized. In poor countries, women with fertility problems may have their gender identity questioned, experience social exclusion or divorce, be suspected of having evil potential and be subject to harassment, especially from their in-laws. In settings where women are subordinated, they are highly likely to be blamed for infertility. Given the very limited access to assisted reproductive treatments in these settings, infertility leads to profound human suffering.

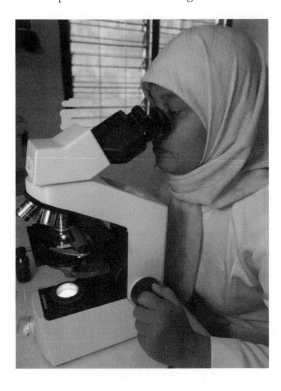

The diagnosis and psychosocial sequelae of infertility and the complex psychological responses to technologically assisted conception are central to the health of people facing these life experiences, and should be considered in research and clinical services. Causes of infertility differ, and in each country an accurate understanding is needed of the fertility problems of the population. In most countries, the prevalence, etiology and mental health effects of fertility problems have not been established, and relatively little is known about the psychological functioning of affected people, especially in developing countries.

There is a need for information on the nature of infertility treatment services in developing countries, and the long-term psychological consequences of infertility, including after the birth of a child. Data are needed on the short- and long-term psychosocial and medical consequences for both donors and recipients of gametes, including women in egg-sharing programmes. There is also a need for long-term comprehensive follow-up of the physical and mental health of offspring of assisted conception, with disaggregation by method of conception. Multiple pregnancies, which are more common after assisted conception, carry greater psychological hazards. The interaction between infertility and multiple gestations in influencing perinatal mental health should be clarified. The short- and long-term psychological effects of fetal reduction in multiple-gestation pregnancy need to be systematically investigated. The potential of psychological treatments to relieve the distress associated with infertility and assisted reproduction should be investigated in randomized controlled trials.

Infertility treatment services in all settings need to be based on evidence about local causes and best practice in treatment, and should include mental health care as a component of routine care. Mental health care should be focused on assisting the person to make a realistic appraisal of the chance of treatment success; providing emotional support in the interval between embryo transfer and pregnancy testing; and assisting the person to make a clear choice about when to stop treatment.

Female genital mutilation

The health effects of female genital mutilation, in areas where the practice is widespread, are just starting to be documented, and many of the existing data come from studies with methodological limitations. Most of the publications are case reports or case series, while only a few studies have compared women who have and have not had FGM. In some articles, the type of FGM is not defined, while in others all types are combined. In addition, the age or developmental stage at which the procedure was performed is often not reported. Many of the investigations have not included clinical examination of the perineum, and classification of FGM status may not be reliable in these circumstances.

Most of the studies examining the complications of female genital mutilation have been done in Africa, but some evidence has been gathered in industrialized countries, among immigrant populations. The adverse physical sequelae of female genital mutilation have been more comprehensively investigated and described than the psychological effects. The most obvious long-term adverse effects of FGM are on gynaecological health, especially sexual and obstetric functioning.

There is an almost complete lack of systematic evidence on the psychological sequelae, including mental health effects, of female genital cutting. It has been suggested that this situation has led to unfounded speculation about the psychological impact of FGM. Some reports have described the conflict faced by young women who want to conform to parental and societal expectations by complying with FGM, but who are thereby exposed to fear, pain, complicated recovery and possible long-term health problems. Chronic depression and anxiety have been observed among women who have had FGM, associated with genital disfigurement, gynaecological dysfunction and specific fears that cysts or scars are cancer or that the genitals are re-growing. Anxiety is also associated with obstructed menstrual flow and both anticipation of, and actual experience of, painful intercourse. It has been suggested that women might be traumatized by the procedure, on the basis of such responses having been observed in women who have undergone mutilating gynaecological procedures for clinical reasons.

Overall, given the severity of physical damage and long-term adverse health effects, it is highly likely that genital cutting has an adverse effect on women's mental health. As long as the practice continues, systematic and comprehensive examination of these effects is urgently needed. Information is also needed on the complex interactions between the social position of women and the pressure to maintain tradition and to adhere to family expectations, and their effects on the psychological response to genital mutilation. The psychological effects of failing to comply with genital mutilation in settings where it is an established traditional practice need to be assessed.

Health professionals in countries where female genital mutilation is practised, or to which women who have experienced genital mutilation migrate, need to have specific knowledge and skills in order to provide appropriate health care. Obstetric health professionals should be trained to provide antenatal, intrapartum and postpartum health care for women who have undergone FGM, especially type III. The care provided needs to be informed by cultural sensitivity, provision of choice, and an appreciation of human rights. Research exploring the possibilities and implications of changing this practice in communities where it is common is urgently needed.

Reference

WHO (2001) *The World Health Report 2001. Mental health: new understanding, new hope.* Geneva, World Health Organization.

Annex

WHO SURVEY QUESTIONNAIRE ON THE MENTAL HEALTH
ASPECTS OF REPRODUCTIVE HEALTH

WHO is currently carrying out a global review of women's mental health as it intersects with their reproductive health with emphasis on STDs/HIV/AIDS, pregnancy and postpartum, miscarriage, unwanted pregnancy/abortion, infertility, peri and post menopause, and domestic and sexual violence.

This involves reviewing the published and unpublished literature on the subject of the last 10 years from developing and developed countries with special emphasis on developing countries, including all epidemiological, clinical and operational research; programme/interventions evaluations, ongoing or completed country project work on the subject, pilot projects etc. On the basis of an analysis and synthesis of such literature, the review document entitled "Implications of Reproductive Health on Women's Mental Health" would provide:

- the most updated information/ knowledge on the epidemiology and ways in which Reproductive health events impact on women's mental health;
- the biopsychosocial factors that create vulnerability to mental problems and those that may be protective; and
- the types of programmes that could mitigate the adverse effects and promote positive mental health; and
- indications of the most feasible ways in which health authorities could advance policies, formulate programs and reorient services to meet the mental health needs of women during their reproductive lives.

In order to assist us in compiling this much-needed review, we would be grateful if you could take some time to answer the following:

Have you carried out research dealing with the epidemiology, determinants and/or outcomes of different reproductive health events during women's lifecycle?

1. **Yes**
2. **No**

If yes, could you please list the topics covered and supply us with copies of any relevant reports/ publications.

Are you currently or have you in the past conducted any research on the determinants and outcomes of women's mental health?

1. **Yes**
2. **No**

If yes, could you please list the topics covered and supply us with copies of the relevant reports/ publications.

Does your research incorporate any focus on the impact of various reproductive health events during the lifecycle on women's mental health?

1. **Yes**
2. **No**

If yes, could you identify the specific areas of reproductive health involved and the aspects of mental health you address? Please supply us with copies of the relevant reports/publications.

Have you been involved in policy development/programmes/services addressing women's mental health? reproductive health? or both?

1. **Yes**
2. **No**

If yes, could you please explain and list the issues covered and supply us with copies of any relevant reports/publications.

What aspects of reproductive/mental health do you believe require increased attention?

Please list topics and explain why you believe further knowledge is necessary?

Please indicate contact details of other sources of information on this subject.

Other comments/suggestions.

We thank you in advance for your collaboration in this important but too often neglected area. All information provided will be carefully reviewed and duly acknowledged if used.

Sincerely

Meena Cabral de Mello
Senior Scientist
Department of Mental Health and Substance Dependence
World Health Organization
CH1211 Geneva 27
Fax +41 22 791 4160
e-mail: cabraldemellom@who.int